DR. MICHAEL HUNTER'S
BREAST CANCER BOOK

*To Monica
My dear have a good
read both as patient and as
as a doctor! Enjoy!*

George

Hope is being able to see that there is
light despite all of the darkness.

Desmond Tutu

DR. MICHAEL HUNTER'S BREAST CANCER BOOK

PUBLISHED BY CANCERINFO, LLC

Any Internet addresses, phone numbers, or company or product information printed in this book are offered as a resource and are not intended in any way to be or to imply an endorsement by the author, nor does the author vouch for the existence, content, or services of these sites, phone numbers, companies, or products beyond the life of this book.

This book is not intended to provide therapy, counseling, or clinical advice or treatment, or to take the place of clinical advice and management from your personal health care provider. Readers are advised to consult their own qualified clinicians regarding medical issues. Neither the publisher nor the author take any responsibility for any possible consequences from any treatment, action, or application of information in this book to the reader.

ISBN 9798370882807

Library of Congress Cataloging-in-Publication Data

Names: Hunter, Michael, author.
Title: Dr. Michael Hunter's Breast Cancer Book / Michael Hunter, M.D.

Subjects: Breast--Cancer--Epidemiology Breast--Cancer--Risk factors
Breast--Cancer--Management

For those who care about men and women who have (or had) breast cancer. You genuinely inspire me.

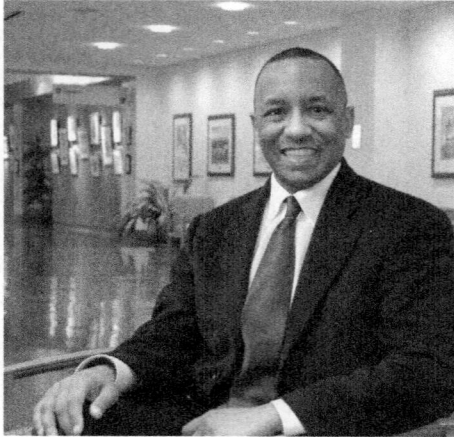

DR. HUNTER

I am a **radiation oncologist** in Seattle (USA) with
degrees from Harvard, Yale, and University of Pennsylvania.

I served on the Board of Komen Foundation of Puget Sound, as a consultant to the Washington Breast, Cervical, & Colon Health Project,
and as a cancer program medical director. You can find me regularly
blogging at www.newcancerinfo.com and www.medium.com.

DR. MICHAEL HUNTER'S

BREAST CANCER BOOK

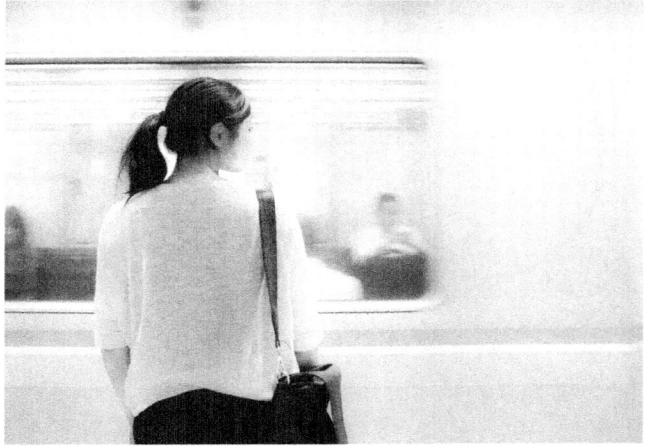

MY MISSION

Surreal. Few words have a greater impact. Many describe the time around hearing "You have breast cancer" as surreal, with many individuals moving from confusion to shock and grief, anger, fear, and despair. Most need time to work through these emotions. Once you do, you should be better able to navigate the journey to becoming better.

Breast cancer is a story with many chapters. No matter where you find yourself in the journey, I designed this book to help you navigate it. Herein, you will find information about why you may have gotten breast cancer (and basic, sustainable lifestyle adjustments that might improve the odds of it never coming back), what it looks like under the microscope, staging (extent of cancer), prognosis, and cancer management. For brevity, I will not address natural medicine approaches, nor focus on psychological well-being in this book. I do hope to be a source of knowledge and support for you.

Contents

BASICS

knowledge

BREAST CANCER is the most common non-skin cancer among women worldwide. In 2022, an estimated 287,850 women in the USA received a breast cancer diagnosis, with an additional 51,400 told that they have non-invasive (in situ) breast cancer. Worldwide, there are 2,261,419 new cases each year, making breast cancer the most common malignancy.

From the 1940s until the 1980s, breast cancer incidence (new cases) rates in the USA increased slightly. In the 1980s, incidence rose greatly (likely due to increased mammogram-based screening) and then leveled off during the 1990s.

Breast cancer incidence declined in the early 2000s. This decline is associated with a drop in menopausal hormone therapy (after the Women's Health Initiative study showed its use increased breast cancer risk). Since 2007, the incidence of breast cancer has remained roughly stable.

MALE BREAST CANCER is uncommon. About 2,710 men received a diagnosis of invasive breast cancer in 2022. For a man at average risk, the lifetime chance of developing breast cancer is about 1 in 833.

Inspire

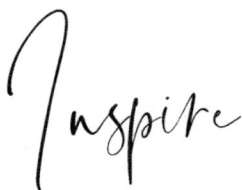

Outcomes improving

Mortality rates improving
Breast cancer death rates in the USA increased by 0.4 percent from 1975 to 1989 but decreased rapidly (a total decline of 39 percent through 2015). The decrease occurred among younger and older women but has slowed among women under 50 since 2007. This drop in mortality appeared to be associated with treatment and early detection improvements.

Not all groups have benefited from these advances equally: There has been a striking divergence in mortality trends among black and white women since the early 1980s. As treatment improved, the gap between whites and blacks increased: In 2015, breast cancer death rates were 1.4 times higher among black American women than their white counterparts.

Risk
While we cannot confidently say why you (or someone you care about) got breast cancer, the disease has many risk factors. We will review these in this chapter, but first, I want to introduce some key definitions:

- *Absolute risk*
  Odds you will develop a specific disease over a certain time

- *Lifetime risk*
  Odds you will develop a disease in your lifetime

- *Risk factors*
  Anything affecting your risk of getting a particular disease

- *Relative risk*
  The ratio of absolute risks

We will also look at factors associated with a lower risk of breast cancer. We sometimes refer to such factors as protective risk factors or just protective factors.

RISK

• You are told that if you take "anti-estrogen" pills (for example, tamoxifen) as a risk-reducing maneuver, your relative risk of breast cancer becomes about 0.5. Your risk of getting breast cancer is half that of someone in your situation who did not take the drug. On the other hand, a relative risk of 3 means that you are three times more likely to get a disease compared to someone with a "normal" risk.

• You hear that a certain drug decreases your risk of death by 25 percent. Sounds like a lot, but 25 percent of what? If your risk of death is 4%, the drug will make it 3 percent (the **absolute reduction** in risk is one percent). If the risk is 40 percent, the drug will reduce it to 30 percent (an absolute reduction of 10 percent).

Why

"Fixed" risk factors

Age

The older you are, the more likely you are to get breast cancer. Less than five percent of women diagnosed with breast cancer in the USA are younger than 40. About half of women with breast cancer or over 60. While the incidence of breast cancers driven by estrogen increases with age, the incidence of estrogen receptor-negative breast cancer increases until age 50, then levels off.

Female
Being a female is a strong risk factor for breast cancer. Men can get breast cancer, but the disease is about 100 times more common among women. Male breast cancer incidence has risen slightly since 1975 (from 1 to 1.3 per 100,000). Moreover, men are more likely than women to have advanced-stage breast cancer due to lower awareness and the lack of screening among men.

Personal history of breast cancer
A personal history of ductal carcinoma *in situ* (DCIS) or invasive breast cancer increases the risk of invasive cancer in the opposite breast. This risk may be on the order of 0.5% per year, but the risk varies by factors such as your age at initial diagnosis, whether you have a so-called breast cancer gene (BRCA), and by the primary cancer hormone receptor status.

Height
The taller you are, the higher your risk of breast cancer. In a study of more than 100,000 women (followed for twelve years), women 5 feet 7 inches (1.75 meters) or taller appeared to be 1.6 times more likely to get breast cancer than women under 5 feet 2 inches (1.6 meters). Every 2 inches (5 centimeters) adds 11 percent risk.

AGE

RISK VARIES BY AGE

	RISK*
20	1 in 1,567 (0.1%)
30	1 in 204 (0.5%)
40	1 in 65 (1.6%)
50	1 in 42 (2.4%)
60	1 in 28 (3.5%)
70	1 in 24 (4.1%)
Lifetime	**1 in 8 (12.4%)**

* Breast cancer risk (for women) over the next ten years.
Your risk may be higher or lower.

Density

Breast density describes the proportions of different breast tissue types. High breast density means more breast and connective tissue than breast fat.

Low breast density means that there is a greater proportion of fat. In 2006, a meta-analysis (study of studies) showed breast density as an independent risk factor for breast cancer. Women with very high breast density may be up to four to five times more likely to get breast cancer than those with low breast density.

Many, but not all, research studies demonstrate a link between breast density and the risk of getting breast cancer. Still, many states in the USA have enacted legislation mandating breast-density reporting to women who have undergone mammography.

Geography

Breast cancer incidence rates around the world vary greatly. Developed countries (such as the United States, England, and Australia) have higher rates than developing countries (such as Cambodia, Nepal, and Rwanda). Within the United States, incidence also varies (here are 2022 data):•

Higher
  Rhode Island, New Hampshire, Connecticut, Hawaii, New Jersey, North Carolina, Massachusetts, Montana, District of Columbia, and Delaware.

  • Lower
  Puerto Rico, Wyoming, New Mexico, Arizona, Utah, Texas, West Virginia, Alaska, Arkansas, Florida, Alabama, California, Mississippi

Worldwide, breast cancer incidence is highest in Belgium, followed by the Netherlands, Luxembourg, France, New Caledonia (France), Denmark, Australia, New Zealand, Finland, and the USA.

Mortality also varies by geography. While variations in mortality rates reflect variations in incidence, the other major contributor to the mortality rate is survival. Breast cancer mortality rates are highest in Barbados, followed by Fiji, Jamaica, Bahamas, Papua New Guinea, Somalia, Mali, Dominican Republic, Syria, and Samoa.

Some factors contributing to these differences include variations in risk factors, access to screening, and treatment. These are, in turn, influenced by socioeconomic factors, legislative policies, and proximity to medical services.

Race

Breast cancer incidence and mortality vary by race and ethnicity among women in the USA. Non-Hispanic whites have the highest risk, followed by African-Americans*, then Asian and Pacific Islanders. American Indians and Alaska natives have the lowest incidences. Here are the numbers from the Komen Foundation (www.komen.org):

Race and ethnicity	Lifetime risk
Non-Hispanic White	14%
Non-Hispanic Black	12%
Asian and Pacific Islanders	12%
Hispanic	11%
American Indians and Alaska Natives	10%

African-American women have the highest breast cancer-related death rate, while Asian-American and Pacific Islander women have the lowest. Between 2008 to 2012, rates of breast cancer diagnosis increased by 0.4 percent per year in African-American women, compared to 1.5 percent per year among women identifying as Asian or Pacific Islanders. The diagnosis rates in the period remained stable among women of white, Hispanic, American Indian, and Alaska Native origins.

American Cancer Society researchers analyzed data from the National Cancer Institute's Surveillance, Epidemiology, and End Results. They found that in 2012 black and white women were diagnosed with breast cancer at about the same rate.

In seven states, the breast cancer rates among black women surpassed those of white women between 2009 and 2012. That increase was seen primarily in the country's Southern region: Alabama, Kentucky, Louisiana, Mississippi, Missouri, Oklahoma, and Tennessee.

---

*Among women under 45, African-American incidence is the highest.

African-Americans - Mortality

African-American women with breast cancer are 1.4 times more likely to die from their cancer compared with white women, despite the former having a four percent lower incidence rate of breast cancer. While socioeconomic factors such as income, health insurance, and access to health services probably contribute to these disparities, they don't fully explain the variant risks. Differences in rates of getting screening mammograms don't explain it either: African-American women and white women now have the same rates of mammogram use. By 2013, among women 40 and older, 66 percent of African-American women and 66 percent of white women had a mammogram in the prior two years.

Investigators at the Harvard Massachusetts General Hospital assessed white and African-American women (with stages I to III breast cancer) diagnosed from 1988 to 2013. These women had their breast cancer tissue submitted to The Cancer Genome Atlas. The researchers then evaluated the association of race and genetic traits with tumor recurrence. Here is what they found:

African Americans had greater genetic variation and more basal gene expression tumors within a given tumor. This pattern suggests more aggressive tumor biology among African Americans than whites. This factor may contribute to the significant racial disparities seen when examining breast cancer outcomes among different racial groups. In addition, socioeconomic and healthcare access disparities may contribute to worse outcomes among African American women.

Immigrants

Immigrants typically see a rise in breast cancer incidence after coming to the United States. For example, women who come to the United States from Asian countries (where breast cancer incidence is four to seven times lower than in the USA) experience a 1.8 times increase in risk after living in the USA for a decade or more. A generation later, the risk for their daughters approaches that of USA-born women.

Turning to Hispanic women, those born in the United States have a significantly higher rate of breast cancer than immigrant Hispanics. However, the longer immigrant women spend in the United States, the greater their risk for breast cancer. This association is especially true for women who immigrate to the USA before the age of 20 years old.

Family

Most women with breast cancer do not have a family history. Only about 13 percent have a first-degree relative (mother, sister, or daughter) with breast cancer. However, a family history of certain cancers (for example, breast, ovarian, or prostate) can increase your risk of breast cancer.

- A first-degree relative (sister, mother, or daughter) has breast cancer: Your breast cancer risk may double.
- Two first-degree relatives have breast cancer: Your risk may triple.

Inherited genetics

Breast cancer susceptibility genes (such as BRCA1, BRCA2, p53, ATM, and PTEN) are associated with only five to 10 percent of all breast cancers. Breast and ovarian cancer appear to be more common among women of Ashkenazi (with ancestors from Central or Eastern Europe) Jewish descent, given a higher prevalence of risk-raising BRCA1 and BRCA2 (BReast CAncer genes 1 and 2) mutations.

Everyone has BRCA1 and BRCA2 genes. Some have inherited mutations in one or both of these genes, increasing the risk of several cancers. One in 40 women of Ashkenazi Jewish descent carries one of these mutations, compared to one in 400 in the general population. Of those with breast cancer, roughly 10 percent will have a BRCA mutation. About five percent of women with breast cancer in the non-Ashkenazi Jewish population carry a BRCA mutation.

Are BRCA mutations limited to individuals of Askenazi Jewish descent? The answer is no; various ethnic and racial groups are also susceptible. For example, young African-American women with a breast cancer diagnosis at age 50 years or younger have a much higher BRCA mutation frequency than that previously reported among young white women with breast cancer, according to a recent United States-based study.

Women who have inherited mutations in the BRCA1 or BRCA2 genes are significantly more likely to develop breast or ovarian cancer, especially at a younger age. About five percent of women with breast cancer in the United States have mutations in a BRCA1 or BRCA2 gene, based on estimates among non-Hispanic white women. Having a BRCA gene mutation can raise your risk of several cancer types, including melanoma, ovarian, breast (including among males), and prostate cancer.

Other genetic factors

• P53 / Li-Fraumeni syndrome

p53 gene mutations can raise your risk of breast cancer, leukemia, and lung and brain cancers. Those with Li-Fraumeni syndrome have a 50 percent breast cancer risk by 60, and p53 mutations may be associated with up to 7 percent of all breast cancers among women under 40. These cancers tend to be estrogen receptor-positive, progesterone receptor-positive, and HER2-positive.

• PTEN/Cowden syndrome (uncommon)

The PTEN gene provides instructions for making an enzyme found in almost all tissues. The enzyme acts as a tumor suppressor; it helps regulate cell division by keeping cells from growing and dividing too rapidly or uncontrolled. PTEN gene mutations can lead to numerous hamartomas (benign, non-cancer growths) and can increase the risk of thyroid, uterus, and breast cancer. Those who have it have a lifetime risk of up to 85 percent.

• Other gene abnormalities

A higher risk of breast cancer is associated with several other gene abnormalities. For example, mutations in ATM, BRIP1, CHEK2, NBS1, PALB2, or RAD50 genes raise breast cancer risk by two to four times. These genes are typically low penetrance (less likely to show) and contribute less to the overall numbers of breast cancer, at least compared to BRCA, p53, or PTEN mutations.

Tobacco

Some studies point to tobacco use slightly raising breast cancer risk. For example, the EPIC study found a 1.06-fold increase in risk at 11 years of follow-up, while the Nurses' Health Study demonstrated a 1.09-fold increase at the 30-year follow-up mark. Meta-analyses (analyses of collections of studies) show mixed results: The Collaborative Group on Hormonal Factors in Breast Cancer demonstrated no increase in breast cancer risk. On the other hand, two other meta-analyses found a 1.12 to 1.13-fold increase in risk.

DES (diethylstilbestrol)

Some pregnant women in the USA received the drug DES between 1940 and 1971 to reduce the risk of miscarriage. Women who take DES during pregnancy have a slightly elevated risk of breast cancer. Those exposed to DES in utero - those whose mothers took DES while pregnant - may have a slightly increased breast cancer risk after age 40.

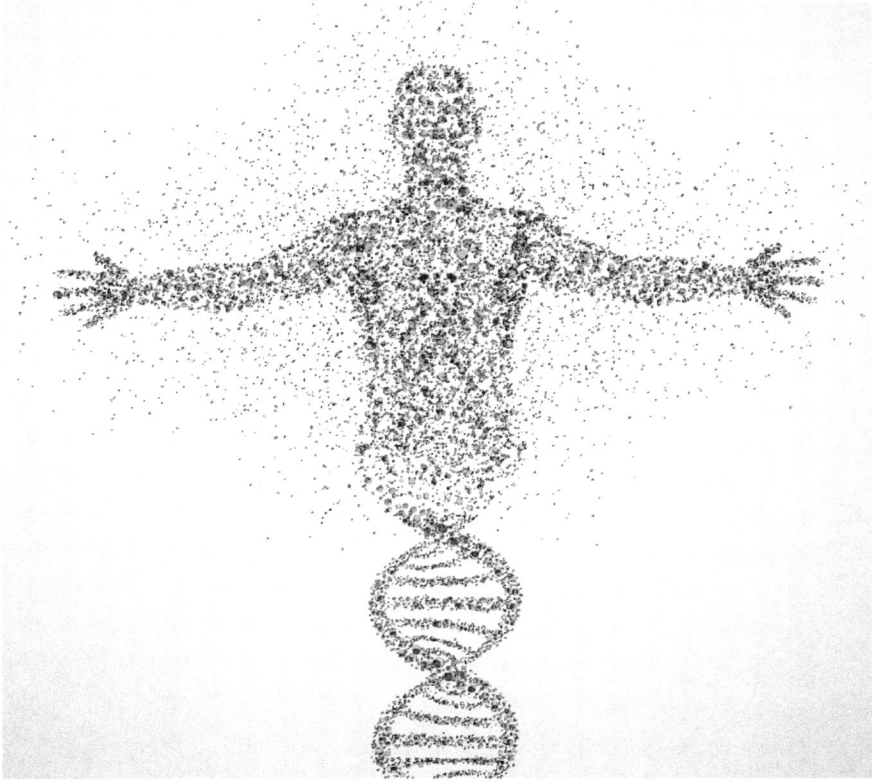

All races and ethnic groups have high-risk genes

Only five to 10 percent of breast cancers are directly linked to the inheritance of known breast cancer susceptibility genes. The overall frequency of pathogenic mutations in known breast cancer predisposition genes is 9.1 percent for non-Hispanic Whites, 9.8 percent for African Americans, 10.2 percent for Hispanics, 7.6 percent for Ashkenazi-Jewish, and 7.5 percent for Asians.

Hyperplasia and other benign breast conditions

Benign breast conditions are not cancers; some increase your risk of getting breast cancer, while others do not.

- Proliferative (fast-growing cells) increase risk

  Usual hyperplasia: May double breast cancer risk compared to women without a proliferative disorder.

  Atypical (ductal or lobular) hyperplasia (ADH; ALH): May increase breast cancer risk by a factor of four or five compared to women without a proliferative condition. Women with atypical hyperplasia may consider taking a risk-lowering pill such as tamoxifen or raloxifene.

- Non-proliferative (cells not fast-growing) don't increase risk unless nearby cells are atypical or DCIS. Non-proliferative conditions include simple cysts, fibroadenomas, and intraductal papillomas. Some studies have found radial scars increase risk, while others have not.

LCIS

When abnormal cells grow inside the breast lobules but have not spread to nearby tissue or beyond, the condition is called lobular carcinoma in situ (LCIS). In situ means "remaining in place." Despite containing the term carcinoma (cancer), lobular carcinoma in situ is not itself cancer. However, LCIS markedly increases your risk of breast cancer in the future in either breast. LCIS does not cause symptoms and typically does not appear on a mammogram. It tends to be incidentally discovered (for example, with a biopsy performed on the breast for some other reason).

The finding of LCIS is associated with a **30 to 40 percent lifetime risk** of developing invasive breast cancer. This risk compares to a chance of approximately 12.5 percent for a woman at average risk in the USA. Another study puts the breast cancer risk at 21 percent over the ensuing 15 years. Management options for those with LCIS may include "anti-estrogen" approaches such as tamoxifen pill use, removal of both breasts, or incorporation of MRI with mammograms for high-risk screening.

Diabetes

The risk of developing breast cancer varies by diabetes type:

Type 1 (insulin-dependent; juvenile) diabetes*: No increase in risk

- Typically occurs before age 40
- The body doesn't produce insulin
- Type 1 diabetes *does not* increase breast cancer risk.

Type 2 diabetes: Increased breast cancer risk

- The body cannot produce enough insulin to function properly, or the cells in the body do not normally react to the insulin it does produce (insulin resistance).
- Risk factors for Type 2 diabetes include being overweight, physical inactivity and eating an unhealthy diet.
- Type 2 diabetes *increases* breast cancer risk: Postmenopausal women 50 years or older who have type 2 diabetes have about a 1.2 to 1.27-fold increase in risk of developing breast cancer. We don't fully understand why breast cancer risk is increased, but many risk factors are similar for type 2 diabetes and for breast cancer.

Gestational (pregnancy-related) diabetes: No increase in risk

- The body cannot produce enough insulin to transfer glucose into cells, causing high blood glucose levels.
- Most can control their diabetes with exercise and diet.
- Gestational diabetes is *not* linked to an increase in breast cancer risk. But, while blood glucose levels usually go back to normal after pregnancy, there is a 35 to 65 percent chance of developing type 2 diabetes in the next 10 to 20 years.

Thyroid cancer

There *may* be an association between thyroid cancer and breast cancer incidence: Several lines of evidence suggest that breast cancer and thyroid cancer occur together in the same female patients more frequently than would be expected by chance. While I do not recommend routine screening for thyroid cancer among those with breast cancer, it seems reasonable to emphasize routine breast cancer screening among those with thyroid cancer.

Risk factors

Hormone-related

Early menarche

Early age at menstrual period onset (menarche) is associated with a higher risk. There is a one-tenth reduction in risk for every two-year delay in the menses onset. The average age of menarche in the USA is 13 (slightly higher for Asians and slightly lower for Hispanics and African-Americans).

Late menopause

A pooled analysis of more than 400,000 women found that for every year older a woman was at menopause, breast cancer risk increased by three percent. A woman who enters menopause after 55 years of age has twice the risk of a woman who did so before 45.

No children

Women without a full-term pregnancy have a 1.2 to 1.7-fold risk increase. A full-term pregnancy reduces your total number of lifetime menstrual cycles. In addition, breast cells are immature and very active until your first full-term pregnancy. Immature breast cells respond to the hormone estrogen: A first full-term pregnancy makes the breast cells more fully mature, with the cells then growing more regularly. Immediately after a full-term pregnancy, a woman's risk of getting breast cancer increases. By a decade later, the pregnancy begins to reduce risk. The initial increase is especially true for women over 35, with a 1.3-fold increase in risk five years after delivery.

Age of first full-term pregnancy

Women who become pregnant later in life are at increased risk of developing breast cancer. The cumulative risk (compared to women with a full-term pregnancy up to age 70) is 20 percent lower, 10 percent lower, and five percent higher among women who delivered their first child at age 20, 25, or 35, respectively.

Modifiable: Reproductive

Birth control pills

If you are currently using birth control pills (or stopped recently), you may have a 1.2 to 1.3-fold increased risk of breast cancer (compared to women who never used oral contraceptives). Once a woman stops taking birth control pills, her risk decreases. A decade or so later, the risk becomes similar to a woman who has never been on the pill. However, most studies are older and look at higher-dose birth control pills. Research continues on more modern forms of the pill, and some forms (mini-pills) may not have an increased risk. In addition, birth control pills may reduce your risk of the uterus and ovarian cancer and reduce the chances of undesired pregnancy. Data regarding Depo Provera, hormone-releasing IUDs, birth control patches, and vaginal rings are limited.

Breast-feeding

Breast-feeding lowers breast cancer risk, especially among premenopausal women. A pooled analysis of 47 studies examining cumulative time spent breastfeeding yielded the following results: For those who breastfeed for less than a year, risk reduction is possible. Breastfeeding a year, and risk slightly decreases, with two years duration giving twice the benefit as one year. Breast-feeding for more than two years provides the most risk reduction.

Hormone receptor-negative breast cancers have no receptors for the hormones estrogen or progesterone (they are estrogen- and progesterone receptor negative). This subtype of breast cancer doesn't respond to hormonal medicines which target hormone receptors and is considered more aggressive than hormone receptor-positive breast cancer.

A meta-analysis (a study that combines and analyzes the results of several earlier studies) found that women who had breastfed for any time had up to 20 percent lower risk of developing hormone receptor-negative breast cancer. The association between breastfeeding and receptor-positive breast cancers needs more investigation.

Other risk factors

Light at night, melatonin, and breast cancer
Melatonin is a hormone involved in sleep cycle regulation. At night, we make more melatonin, leading to sleep. Exposure to light at night can suppress melatonin production. Lowering melatonin increases estrogen, potentially increasing your breast cancer risk.

Radiation exposure in youth
Significant radiation exposure early in life (for example, radiation therapy to the chest area for childhood cancer) increases the breast cancer risk significantly. If you have had therapeutic irradiation to the chest region, ask a valued healthcare professional about recommended screening. Later in this chapter, we will turn to some potential risk-reducing maneuvers.

Hormone replacement therapy (HRT)

- **Combination estrogen/progesterone increase risk**

  Breast cancer risk *increases* within the first five years of combination estrogen/progesterone use. Combination hormone use, through 18.3 years of follow-up, increased breast cancer incidence by nearly 1.3 times and continued to raise risk through the follow-up of 18.3 years.

- **Estrogen alone reduces breast cancer risk**

  The Women's Health Initiative updated analysis showed that estrogen-only hormone replacement therapy significantly *reduced* breast cancer incidence (by about one-quarter) and mortality, with these favorable effects lasting for over 15 years after discontinuing use. Researchers presented this new evidence at the San Antonio Breast Cancer Symposium on December 13, 2019.

On the other hand, a 2019 meta-analysis of 58 studies discovered that both estrogen-only HRT and combination HRT increased breast cancer risk. A meta-analysis combines and analyzes the results of several earlier studies.

HORMONE REPLACEMENT

RISK WITH ESTROGEN + PROGESTERONE

	Extra cases per 10,000 women
Breast cancer	**9**
Deep vein thrombosis (clots)	4
Pulmonary embolism (lung clots)	4
Stroke	5

	Fewer cases per 10,000 women
Uterus (endometrial) cancer	3
Hip fracture	5

Changeable: Estrogen-related factors

Weight gain after menopause increases risk

Before menopause, extra weight is protective, as blood levels of estrogen are lower among overweight people. Being overweight becomes harmful after menopause: The risk of breast cancer may be nearly 1.6 times higher than for normal-weight post-menopausal women. In one recent study, researchers reported that overweight or obese post-menopausal women had an increased invasive breast cancer risk compared with women of normal weight, with a greater risk for more severe obesity.

Very obese women appear to have an increased risk for estrogen- and progesterone-driven breast cancer but *not* for other types. These women were also at increased risk for larger tumors and death. Women with a baseline Body Mass Index (BMI) of under 25 who gained more than 5% of their body weight over the years of the study also had an increased risk for breast cancer. However, women already overweight or obese did not.

Alcohol

Alcohol consumption increases cancer risk in general: In 1988, the International Agency for Research on Cancer (IARC) declared that alcohol is a carcinogen. A recent study showed a dose-response relationship between alcohol consumption and the risk of getting breast cancer among premenopausal and post-menopausal women.

In the European Prospective Investigation Into Cancer and Nutrition (EPIC) study, 334,850 women ages 35 to 70 were recruited in 10 European countries and followed for an average of 11 years. Here are the results:

- Alcohol was associated with risk: Every 10 grams/day increase in alcohol intake raised the risk by 4.2 percent.
- Risk appeared elevated for *both* hormone receptor-positive and hormone receptor-negative breast cancers.
- Risk appeared higher among women who started drinking before their first full-term pregnancy.

Current evidence is sufficient to conclude that **alcohol is causally related to breast cancer development.**

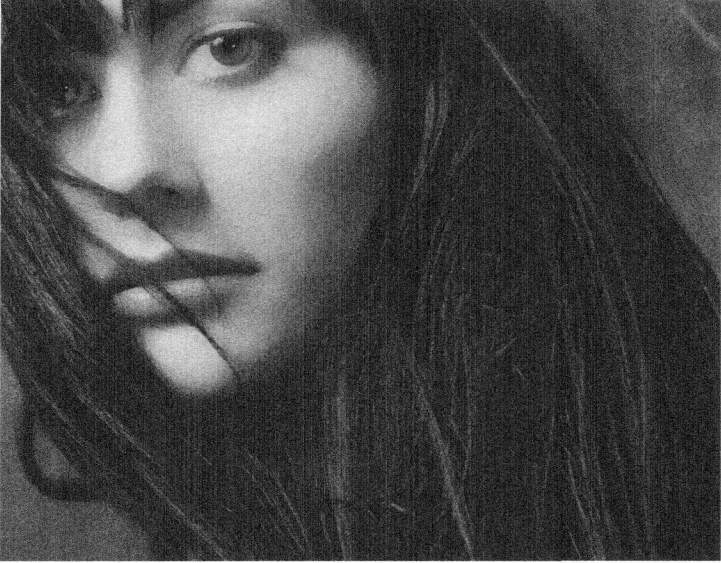

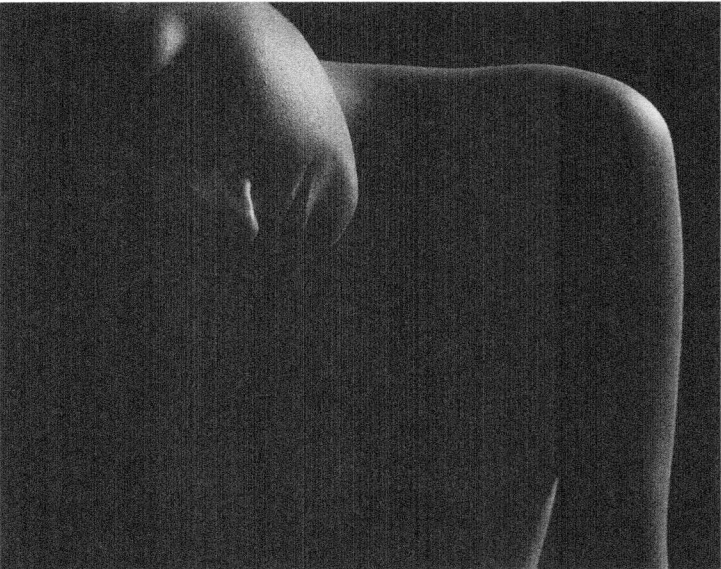

Changeable: Diet

Diet

A Mediterranean diet (rich in plant foods, fish, and olive oil) is associated with better heart health. A Spanish study suggests it may also reduce the risk of developing breast cancer. Investigators randomly assigned more than 4,200 women, ages 60 to 80, to eat either a Mediterranean diet supplemented with extra virgin olive oil or nuts versus a low-fat control diet. The women who joined the study from 2003 to 2009 were all at high risk for heart disease, and their average body mass index was 30 (considered obese; obesity is itself a risk factor for the development of post-menopausal breast cancer). Less than 3 percent had used hormone therapy, and the average age was 68.

The Mediterranean plus olive oil group had a 68 percent lower risk of developing breast cancer over a five-year follow-up period than the control diet group. While the Mediterranean diet with nuts reduced risk, the results were not statistically significant. There are some limitations to the study, including the fact that breast cancer was not the primary subject of the research. In addition, it is unknown whether the olive oil was beneficial on its own or only when taken with the Mediterranean diet.

How much olive oil?

Women in the study consumed four tablespoons daily, using it as a spread for salads and cooking. Those in the nut consumption group ate about an ounce of nuts daily, half walnuts and half split between hazelnuts and almonds. While the results seem promising, we need longer follow-up and validation studies. Still, this PREDIMED study adds to growing support for the health benefits of a Mediterranean-type diet.

A systematic review suggests that the Mediterranean diet pattern (and diets composed largely of vegetables, fruit, fish, and soy) is associated with a decreased risk of breast cancer. Researchers found no association between traditional dietary patterns and the risk of getting breast cancer. Only one study showed an increase in risk associated with the Western dietary pattern. I am unaware of the effect of any diet on the prognosis for those who already have breast cancer. However, I recommend adherence to a balanced diet, including copious fruits and vegetables (and limiting highly processed foods).

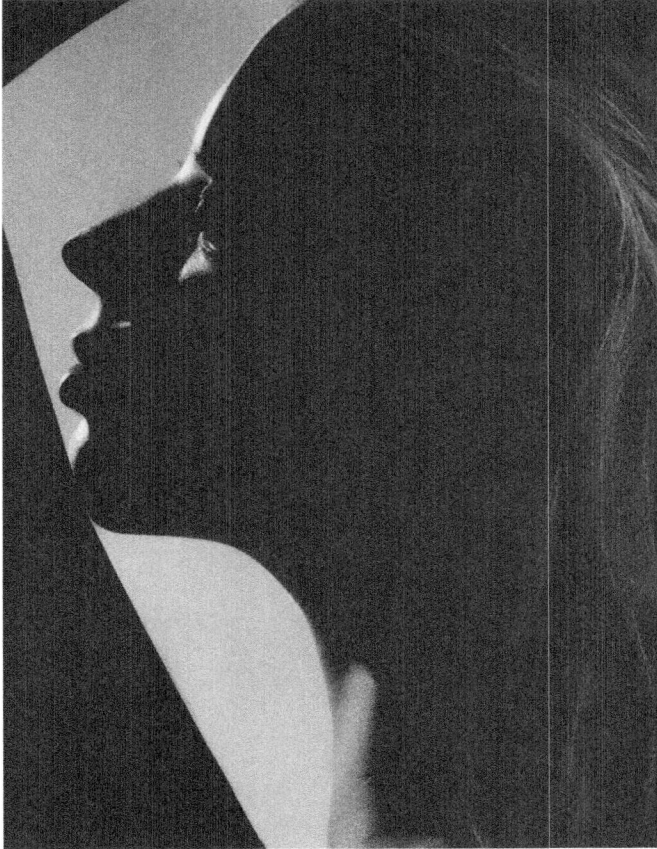

Changeable: Diet

Low-fat diet

You may ask this question: Can a dietary intervention prevent breast cancer deaths? The answer may be yes, according to information presented at the American Society of Clinical Oncology National Meeting in 2019. An analysis of long-term follow-up of women enrolled in the Women's Health Initiative (WHI), a United States National Institutes of Health study of 48,385 post-menopausal women. The participants had no personal history of breast cancer. The WHI study randomized women to a low-fat dietary intervention or a normal diet.

After more than eight years, the women in the low-fat group lost about 3 percent of their body weight on average but did not have a statistically lower risk of invasive breast cancer. Now, we have a longer follow-up.

After a cumulative median follow-up of 19.6 years, a significant reduction in breast cancer-related deaths has emerged: Those on a lower-fat diet had a relative 15 percent reduction in all-cause mortality and a 21 percent lower risk of breast cancer mortality. The diet is a reasonable, balanced approach that cuts fat intake to about 20 to 25 percent of calories and increases fruits, grains, and vegetables. This diet is similar to DASH, a strategy designed to treat high blood pressure.

Modifiable: Blue light at night

Exposure to light

Light at night is bad for your health, and exposure to blue light emitted by electronics and energy-efficient light bulbs may be especially so. Here is an excerpt from the Harvard Health Letter:

> "Until the advent of artificial lighting, the sun was the major lighting source, and people spent their evenings in (relative) darkness. Now, evenings are illuminated in much of the world, and we take our easy access to all those lumens for granted. But we may be paying the price for basking in all that light. Light throws the body's biological clock—the circadian rhythm—out of whack at night.

Night shift

Many (but certainly not all) studies have linked working a night shift to a higher risk of breast and prostate cancer, diabetes, heart disease, and obesity. It's not entirely clear why nighttime light exposure seems so bad for us. Light exposure drops melatonin, which influences our awake/sleep rhythms. Some early evidence suggests lower melatonin levels might explain the association with cancer.

Type of light: The blues

Melatonin is a hormone in your body that plays a role in sleep. The production and release of melatonin in the brain are connected to the time of day, increasing when it's dark and decreasing when it's light. Melatonin production declines with age. While the light of any color can suppress melatonin, blue light/wavelengths (beneficial during daylight hours because they boost attention, reaction times, and mood) seem to be the most disruptive at night. \

Exposure to electronics with screens (and energy-efficient lighting) increases our exposure to blue wavelengths, especially after sundown. Harvard researchers examined the effects of 6.5 hours of blue light exposure with exposure to green light of comparable brightness. The blue light suppressed melatonin for about twice as long as the green light and shifted the natural 24-hour cycle by twice as much (3 hours vs. 1.5 hours).

Changeable: Lifestyle

Physical Activity

Physical activity may lower the risk of breast cancer, especially for women who have gone through menopause. Exercise can lower estrogen levels, fight obesity and boost immune system cells that attack tumors.

  • Before you start an exercise program, please consult a valued healthcare provider. This input is especially important if you have been inactive for a long time, are overweight, have a high risk of heart disease, or have a high risk of other chronic health problems.
  • **Include physical activity in your daily routine.** Aim for the minimum of the equivalent of a brisk walk for 30 minutes daily.

Weight

  • Gaining weight after menopause increases breast cancer risk.
  • Weight gain of 20 pounds or more after age 18 *may* increase your risk of breast cancer.
  • If you have gained weight, losing weight may lower your risk of breast cancer. Aim for a body mass index (BMI) of 20 to 25.

Breast-feeding

Breast-feeding can *lower* breast cancer risk.

Alcohol

Alcohol increases breast cancer risk: The more you drink, the higher your probability of developing breast cancer. If you drink alcohol, aim for less than one standard drink a day, on average. Getting enough folic acid may lower the risk linked to drinking alcohol, but the evidence here is not high-level. You can find folic acid in multivitamins, oranges, orange juice, green vegetables, and fortified breakfast cereals.

RISKS

	Lower	Higher	RR*
BRCA mutation	Negative	Positive	3 - 7x increase
Mother or sister with breast CA	No	Yes	2.6
Age	30 to 34	70 to 74	18
Age at menarche	Over 14	Less than 12	1.5
Age at first birth	Under 20	Over 30	1.9 to 3.5
Age at menopause	Under 45	Over 55	2
Use of contraceptive pills	Never	Past/current	1.1 to 1.2
Estrogen + progestin	Never	Current	1.2
Alcohol	None	2 to 5/day	1.4
Breast density	0	75 or higher	1.8 to 6
Bone density	Lowest quartile	Highest quartile	2.7 to 3.5
History of benign breast biopsy	No	Yes	1.7
History of atypical hyperplasia	No	Yes	3.7

Protective

Breast-feeding (months)	16 or more	0	0.7
Full-term pregnancies	5 or more	0	0.7
Exercise	Yes	No	0.7
Postmenopausal BMI	Under 22.9	Over 30.7	0.6
Ovaries removed before age 35	Yes	No	0.3
Aspirin	More than once weekly, 6+ months	Non-user	0.8

* relative risk

Triple negative

Triple-negative breast cancer (TNBC) is a term that we often apply to cancers that are low in the expression of estrogen receptors (ER) and progesterone receptors (PR), as well as human epidermal factor receptor 2 (HER2). TNBC often behaves more aggressively than other breast cancer types. Triple-negative breast cancer accounts for about 20 percent of breast cancers worldwide. It is more common among women younger than 40 than estrogen- or progesterone-receptor-positive breast cancer. The risk of TNBC is about doubled among those under 40 compared with women over 50. Let's look at some of the risks unique to triple-negative breast cancer:

Inherited breast cancer genes

Up to 20 percent of patients with triple-negative breast cancer have a breast cancer gene (BRCA) mutation, particularly in BRCA1. By contrast, less than six percent of all breast cancers are linked to BRCA. Generally, if you have TNBC and are 60 years or younger, you should have genetic testing.

Race

African-Americans have a significantly higher risk of triple-negative breast cancer than non-African-American women.

Pre-menopausal

TNBC is more common among premenopausal women.

Maternal

According to some (but not all) studies, breastfeeding may lower TNBC risk. Limited data also suggest that younger age at first pregnancy may increase the risk of TNBC. Finally, those who have had no full-term pregnancies may have a higher risk; on the other hand, some studies hint that having three or more births may increase the risk of TNBC, but there is no compelling evidence.

Other hormonal factors

Some (but not all) studies have linked other hormonal factors (early age to start menstruating, ongoing hormone replacement therapy, oral contraceptive use) to triple-negative breast cancer.

TRIPLE-NEGATIVE BREAST CANCER

The most common receptors known to fuel most breast cancer growth – estrogen, progesterone, and HER-2 – are not present in the cancer cells.

If we think of cancer cells as houses, the front door has three types of locks (receptors). One lock is for the female hormone estrogen. Another is for the female hormone progesterone. The third lock is a protein called human epidermal growth factor.

For breast cancer with any of these three locks, we have a few keys (such as blocking the estrogen receptor) to kill cancer or to stop it from dividing.

If you have triple-negative breast cancer, the three locks are missing. So doctors have fewer keys for treatment. Fortunately, chemotherapy (and sometimes immunotherapy) can be effective options.

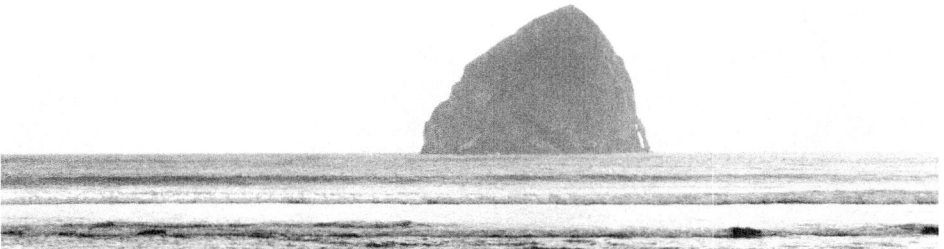

Male breast cancer

Risk factors

Aging is a significant risk factor for male breast cancer. The risk of breast cancer increases with age. The average age at diagnosis is 68.

Family history; genes

Breast cancer risk increases if blood relatives have had breast cancer. About one in five men with breast cancer have a close male or female relative with the disease. Men with a mutation (defect) in the BRCA2 gene (BReast CAncer gene 2) have an elevated lifetime risk of about six in 100. BRCA1 mutations also raise breast cancer risk to about one in 100. Although gene mutations are most often found in members of families with many cases of breast and/or ovarian cancer, they can occur in men with breast cancer who do not have a strong family history. Mutations in CHEK2 and PTEN genes also raise the risk.

Klinefelter syndrome

Klinefelter syndrome is a congenital condition (present at birth) that affects one in 1000 men. Normally the cells in mens' bodies have a single X chromosome along with a Y chromosome, while the cells of women' have two X chromosomes. Men with Klinefelter syndrome have cells with a Y chromosome plus at least two X chromosomes (and sometimes more). These men typically have smaller than normal testicles. Many are infertile, as they can't produce functioning sperm. Compared with other men, they have lower levels of male hormones (androgens) and more estrogens (female hormones). Given this, many develop gynecomastia (non-cancer male breast growth).

Some studies have found that men with Klinefelter syndrome are more likely to get breast cancer: One study reported a breast cancer risk of one in 100. Estimating risk is tough, as the numbers of individuals with the condition are small. The risk may be higher, but it is still low overall because this is an uncommon cancer, even among men with Klinefelter syndrome.

Estrogen

Estrogen-related drugs were once used as hormonal therapy for men with prostate cancer. Estrogen may slightly increase breast cancer risk. Transgender individuals who take high doses of estrogen as part of a sex reassignment may also have a higher breast cancer risk. Unfortunately, we don't have any studies of breast cancer risk among transgender individuals, so the actual breast cancer risk is unclear.

Alcohol

Heavy consumption of alcoholic beverages increases breast cancer risk among men. This increase may be because of its effects on the liver. The liver binds proteins that carry hormones in the blood that affect hormone activity. Men with severe liver diseases such as cirrhosis have relatively low levels of male hormones and higher estrogen levels. They have a higher rate of benign male breast growth (gynecomastia) and a higher risk of developing breast cancer.

Obesity

Obesity is a likely risk factor for male breast cancer. Fat cells convert male hormones (androgens) into female hormones (estrogens). Obese men have higher levels of estrogen in their bodies.

Testicular conditions

Certain conditions, such as having an undescended testicle, having mumps as an adult, or having one or both testicles surgically removed, may slightly increase male breast cancer risk.

Certain occupations

There may be an increased risk among men who work in hot environments such as steel mills. Exposure to higher temperatures for long periods can affect the testicles, affecting hormone levels. Men heavily exposed to gasoline fumes may also have a higher risk.

While male breast cancer has been on a slow rise since 1975, **male breast cancer death rates have dropped** by about 1.8 percent per year since 2000.

Breast cancer risk

Tools

Risk assessments educate patients about cancer risk, determine if genetic testing is indicated, and help decide when breast cancer screening with mammograms should start. High-risk patients may be offered screening breast magnetic resonance imaging (MRI) in addition to annual mammograms and chemo-prevention to help reduce breast cancer risk.

There are various risk-prediction models for breast cancer. We may conveniently stratify women into one of three risk groups for the development of breast cancer:

> • **Average risk (75% of women):** No family history of the disease and no significant personal risk factors (for example, a previous biopsy of the breast) that would constitute a higher risk. Those in the average risk group have a 12 percent chance of developing breast cancer.

> • **Women with hereditary breast cancer** risk and a genetic mutation known to confer a high lifetime risk (12 percent of women).

> • **Moderate risk:** Women with a family history of breast cancer not associated with known genes or women who have had a breast biopsy that shows a precancerous change.

Several credible online tools are available to help women, and their care providers better understand breast cancer risk. Such knowledge may help inform your decision-making regarding breast cancer risk reduction strategies, genetic counseling/testing options, and screening options for the earlier detection of breast cancer. Alas, no tool can predict your risk with certainty, and each test has strengths and limitations. Let's look at some of these tools.

Your Disease Risk (www.yourdiseaserisk.wustl.edu) is a wonderful website from Washington University (USA) that offers both educational material and a risk assessment tool for breast cancer (and other diseases as well). It puts you into above-average, average, or below-average risk categories compared to the general population. I like this easy-to-use tool. The tool was developed using data for the USA and estimates your risk relative to the US general population. In addition, the tool only considers limited information about your family history of breast cancer, which could lead to underestimating risk for some patients.

Risk assessment tools for health professionals
Many of these tools are accessible to you online. Still, if you choose to explore any of them, please discuss your results with a valued healthcare provider.

What	Factors	Notes
Gail model	Previous breast biopsies (and whether atypia is present); reproductive history (age at start of menstruation and age at first live birth of a child); family history of breast cancer among first-degree relatives (e.g. mother; sister; daughter)	• Only considers limited info about family breast cancer history • Does not include factors such as use of hormone replacement therapy, breast density, and lifestyle factors such as smoking, alcohol use, diet, or physical inactivity
Breast Cancer Risk Assessment Tool	Age; age at first menarche; age at first live birth of a child; family and personal history of breast cancer;	• A 5-year risk of 1.67% or higher is considered high risk for developing breast cancer
IBIS (Tyrer-Cuzick) Breast Cancer Risk Evaluation Tool	Age; age at first live birth of a child; age at first period; age at menopause; height and weight; prior risk-increasing benign biopsy of breast; use of hormones; comprehensive family history	• Does not include risk factors associated with lifestyle or breast density • Genetic counseling advised when the model predicts a 10% or higher chance that you have a mutation of BRCA

At high risk?

Prophylactic bilateral mastectomy

Today, many high-risk women are choosing to have surgical removal of both breasts to reduce their risk of developing breast cancer in the future. While such a radical move indeed reduces the risk, it remains unclear as to whether it has a significant impact on survival odds. Still, some choose the removal of both breasts as they feel the complications associated with the surgery are worth the benefits (psychological, desire for symmetry, reduced need for future mammogram surveillance).

The primary goal of bilateral prophylactic (risk-reducing) mastectomy is to reduce breast cancer risk. Here are estimated risks based on various factors:

Genetic risk factors	Lifetime risk
BRCA1	81 percent
BRCA2	85 percent
p53	24 percent
PTEN	25 percent

Non-genetic risk factors	Relative risk
Classic LIN*	7 to 11 times
ADH/ALH*	4 to 5 times
Proliferative change, without atypia	1.9 times

* LIN   lobular intraepithelial neoplasia
  ADH   atypical ductal hyperplasia
  ALH   atypical lobular hyperplasia

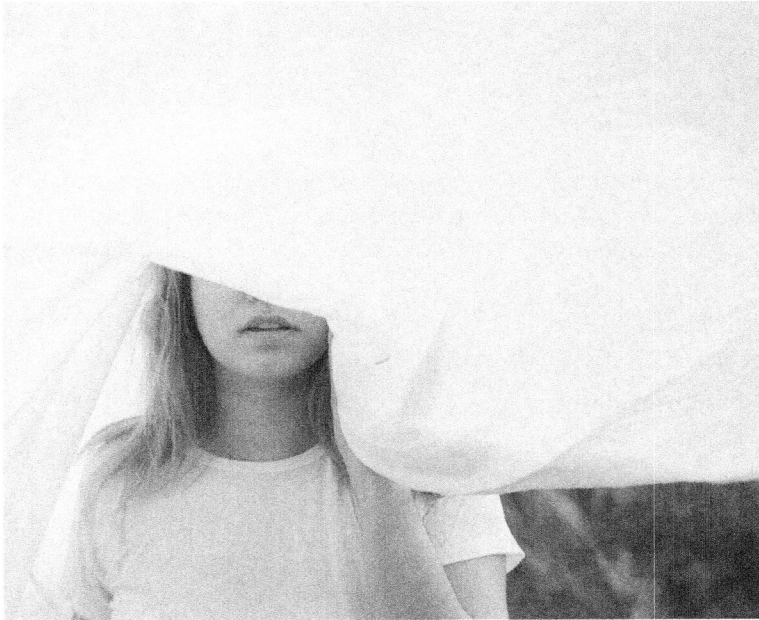

High risk? Consider:

	Relative risk drop
Tamoxifen (pills)	37-49 percent
Raloxifene (pills)	56-59 percent
Exemestane (pills)	65 percent
Removal of both ovaries	53 percent
Removal of both breasts	90 to 100 percent

Key points

Risk

Breast cancer remains the most common (non-skin) cancer among women in the United States. Fortunately, mortality from breast cancer continues to decline. We may conveniently divide risk factors into one of three major groups:

- Inherited genetics
- Hormone-related (including reproductive factors)
- Environmental

Action list

Many risk factors are not easily modifiable. Still, let's focus on the potentially changeable ones:

- **Physical activity:** Aim for the equivalent of a brisk walk for 150 minutes per week (for example, 30 minutes for five days per week)

- **Weight:** Shoot for a Body Mass Index (BMI) of 20 to 25

- **Alcohol:** Be prudent, limiting consumption to no more than three to seven standard drinks per week (and not more than three at any given time)

- **Diet:** Preferred diets include ones that are relatively low in fat, and rich in fruits and vegetables. Very limited evidence suggests that there may be some value to adding extra virgin olive oil into your diet, per haps as much as four tablespoons per day!

- **Anti-estrogen (endocrine) therapy:** If you are on these pills, don't forget to take them as prescribed. Many patients are non-compliant.

- **Hormones:** Long-term use of estrogen and progestin *in combination* as menopausal hormone replacement therapy increases the risk of breast cancer.

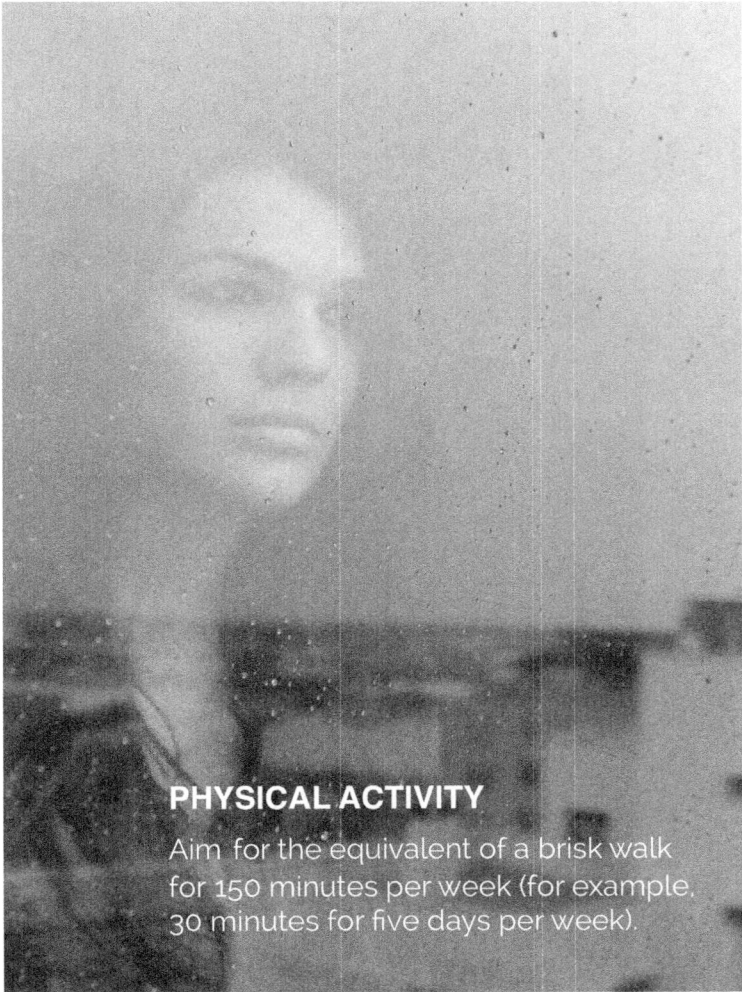

PHYSICAL ACTIVITY

Aim for the equivalent of a brisk walk for 150 minutes per week (for example, 30 minutes for five days per week).

2
IMAGE

Tools

mam•mo•gram Images of the breast obtained using X-rays.

Mammograms are the foundation of screening for women at average risk of getting the disease. Several randomized trials comparing screening mammograms versus no screening mammograms have shown that this imaging test decreases the odds of dying from breast cancer. Digital mammograms and tomosynthesis (3-D mammograms) are more recent innovations.

ul•tra•sound Images of the breast, obtained using sound waves.

Ultrasound is commonly used as a diagnostic follow-up when mammograms reveal something concerning. While not   generally used as a screening tool for women at average risk, some centers will incorporate ultrasound into screening for highly select women with increased breast density.

MRI Breast images of the breast obtained using powerful magnets.

Magnetic resonance imaging (MRI) is used for breast cancer diagnosis and staging. In addition, MRI may be added to mammograms for screening women at high risk. Breast MRI uses magnetic fields and an intravenous (IV) contrast agent to create images of the breast.

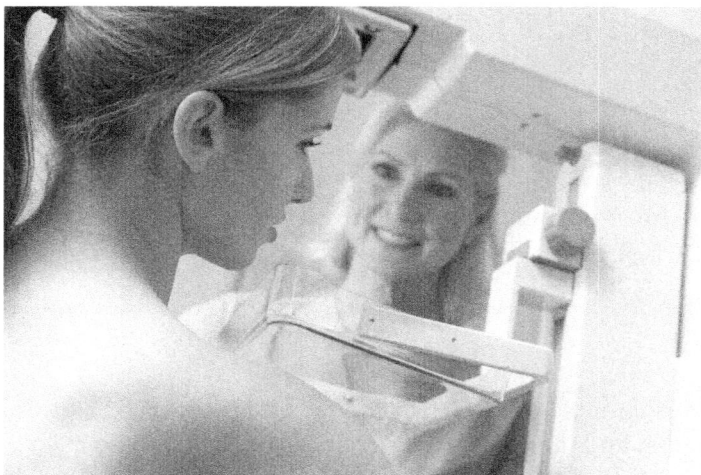

Mammograms

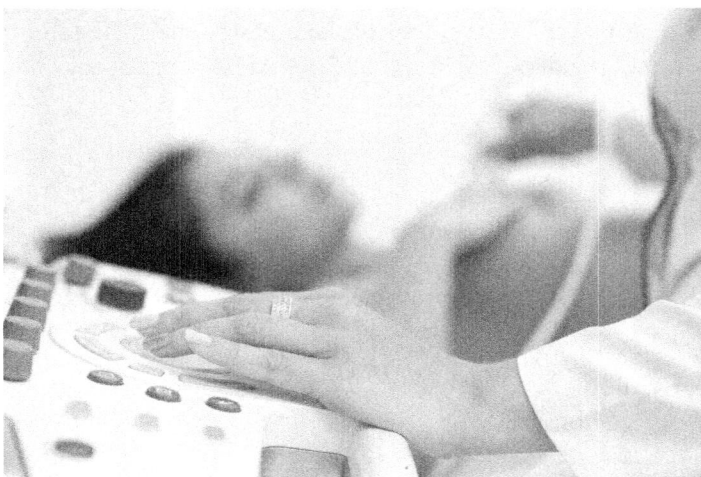

Ultrasound

Mammograms

to·mo·SYN·the·sis

A form of digital mammogram that creates a **3-D** picture of the breast using X-rays.

What

A regular mammogram typically takes two X-rays of each breast (one from top to bottom and the other from side to side). Digital tomosynthesis takes multiple X-ray pictures of each breast from many angles. The breast is positioned similarly to standard mammograms, but less pressure is applied. The X-ray tube moves in an arc around the breast, while multiple images take approximately seven seconds. The imaging device then sends information to a computer to create clear 3-D images of the breast. These multiple pictures create a layer-by-layer look at the breast tissue — one millimeter at a time — removing tissue overlap that may hide cancers or mistake dense breast tissue for cancer.

Why

Results with tomosynthesis are quite promising. Tomosynthesis can make breast cancers easier to see, especially in dense breast tissue, and may reduce the chances you will be called back for additional studies.

Better detection, fewer recalls

In one large study, researchers looked at data from 13 medical centers before and after they began using tomosynthesis. Digital mammograms with tomosynthesis detected one additional cancer for every 1,000 scans and resulted in 15% fewer false alarms – women called back for more tests, only to discover they did not have cancer. Researchers did not design the study to determine whether mammograms using tomosynthesis can save more lives than standard digital mammograms. The bottom line? Investigators found that the use of tomosynthesis ("3-D") mammograms was associated with:

- Improved cancer detection rates, especially invasive cancers
  - A decrease in callbacks, which may lessen anxiety for patients

No access to tomosynthesis?

Dr. Robert Smith, American Cancer Society senior director of cancer screening, offers that the study described above does not mean all women should seek out 3-D mammograms. Although the study showed an important improvement in cancer detection rates, the improvement was small. The more dramatic finding, he observes, was having a lower chance of being called back for additional testing; that is, compared to standard mammograms, tomosynthesis resulted in fewer false positives.

Step into the forest

I love this analogy from www.breastcancer.org: Traditional mammograms take only one picture, across the entire breast, in two directions: Top to bottom and side to side. It's like standing on the edge of a forest, looking for a bird somewhere inside. To better find the bird, take ten steps at a time through the forest and look all around you with each move. Welcome to the world of the 3-D mammogram, tomosynthesis. A radiologist analyzes your exam results and sends a report to your physician. For non-emergency situations, it usually takes a day or so to interpret the report and deliver the results.

Did you know?

The Food and Drug Administration (FDA) approved breast tomosynthesis in February, 2011. By the following month, the Harvard Massachusetts General Hospital breast imaging team performed the first clinical breast tomosynthesis exam in the United States.

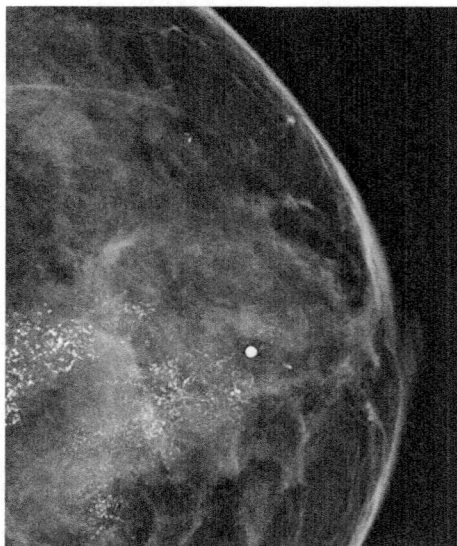

Mammogram
Malignant (cancer)
calcifications

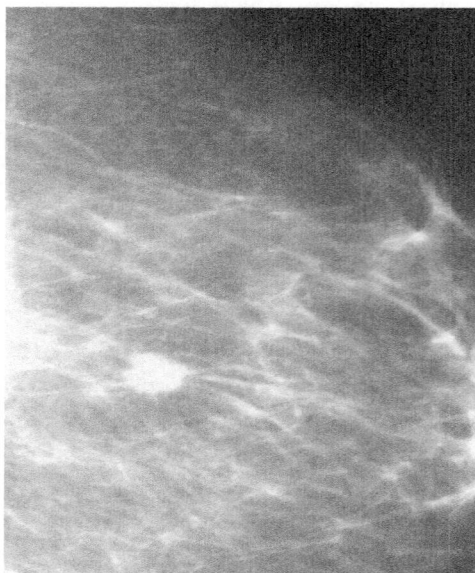

Mammogram
Mass (cancer)

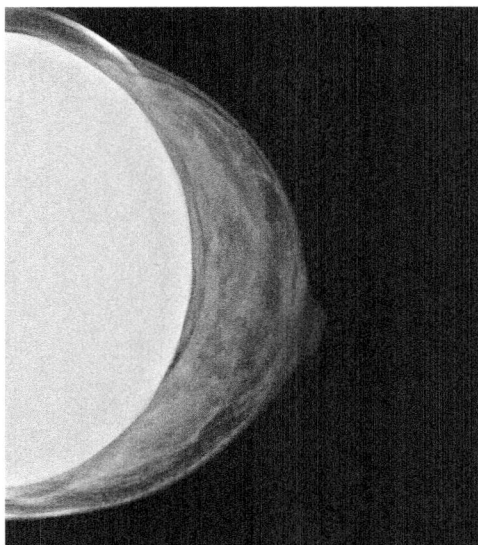

Mammogram
Implant obscures
some tissue
(displacement views can
help)

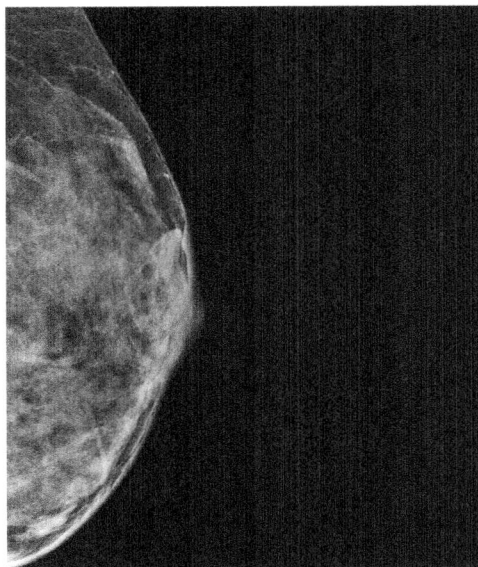

Mammogram
Cancer calcifications
Implant displacement
(pushed away) view

Screen

screen·ing [skrēn´ ing]
Looking for cancer before a person has any symptoms.

Shared decision-making among patients and healthcare providers is critical to optimizing your care. Growing evidence points to a potential for over-diagnosis with screening and the fact that we may have underestimated the potential harms of screening individuals not at high risk for developing breast cancer. In this chapter, I will attempt to illustrate the trade-offs between the potential benefits and harms of screening for breast cancer.

Benefits

Researchers have conducted multiple clinical trials involving over 600,000 women in the USA, Canada, the United Kingdom, and Sweden. The combined results point to a **reduction by one-fifth of the odds of dying of breast cancer.** Still, there have been numerous criticisms of the methods of the studies. Many patients in the studies "crossed over" to getting screened. On the other hand, might the reduction in breast cancer mortality be better with more modern imaging techniques?

Harms

Breast cancer screening can result in false positive results: The test says cancer may be present when it is not. We also have a risk of over-diagnosis: Here, the test finds something clinically insignificant. Low-grade DCIS (ductal carcinoma in situ) may be an example. Unfortunately, it is not always possible to distinguish cancers that are biologically insignificant from those that are potentially dangerous. Thus, we tend to treat all cancers.

Controversy

The odds of dying of cancer spreading (metastasizing) to distant sites are about one-third lower than in the 1980s. One model calculates that about half of this reduction is due to better systemic therapy, such as chemotherapy and endocrine therapy; the other half is due to screening and local therapies.

Skip mammograms?

Screening tools are more likely to have value when applied to individuals at higher risk of developing cancer and for whom the early intervention is more effective than later treatment. So, how do we decide at what age a woman (at average risk for breast cancer) should begin mammograms?

Randomized trials show that mammograms reduce breast cancer mortality in those most likely to develop breast cancer. For those without a risk-raising genetic mutation such as BRCA (BReast CAncer gene), those under 40 are at low risk for breast cancer. Risk rises between 40 and 45 and rises more steeply for those between 45 and 65. There are two groups of individuals for which mammograms would not likely provide value:

- Average-risk women under 40 years old
- Women with a limited life expectancy

Groups such as the American Cancer Society, the National Comprehensive Cancer Network (NCCN), and the US Preventative Task Force attempt to make screening recommendations by weighing potential benefits and harms (including unnecessary biopsies).

Shared decision-making

A care provider should help you make an informed, values-based decision about whether (and how often) to have screening for breast cancer. I hope this chapter will help improve your knowledge about the pros and cons of screening and encourage you to structure your breast cancer screening actively. First, however, let's explore the screening tools.

Age

Screening benefits (including a reduction in breast cancer mortality) and harms (false positives and over-diagnosis) vary by age. For example, the ability of mammograms to detect cancer is higher among older women in general:

	Sensitivity
The early 40s	73%
The early 60s	85%

In addition, breast cancer incidence rises with age in general. Age and life expectancy, therefore, play an important role in determining mammogram efficacy. When should you begin getting mammograms?

• Under 40?

The expert guidelines are conflicting for women (at average risk) 40 years old or older. Should you start screening at 40? 45? 50? We start with this fact: The number of lives saved by screening is lower for younger women than for older women. This finding is due, at least in part, to the fact that breast cancer incidence is lower among the younger group. In addition, the sensitivity (the disease is there, and the test finds it) and specificity (the disease is not there, and the test gets it right) is lower in younger women.

• Over 40 years?

For women (at average risk) who are 40 years old or older, the expert guidelines are conflicting. Should you start screening at 40? 45? 50? We start with this fact: The numbers of lives saved by screening are lower for younger women than they are for older women. This is due, at least in part, to the fact that breast cancer incidence is lower among the younger group. In addition, the sensitivity (the disease is there, and the test finds it) and specificity (the disease is not there, and the test gets it right) is lower with younger women.

A meta-analysis (an analysis of a collection of studies) of eight randomized trials demonstrated a **15 percent relative reduction in breast cancer mortality** among women ages 39 to 48 who were randomized to have screening mammograms.

Let's look at age differently: How many women (at average risk) do we need to screen to prevent one woman from dying?

	Number Needed to Screen
Ages 30 to 49	1,904
Age 50 to 59	1,339

Age: When to stop mammograms

There is no general agreement on the right age to stop having screening mammograms. It is not unreasonable to continue screening if you have a life expectancy of at least 10 years, irrespective of your age. Screening mammograms can lead to earlier stage presentations, but may not meaningfully improve your survival odds. Why? If you are older, you have competing risks such as heart attack and stroke. In addition, screening mammograms may find breast disease (such as low-grade ductal carcinoma *in situ* or DCIS) that is not clinically meaningful.

Unfortunately, none of the 8 randomized trials included women 75 and older. Observational studies suggest a *possible* decrease in breast cancer mortality among healthy women 80 and older who are regularly screened with mammography; however, these studies are limited by various biases (lead time, length time, and selection types).

American Cancer Society Guidelines for women at average breast cancer risk

For screening, average risk means that you have no personal history of breast cancer, a strong family history of breast cancer, or a genetic mutation known to increase the risk of breast cancer (for example, in a BRCA gene) and have not had chest radiation therapy before the age of 30.

- **Women between 40 and 44** have the option to begin screening with a mammogram every year.
- **Women 45 to 54** should get mammograms every year.
- **Women 55 and older** can switch to a mammogram every other year or choose to continue yearly mammograms.

Mammogram frequency uncertainty

We need more data on the optimal frequency for screening mammograms. Some advocate for yearly mammograms, while others suggest screening every two years. Here are some research findings from the Breast Cancer Surveillance Consortium:

- Premenopausal women who had every two-year screening had less favorable cancers (Stage IIB and higher).

- Women using menopausal hormones who were screened every two years had less favorable cancers.

- Postmenopausal women not on hormones did equally well with screening mammograms annually or every two years.

Harms in more detail

While mammograms reduce the chances of dying of breast cancer, there are some potential harms associated with screening:

- Insignificant cancers

Diagnosis of cancers that would otherwise never have caused symptoms or death can expose you to immediate risks (surgical deformity or toxicities from radiation therapy, hormone therapy, or chemotherapy) and late side effects (for example, arm swelling). Although management is typically tailored to individual tumor characteristics, there is no reliable way to distinguish which cancer would never progress in an individual patient; therefore, some treatment is nearly always recommended. Incidence studies in the USA found that at least 20% of screen-detected breast cancers are over-diagnosed.

- False-Positives

About 10 percent of women will be recalled from each screening examination for further testing, and only 5 percent called back will have cancer. These extra tests have financial costs and can also cause anxiety. False positives are more common among younger women, those with previous biopsies of the breast, a family history of breast cancer, estrogen use, an increased time interval between screenings, no comparison of the current mammogram with previous ones, and a radiologist's tendency to call mammograms abnormal.

• Mammogram-Induced Breast Cancer

The breast dose associated with a typical two-view mammogram is approximately four mSv (milli-Sieverts). Latency is at least eight years, and the increased risk is life-long. In theory, annual mammograms in women aged 40 to 80 may cause up to one breast cancer per 1,162 women. The reduction in death thanks to screening mammograms greatly outweighs the risk of death due to radiation-induced cancers.

As medical questions often have no clear-cut answers, transparent information is critical to decision-making. In this context, I present a fact box developed at the Harding Center for Risk Literacy. In the table, the numbers refer to 1,000 women over 50 who participated in screening for ten years or more (screening group), compared to 1,000 women of the same age who did not participate in screening during the same period (control group).

Breast Cancer Early Detection by Mammography

For women 50 years or older who did or did not participate in screening for about 10 years (results for every 1,000 women)

	No Screening	Screening
Benefits		
How many **died from breast cancer?**	**5**	**4**
How many died from all types of cancer?	21	21
Harms		
How many had false alarms or biopsies	-	100
How many with non-progressive cancer had unnecessary partial or complete breast removal?	-	5

Risk

Many factors determine breast cancer risk. Some are genetic and relate to family history, and others are based on personal factors such as reproductive and medical history. We have several tools to calculate your risk of developing breast cancer. Although these tools can estimate your risk, they cannot tell whether or not you will get breast cancer.

Gail model

The most commonly used tool to calculate breast cancer risk is the Breast Cancer Risk Assessment Tool, also known as the Gail Model tool. This simple tool incorporates variables such as age, race, history of breast disease, age at onset of menses, family history, and the number of full-term pregnancies. It calculates a woman's risk of developing breast cancer within the next five years and her lifetime (up to age 90). You can find this easy-to-use tool here:

Limitations

The Gail Tool does not give a good estimate of risk in some women, including those with:

- A personal history of invasive breast cancer, ductal carcinoma *in situ* (DCIS), or lobular carcinoma *in situ* (LCIS);
- A strong family history of breast cancer, who may have an inherited gene mutation (such as BRCA1);
- The original model was based on data from white women. The current model better estimates the risk for African-American, Asian-American, and Pacific-Islander women. However, it's still not clear how well the model works in other racial/ethnic groups.

Other tools use family history to estimate breast cancer risk. These include BRCAPRO, IBIS (which uses the Tyrer-Cuzik model), and BOADICEA. Such tools can be particularly useful for women with one or more relatives with breast or ovarian cancer.

SCREENING MAMMOGRAMS
NUMBER TO PREVENT ONE BREAST CANCER DEATH

Age	False positive*	Need biopsy*	DCIS or invasive cancer*	Number needed to be screened
40-49	98	9	3	**1,904**
50-59	87	11	5	**1,339**
60-69	79	12	7	377
70-79	69	12	8	?
80-89	59	11	2	?

* The estimates are for a single screening for a woman at *average* risk.

Exam

Clinical breast examination (CBE)

CBE by a healthcare provider has yet to be well-tested. One Canadian clinical trial used a clinical breast exam in conjunction with mammography and was the comparator modality versus mammography in another trial. It would be challenging to assess the value of CBE as a screening modality when used alone.

And there are potential harms: In the community, the false-positive rate is one to twelve percent. In addition, there can be so-called false negative results, leading to potential false reassurance and delay in cancer diagnosis. In fact, of women with cancer, up to approximately 40 percent will have a clear CBE. Sensitivity (the exam finds cancer when it is there) increases over time.

Breast self-exam

Breast self-exam (BSE) has been compared with no screening activity and has not been shown to reduce breast cancer mortality. Two large, randomized trials (China; Russia) have examined BSE. Neither showed improvements in outcomes among those that performed regular breast self-examinations:

- *Shanghai:* From 1989 through 1991, 266,064 women associated with 519 factories in Shanghai were randomly assigned to a breast self-exam instruction or not. Initial instruction in BSE was followed by reinforcement sessions one and three years later, BSE under medical supervision at least every six months for five years, and ongoing reminders to practice BSE monthly. Intensive instruction in BSE did not reduce mortality from breast cancer.

- *St. Petersburg:* No benefit to breast self-examination.

Limitations

Breast self-exam has potential harms: In the Chinese study, the biopsy rate was 1.8% among the study population (compared with 1% in the control group), with no improvement in cancer detection with screening. Still, breast exams (by you and a medical professional) seem reasonable in countries where regular imaging is not done.

Screening: Emerging tools

Ultrasound

Many tools for the early detection of breast cancer are under investigation. Some are already used in diagnosis and staging and are widely available. But should we use ultrasound for routine screening? Mammograms combined with breast ultrasound may find slightly more breast cancers than mammograms alone for women with dense breasts.

However, mammography plus breast ultrasound leads to more false positive results than mammography alone. Ultrasound is not routinely used for screening among women at average risk for breast cancer. If you don't have access to 3-D mammograms and have dense breast tissue, an elevated cancer risk, or implants, adding screening ultrasound to a regular mammogram can improve cancer detection.

Tomosynthesis (3-D) mammograms

Computer software combines multiple 2-D X-ray images to create a three-dimensional (3-D) image. Radiologists must have special training to read these 3-D images. Combining 2-D mammography with breast tomosynthesis can increase the odds of finding breast cancer, particularly if you have dense breasts or are still menstruating. Tomosynthesis can also lower the "call-back" rate.

Nuclear medicine breast imaging

Nuclear medicine breast imaging (or molecular breast imaging) uses short-lived radioactive agents given through an IV. Breast tissues absorb these agents. Breast cancer cells absorb more substances than healthy cells, and a special camera can image cancer cells. Nuclear medicine breast imaging is under study for use in breast cancer screening, diagnosis, and staging.

Examples include breast-specific gamma imaging (BSGI) and positron emission mammography (PEM). A special camera tracks the gamma-ray-emitting agents used in BSGI. For the PEM, a clinician injects radioactive sugar. Cancer cells consume more of this "hot" sugar than normal cells. Unfortunately, a radiation dose is 15 to 20 times higher than a mammogram dose.

Thermography

Thermography (digital infrared imaging devices) uses infrared light to measure temperature differences on the breast surface. Breast cancer can cause abnormal heat patterns that can theoretically be detected. However, there is no solid scientific evidence that thermography measures of heat can help find breast cancers. We have no randomized controlled trials evaluating its impact on early detection or mortality.

> ⚠️ Thermography is FDA-approved for the detection of breast cancer but is not approved as a *sole* screening tool for screening. It's approved for use with mammography. The FDA warned that thermography should not be used as an alternative to mammograms for breast cancer screening or diagnosis in a safety communication issued on February 25, 2019.

Breast MRI for women with dense breast tissue

Breast magnetic resonance imaging (MRI) uses magnetic fields to create a breast image. There is no ionizing radiation. It is more invasive than mammograms, as MRI requires a contrast agent given through an IV before the scan. Breast MRI is often used for select individuals' breast cancer diagnosis and staging. It is also used in breast cancer screening for women at higher risk.

MRI evaluates the blood flow pattern through the breast tissues, looking for areas where blood rapidly pools and then washes away; this occurs at cancer sites because of angiogenesis, or the formation of new blood vessels, as directed by the cancer.

Mammography plus breast MRI is under investigation for screening average-risk women with dense breast tissue: MRI does not care about your breast density, so that it can outperform mammograms and ultrasound. If you have very dense breasts, you may want to ask your healthcare provider about adding MRI to mammogram screening.

Alas, breast MRI is associated with a relatively high chance of a false positive (the test indicates that cancer is present when in reality it is not; this leads to additional studies and biopsies), is expensive, and not a particularly enjoyable experience (you need to lie face down in what can be a claustrophobia-inducing tube, with clanging noises ringing out).

Screening: High-risk

Experts use your personal and family medical histories, genetic tests, life-style and exposures, and other factors to assess risk and recommend breast screening and risk management. If you are at higher risk of breast cancer, you may need to be screened earlier, more often, and with additional imaging tools than women at average risk. Let's examine some factors that may place you in the high-risk category.

Some inherited genetic conditions can markedly raise your risk of developing breast cancer. These include having a breast cancer gene mutation (BRCA1 or BRCA2) or a first-degree relative with such a mutation. A strong family history of breast cancer (for example, your mother and/or sister) developing at age 45 or younger can increase your risk. Li-Fraumeni, Cowden, and Bannayan-Riley-Ruvalcaba syndromes are associated with genetic changes that can put you in the high-risk category. This connection holds if you or a first-degree relative has one of these syndromes or a p53 or PTEN gene mutation.

A personal history of invasive breast cancer or ductal carcinoma in situ (DCIS) can also raise your risk significantly, as can a personal history of lobular carcinoma in situ (LCIS) or atypical hyperplasia (atypical ductal hyperplasia (ADH) or atypical lobular hyperplasia (ALH)). Finally, a personal history of radiation treatment to the chest region (especially if this occurred before age 30) puts you into the high-risk breast cancer category. To understand your breast cancer risk and the actions you can take to manage it, please consult with medical experts with advanced risk assessment and cancer genetics training.

Is there a role for MRI in breast cancer screening?

MRI can improve cancer detection but increases callback and biopsy rates (which can increase anxiety levels). Those with a lifetime breast cancer risk of over 20% should consider combining MRI and mammography. The current American Cancer Society recommendations for breast MRI screening don't address the timing of MRI in conjunction with mammograms.

RISK GROUPS

High-risk 30%+	• BRCA mutation • Other hereditary cancer syndromes (for example, Li-Fraumeni Syndrome; Cowden Syndrome)
Intermediate risk 20-29%	• Breast biopsy shows *atypical* hyperplasia, or lobular carcinoma *in situ* (LCIS) • A calculated risk of 20% to 29% based on family history, personal health history, or certain genetic markers
Average risk 10-13%	• None of the above factors

Screening MRI timing to optimize performance is controversial. The American College of Radiology offers that premenopausal women should have their breast screening MRI scheduled between days 7 and 14 after the first day of their menstrual cycle; however, data supporting this recommendation are sparse. A study of screening MRI in 244 premenopausal women found that the menstrual cycle phase did *not* significantly affect performance.

Not everyone can have an MRI. Some conditions may make you a poor candidate for an MRI. These include:

- Pregnancy.
- An allergy to gadolinium-based contrast.
- Having certain implanted devices (for example, pacemakers).
- Your kidney function is inadequate.
- You have uncontrolled anxiety or claustrophobia.

MRI and mammogram

Mammograms use very low doses of radiation to make X-ray images of the breast. X-rays do not penetrate dense breast tissue very well, making mammography more challenging. Compared with mammograms, MRI is more sensitive in finding abnormalities within the breasts. MRI scans use radio waves and strong magnets instead of X-rays. The radio wave energy is absorbed and released in a pattern determined by the tissue type. A computer then translates this pattern into a highly detailed image. For a breast MRI, a contrast liquid (gadolinium) is injected into a vein before or during the scan to allow better visualization of the details.

For the MRI, you lie inside a narrow tube with your face down on a platform designed for the procedure. This platform has openings for each breast. This position allows for imaging without compressing the breasts. You have to stay still for the imaging procedure.

Several prospective, non-randomized studies have examined the efficacy of adding breast screening MRI to annual mammograms for women at high risk of developing breast cancer. These studies included women with BRCA gene mutations or a strong family history of breast cancer. Despite differences in patient population and MRI technique, these studies showed MRI is more sensitive to detecting breast cancer than mammograms.

Limitations

MRI can detect smaller tumors than mammograms, but MRI has important limitations: Call-back rates are higher for MRI, ranging from 8% to 17% for imaging and 3% to 15% for biopsy. Subsequent rounds of screening typically have lower call-back rates.

Early detection

Regular screening tests (along with appropriate health management) can reduce your chance of dying from breast cancer. Screening tests can find breast cancer early when the chances of survival are highest. Here are some elements of a personal action plan:

- *Watch for symptoms*

  Breast cancer warning signs vary among women. It is best to see a healthcare provider if you are unsure about a concerning finding. Common symptoms include a change in the look or feel of your breast or nipple or a nipple discharge.

- *Know your breasts*

  Breast self-exam (BSE) seemed promising when first introduced. However, studies on its effectiveness at finding breast cancer early and improving survival suggest it may not offer the same benefits as other screening tests such as a clinical breast exam (by a health provider), mammogram, or a breast MRI (for those at higher risk of getting breast cancer).

- *Know screening recommendations*

  Breast cancer screening can help find breast cancer early when the chances of survival are highest. Women at higher risk may need breast cancer screening earlier and more often than other women. Breast cancer screening is not recommended for most men.

MRI may used for staging patients with known cancer. The imaging test can evaluate extent of cancer or the presence of multifocal or multicentric cancer in the same breast, and to screen the opposite breast.

MRI AND SCREENING

	Holland	Canada	UK	Germany	USA
Sensitivity (%)*					
MRI***	80	77	77	91	100
Mammograms	33	36	40	33	25
Ultrasound	N/A	33	N/A	40	N/A
Specificity (%)**					
MRI	90	95	81	97	95
Mammograms	95	>99	93	97	98
Ultrasound	N/A	96	N/A	91	N/A

N/A = not applicable

*$**$Sensitivity (true positive rate) measures the percentage of correctly identified cancers.

**Specificity (true negative rate) measures the percentage of healthy people correctly identified as not having breast cancer).

***MRI looks at both breasts. Breast MRIs are performed with intravenous contrast. The expert imaging team should have the ability to perform MRI-guided needle sampling (or image-guided localization of MRI-detected findings.

False-positive findings (the test says there is cancer, but in actuality there is not) on MRI are common. Surgical decision should not be based solely on MRI findings. Additional tissue sampling of areas of concern identified by MRI is recommended.

If you have an abnormal mammogram or a concerning physical finding,

what's next? Follow-up typically begins with less invasive tests such as *diagnostic* mammograms or breast ultrasounds. The radiologist examines the images to determine whether the abnormal finding looks suspicious:

- *Not suspicious-appearing*

If the lesion doesn't look like cancer on imaging, you may not need any more testing. An example is a simple cyst.

- *Suspicious-appearing*

A tissue sampling (biopsy) is typically done for suspicious lesions, often using a needle. The concerning tissue is sent to a pathologist to examine it for cancer.

Most calcifications seen on mammograms are *not* cancer. However, calcifications are sometimes a sign of cancer. We may conveniently classify calcifications into one of 3 categories:

1) Benign
2) Intermediate concern
3) Higher probability of cancer

Benign calcifications are typically larger, coarser, and round with smooth margins. They may be scattered or diffuse. Malignant calcifications are typically grouped or clustered, pleomorphic (varying in size and shape), fine, and with linear branching.

Mammogram: Screening versus Diagnostic

Individuals with no symptoms or signs of breast cancer have screening mammograms. Screening mammograms try to find breast cancer when it is too small to be felt by you or your care provider. Those with a known breast problem (such as a lump or nipple discharge) have diagnostic mammograms.

We sometimes use diagnostic mammograms for patients without breast problems with a history of breast cancer management. During a diagnostic mammogram, a radiologist immediately reviews the images; you may have more imaging if there is a concerning area.

74

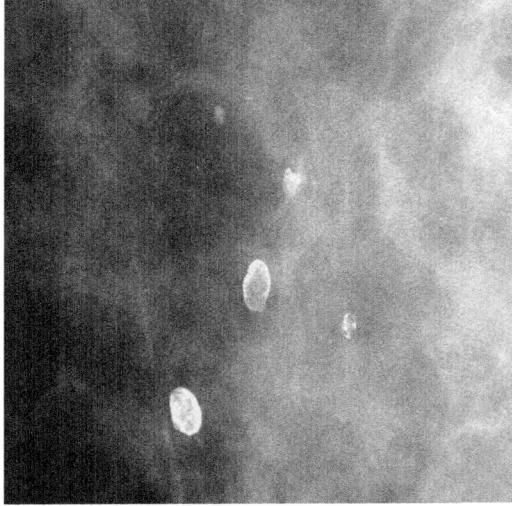

Benign (not cancer) calcifications

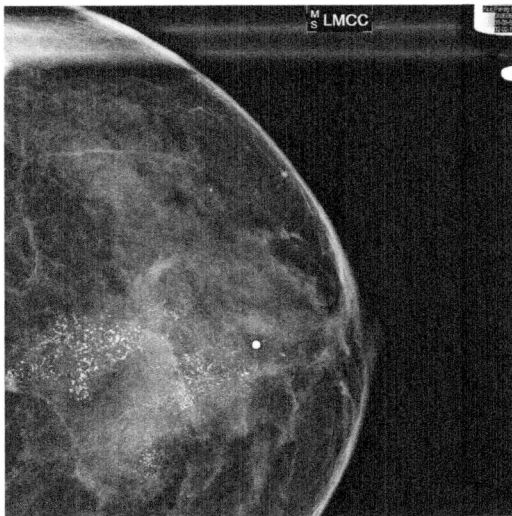

Concerning calcifications

Diagnostic mammograms

Sometimes, a radiologist asks for special images (spot or magnification views) to evaluate a small area of concern. The doctor may interpret the diagnostic mammograms in one of three ways:

- **Not cancer:** An area that looked abnormal on a screening mammogram appears normal. You typically then return to routine annual mammograms.

- **Probably not cancer:** An area that looked abnormal on a screening mammogram is probably not cancer, but it is common to come back in 4 to 6 months to re-check.

- **Looks like it may be cancer:** You need a biopsy.

Special case: Women under 30 with symptoms

For women under 30, most breast lumps are benign (not cancer). The first step is a clinical breast exam (CBE), a physical exam performed by a skilled healthcare provider. The clinician should carefully feel your breasts and underarm area for abnormalities. Examples of abnormal findings include:

- A dominant lump in the breast or underarm area
- Change in breast size or shape
- Dimpling or puckering of the skin
- Pulling in of the nipple or other breast parts
- Nipple discharge
- Pain
- Swelling, redness, warmth, or darkening of the breast

Additional evaluation may include a breast ultrasound (and, for selected women, a mammogram). Selected women may require a biopsy to determine whether a lump is breast cancer.

MAMMOGRAMS

BI-RADS Category	
1 Negative	No significant abnormality.
2 Benign	No sign of cancer, but the reporting radiologist chooses to describe a finding thought benign (such as benign calcifications).
3 Probably benign	98% chance *not* cancer. May be suggested to repeat imaging in 6 months, and regularly thereafter to ensure stability.
4 Suspicious	Findings do not definitely look like cancer, but could be. Radiologist concerned enough to recommend a biopsy.
5 Highly suggestive of cancer	High chance (over 95 percent) cancer present. Biopsy is strongly recommended.
6 Known cancer	May be used to assess response to treatment.

*We use a standard system to describe mammogram findings and results. This system (called the Breast Imaging Reporting and Data System or BI-RADS) sorts results into categories as above. By categorizing in this way, the radiologist can describe the mammogram findings using the common terminology. This makes accurate communication of test results easier.

Breast density

Breast density may be reported on your mammogram report but is often subjective. In addition to a BI-RADS system describing our level of suspicion (please see the table to the right), the BI-RADS system also classifies breast density:

> • *Almost entirely fatty*
> Because fatty breasts have little fibrous and glandular tissue, the mammogram would likely be able to see anything abnormal.

> • *Having scattered fibroglandular density*
> There are a few areas of fibrous and glandular tissue in the breast.

> • *Heterogeneously dense*
> The breast has more areas of fibrous and glandular tissue throughout the breast. This tissue type make finding small masses more challenging.

> • *Extremely dense*
> The breast has a lot of fibrous and glandular tissue. This tissue type can make it harder to see cancer, as cancer can blend in with normal tissues (like finding a snowball in a snow field).

Dense breasts have a significantly higher risk of developing breast cancer. But does the presence of dense breasts (among those with breast cancer) affect the risk of dying of the disease? To examine the relationship between breast density and breast cancer mortality, researchers analyzed data from the Breast Cancer Surveillance Consortium (BCSC), a population-based registry of breast imaging facilities in the USA. They limited data collection to the five BCSC registries that consistently collect data on body mass index (BMI) to be able to adjust for such factors.

After adjusting for other health factors, the analysis showed that the overall group of patients with high-density breasts did not have a higher risk of death from breast cancer than those with lower-density breasts. However, subgroup analysis suggested that there might be an increased risk of breast cancer death among women with low density (BI-RADS 1) who were either obese (2-times increase in risk) or had primary cancers measuring 2 centimeters or greater (1.55-times increase in risk).

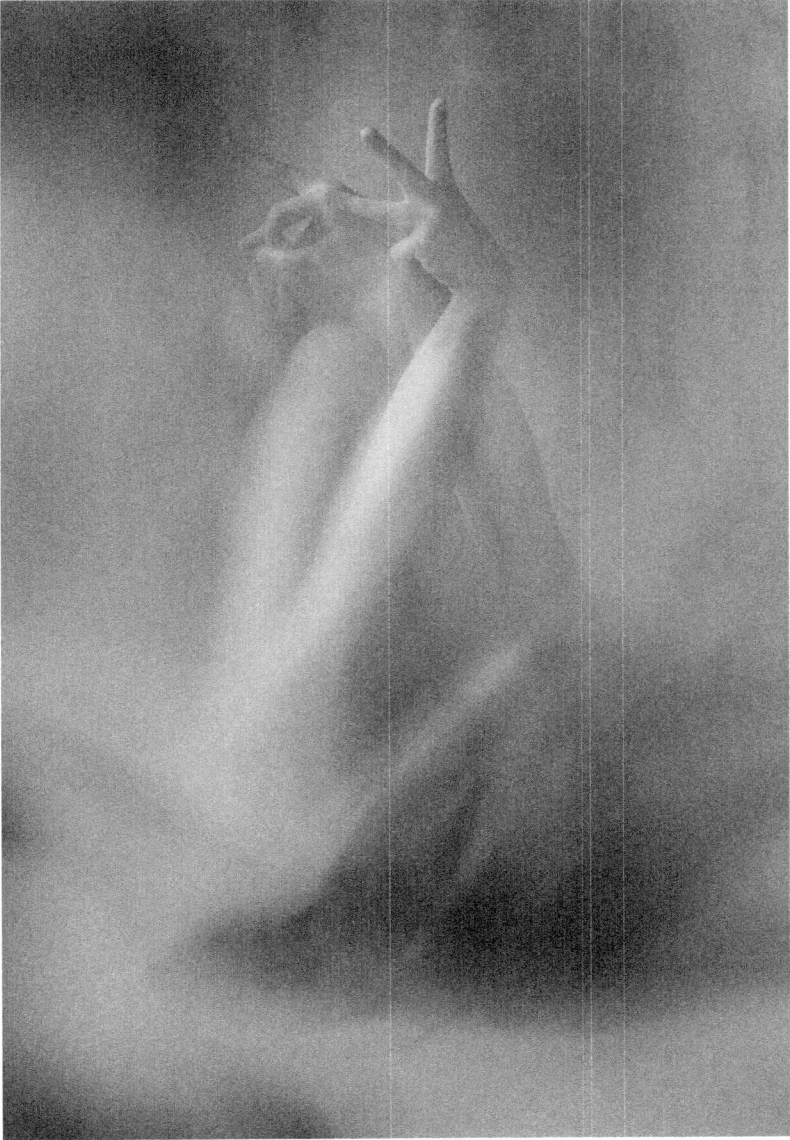

BIOPSY

3

Biopsy types

An outpatient needle biopsy is typically a fairly simple procedure and is generally preferred to a surgical biopsy. Women with abnormal mammograms may have a surgical biopsy rather than the much safer and less invasive needle biopsy. About 20% of biopsies in the USA turn out to be cancer. In countries like Sweden (where only the most suspicious lesions have a biopsy), about 80% of biopsies turn out to be malignant (cancer).

Least invasive

A needle biopsy uses a hollow needle to remove samples of tissue or cells from the breast. The material goes to a pathologist, who studies these samples under a microscope to see if they contain cancer or other concerning findings. There are two types of needle biopsies:

- **Core needle biopsy**
You may have a core needle biopsy if you have a palpable breast lump. This biopsy form is sometimes used for a non-palpable lesion but is visible on imaging. A core needle biopsy can be quite accurate and is less invasive than surgery. A core needle biopsy removes a narrow cylinder of tissue. While there is a small chance of bruising or infection, it is generally accurate and (if cancer is present) can provide information about the cancer type, grade (aggressiveness), and receptor status (Is the cancer driven by estrogen? Progesterone? HER2?)

- **Fine needle aspiration (FNA)**
FNA removes cells from a suspicious lump and is used for palpable lumps. The needle used is thinner than the ones used for core needle biopsies. While core needle biopsy is often the first choice for palpable masses, FNA is sometimes done as a quick means of sampling a breast lump felt during a clinical breast exam or a concerning underarm (axillary) lymph node. The false positive rate is about 1 to 2%. The false negative rate can be 40 percent, so if the FNA does not show cancer, your care team may recommend obtaining more tissue (depending on what the FNA demonstrates).

Most invasive

Most health care providers will first try to figure out the cause of a breast abnormality by doing a needle biopsy. Less commonly, a surgical biopsy is needed. A surgical (or open) biopsy is done by cutting the breast to take out all or part of the lump so it can be looked at under a microscope. The vast majority of open breast biopsies are performed with either local anesthesia alone or local anesthesia combined with intravenous sedation. General anesthesia is typically used for more complex situations; for example, when multiple abnormalities must be removed and local anesthesia would be insufficient.

Incisional biopsy

An incisional biopsy removes only part (but more than a needle biopsy) of the suspicious area, enough to make a diagnosis. It is only done if the tumor is too big to be removed with an excisional biopsy. Incisional biopsies are not commonly performed.

Excisional biopsy (lumpectomy)

An excisional biopsy removes the entire abnormality in the breast. A surgeon typically does it in an operating room (OR). Your surgeon will use local anesthesia to numb the area that will be sampled. You will also need sedation via an intravenous line. Typically, the procedure is an outpatient one: Most individuals do not have to stay in the hospital overnight.

Before surgery, a wire-localization or needle-localization procedure may be performed if the abnormal area cannot be felt. A radiologist uses mammograms, ultrasound, or other imaging to guide a very thin wire into the suspicious area of the breast. The surgeon can then use this wire to find your area of concern during surgery.

In the operating room, the breast tissue that is removed is usually X-rayed. This process lets the surgeon and radiologist match the suspicious areas on the mammogram with those in the biopsy to ensure the correct tissue has been removed. If the areas do not match, the surgeon may try to remove the correct tissue again or wait for another biopsy.

Excisional biopsy (continued)

The incision should be long enough to provide adequate exposure and to ensure that the mass can be removed as a single specimen with a small margin of grossly normal tissue. The surgeon should orient the specimen, and the pathologist should ink all margins. Although an excisional biopsy aims to diagnose cancer, sometimes the surgeon may be able to remove the cancer fully. In these cases, excisional biopsy may be the only breast surgery needed to treat the cancer. For others, lymph nodes may also need removal (in a second surgery later).

Results

After the tissue is removed, the material is sent to a doctor known as a pathologist. The pathologist examines the tissue, including with a microscope, and determines whether the tissue contains cancer. A pathology report (including the diagnosis) is issued and sent to the ordering physician. The report may have material added later, so there can be more than one report for a single biopsy session.

Your pathology report provides your diagnosis. Most initial information comes within 7 to 10 days after your surgery, and you will usually have all the results within a few weeks. Your doctor can let you know when the results come in. If you don't hear from your doctor, call the office. A physician (such as your radiologist, surgeon, or oncologist) will review the report's main findings and answer any questions you may have. The report is prepared for healthcare providers, making the language confusing for the patient. Still, understanding the report's basic parts can help you be a better consumer. Because each individual's breast cancer is unique, it's important to understand the underlying biology of your cancer to personalize your management plan.

⚠ Ask for a copy of your pathology report for your records.

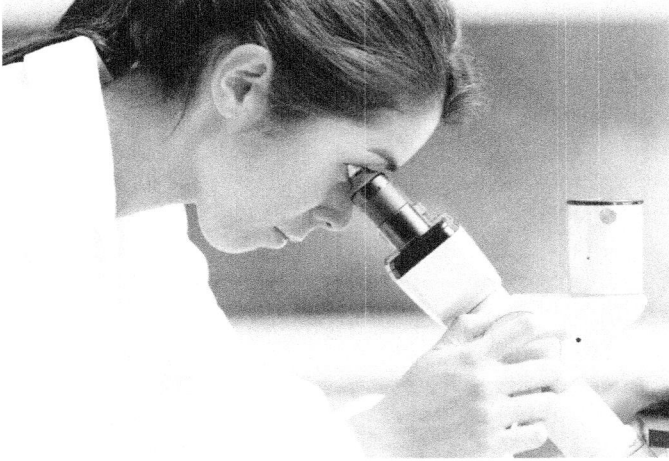

1 **Pathologist** receives biopsy material.

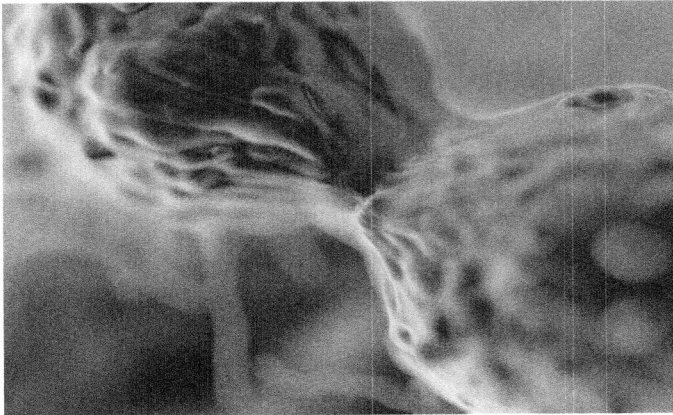

2 Tissue examined under a microscope.

Basics

Cancer is a condition in which cells do not die at the normal rate. A tissue mass (tumor) can form as cell growth exceeds cell death. Breast cancer happens when cells in the breast divide and grow abnormally. Many (but not all) breast cancers grow slowly and are not detected until 10 to 15 years before we can detect them. Up to 75% of breast cancers begin in the milk ducts, while 10 to 15% begin in the lobules. The remainder starts in other breast tissues. Benign means, not cancer.

Non-invasive or invasive?

We may conveniently divide breast cancer into two categories: Invasive versus non-invasive breast cancer. The latter is called ductal carcinoma in situ (DUK-tul kar-sin-O-ma in SY-too) or DCIS. Only about 20 to 25% of breast cancer is non-invasive.

  • Ductal carcinoma *in situ* (DCIS)

  Abnormal cells are confined to the milk ducts. In situ means "remaining in place." With DCIS, the cancer cells are contained within the milk ducts. Many clinicians believe we should not think of DCIS as true cancer (as it cannot spread in its pure form), but the classification has not yet changed.

  Please note that lobular carcinoma in situ (LCIS) is not cancer, but it can raise the future risk of getting cancer in either breast.

  • Invasive breast cancer

  Abnormal cells inside the milk ducts have escaped through the duct wall into the nearby breast tissue. While most of the time, cancer does not spread to nodes or distant organs, it can travel (through the bloodstream or lymphatic vessels) from the breast to anywhere in the body, including the bone, lungs, and liver. We call this metastasis (meh-TAS-tah-sis).

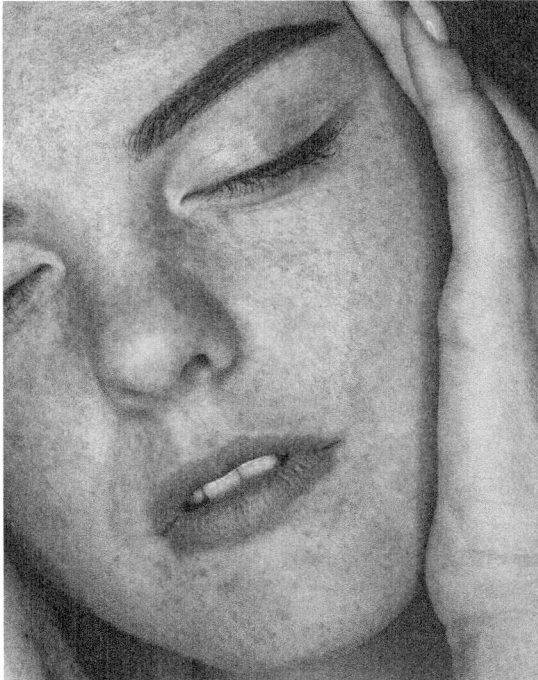

PATHOLOGY 1

- NON-INVASIVE (IN SITU)
- BENIGN (NOT CANCER) LESIONS

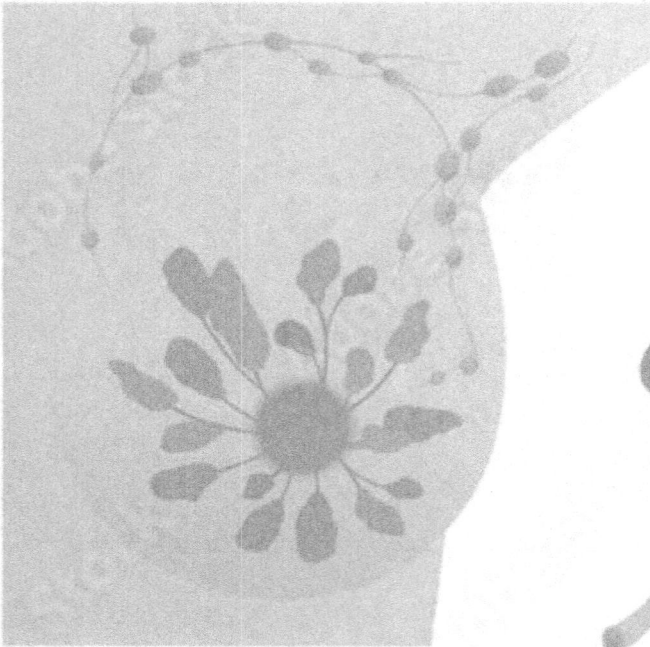

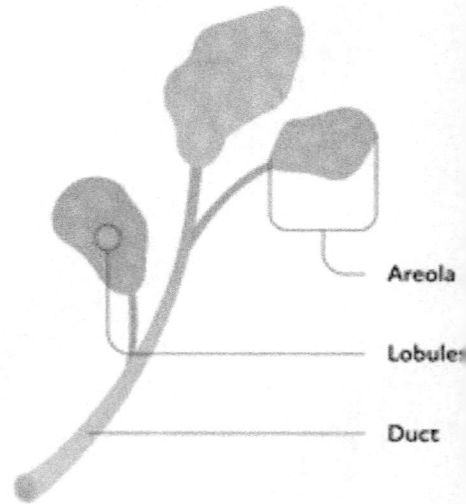

Areola

Lobules

Duct

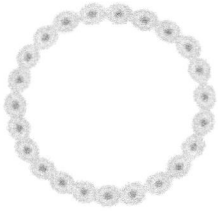

Normal Duct Cells

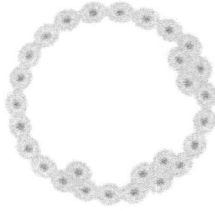

Hyperplazia

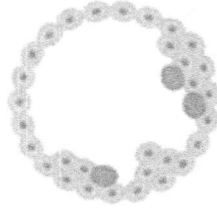

Hyperplazia
with atypical cells

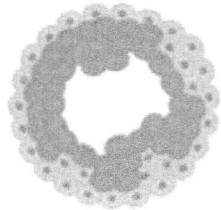

DCIS (ductal
cancer in situ)

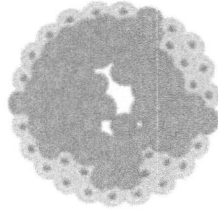

DCIS with
microinvasion

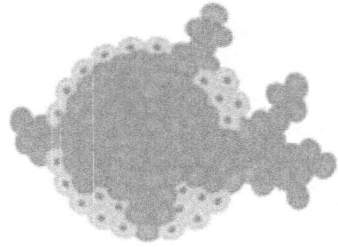

IDC (invasive
ductal cancer)

DCIS (ductal carcinoma in situ)

Biopsy

After a breast biopsy or surgery, a doctor specializing in specimen analysis examines the removed tissue with a pathologist. They examine the cells and tissue grossly and then under a microscope. You can find the pathologist's observations and thoughts in your pathology report. Typically, this report is issued several days after the pathologist receives the tissue. The information in the pathology report is critical to optimizing your management.

Basics

Ductal carcinoma *in situ* (DCIS) is not breast cancer, as many commonly understand it. Non-invasive "cancers" stay within the milk ducts or milk lobules in the breast: The abnormal cells in DCIS have not spread outside the milk ducts (in situ means "remaining in place") into other parts of the breast or to other parts of the body.

DCIS is not lethal in its pure form because it stays confined to the duct. However, DCIS is important because it can be a precursor of potentially deadly invasive breast cancers: Without treatment, DCIS may develop into an invasive breast cancer (which can then potentially spread to regional nodes or even metastasize to distant parts of the body, such as the bones, lungs, liver, or other sites).

Ductal carcinoma *in situ* encompasses a wide spectrum of diseases ranging from low-grade lesions that are not life-threatening to high-grade lesions that may hide bits of invasive breast cancer. The growth of abnormal cells bounded by the basement membrane of the breast ducts characterizes DCIS. DCIS is also known as intraductal (within the milk ducts) carcinoma. You may also hear the terms "pre-invasive" or "pre-cancerous" to describe it.

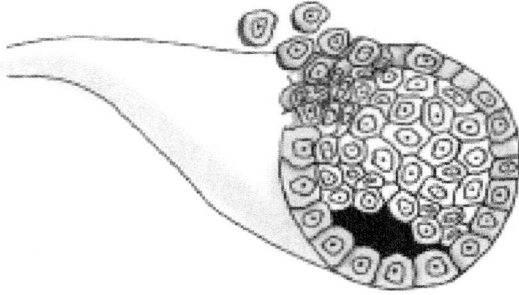

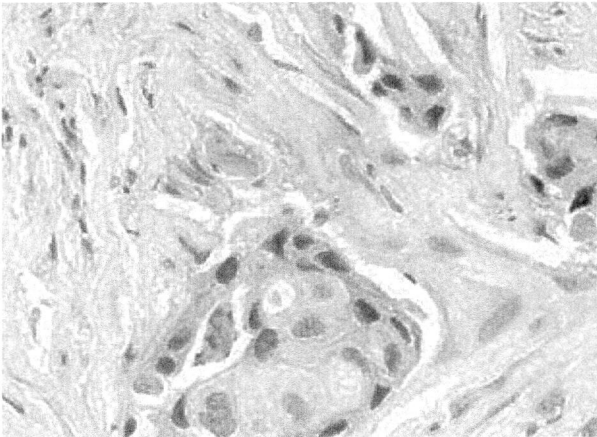

DCIS

The milk ducts contain abnormal cells. In situ ("remaining in its original place") means the cells have not left the milk ducts to invade nearby breast tissue.

DCIS

Before widespread screening mammograms, clinicians usually diagnosed ductal carcinoma in situ (DCIS or intraductal carcinoma) by surgically removing a suspicious breast mass. While first described in 1893, DCIS was rarely diagnosed before the 1980s. Today a quarter of breast cancers diagnosed in the USA are DCIS, a non-invasive breast cancer.

The recognition of DCIS as a specific disease distinct from invasive breast cancer occurred gradually, primarily during the first half of the 20th century. It was rare during that time, accounting for only one to two percent of newly diagnosed breast cancers, and was usually detected when it formed a large palpable mass. Mastectomy became the standard therapy and cured the rare patient who presented with DCIS. With the rise of screening mammograms at the tail end of the 20th century, radiologists had the tools to catch this early-stage breast cancer. Ductal carcinoma in situ sometimes produces calcium deposits in the ducts. This mammogram-detected calcium (rather than a mass) leads to the diagnosis of DCIS for up to one in four individuals with DCIS.

We believe that invasive breast cancer evolves through a non-obligatory series of increasingly abnormal "stages" over long periods, probably decades in many cases. There have been innumerable studies of the biological and molecular features of DCIS, especially since the 1970s. The cells of DCIS and invasive breast cancer are highly similar at the cellular and molecular levels, even though only one is invasive. There are similarities at the genetic level: We can subdivide invasive breast cancer and its non-invasive counterpart DCIS by molecular characteristics (based on features such as estrogen and progesterone receptor status (ER, PR), HER2, and grade).

Does all DCIS eventually progress to become invasive? We believe that not all DCIS will become invasive, but we don't know what percentage will do so. Historically, some DCIS cases did not have treatment; for example, there are limited studies of patients with DCIS that were originally misdiagnosed as benign and did not have surgical removal. These retrospective studies suggest that in the modern era, at least a third or more DCIS cases will eventually progress to invasive breast cancer if undetected.

DCIS

Size and type

The pathology report should address the size of the DCIS, preferably as measured under a microscope. The DCIS can affect your management recommendations. There are different patterns of low-grade (less aggressive-appearing) and moderate-grade DCIS, as viewed microscopically:

- **Papillary** (abnormal cells protrude inwardly from the duct wall)
- **Cribriform** (pierced with small holes as in a sieve. The tumor appears to have open spaces or small holes inside.)
- **Solid** (abnormal cells fill the ducts)

High-grade DCIS, sometimes described as "comedo" or comedo necrosis. Comedo means that there are areas of dead (necrotic debris) abnormal cells inside the breast milk duct. As the cells divide rapidly, they can't get enough nourishment, and these starving cells die, leaving areas of necrosis. Less common variants include the "clinging" carcinoma, intraductal signet ring carcinoma, and cystic hypersecretory duct carcinomas.

Classification

There are many DCIS classification schemes. These often focus on the presence or absence of necrosis (cell breakdown) and characteristics of the cell nucleus (the nucleus stores the cell's DNA and coordinates cell activities). On the previous pages, you saw a division of DCIS types based on the architectural pattern: Solid, cribriform, papillary, and micropapillary are examples. Today, the nuclear grade is emphasized and is reported as low, intermediate, or high.

- Nuclear grade a (low-grade)
  Cells close to normal and grow slowly.

- Nuclear grade 2 (intermediate grade)
  Cells appear abnormal and grow faster than normal.

- Nuclear grade 3 (high grade)
  Cells appear very abnormal and grow fast.

DCIS

Margins; estrogen receptors (ER)

Margins

During a surgical biopsy or breast-conserving surgery, your surgeon removes the DCIS and a surrounding zone of normal-appearing tissue. We refer to this healthy-looking tissue as the surgical margin. If you have no DCIS cells in the margin, your surgeon has likely removed all of the DCIS, and we call the margins "negative" or uninvolved. If the margin is not clear, you may need to do more surgery to ensure that all of the measurable DCIS is out. Optimal margins for DCIS are two millimeters, although not mandatory.

Estrogen receptors

The pathologist will test your DCIS for hormone receptor(s). These tests determine if your DCIS has receptors for the hormone estrogen. A positive result means that estrogen fuels the growth of abnormal cells. If the DCIS is estrogen receptor-positive (ER+), your doctor may recommend treatments to block the effects of estrogen or to lower your body's estrogen levels.

Normal breast tissue uniformly expresses estrogen receptors (ER) and progesterone receptors (PR). ER levels are higher in DCIS lesions that are less aggressive-appearing under the microscope. One review showed estrogen receptor expression in 83% of well-differentiated DCIS, 74% of poorly differentiated DCIS, 91% of DCIS lesions with no necrosis, and 37% of DCIS lesions with significant necrosis.

HER2

Some cancers have a gene mutation that leads to the excess creation of the HER2 protein. The presence of HER2 can promote cell growth. HER2 overexpression is seen more frequently in DCIS (particularly high-grade DCIS):

	HER2 +
• DCIS	50-60%
• Invasive ductal carcinoma	25-30%

While we do not routinely test DCIS for HER2, some data suggest that HER2-overexpressing DCIS is much more likely to be associated with invasive breast cancer (compared with DCIS without overexpression). A University of Pennsylvania study discovered 37 percent of DCIS that had overexpression of HER2 had early invasive breast cancer associated with it. The chances of finding an associated invasive cancer increased by 6.4 times with HER2 overexpression.

DCIS: Are you sure?

The distinction between low-grade DCIS and atypical lesions that are not yet DCIS is primarily based on disease extent. The lesions may have similar histologic characteristics under the microscope. Perhaps not surprisingly, pathologists may misdiagnose breast tissue. A recent American study involved 115 pathologists and 240 breast biopsy specimens. Researchers matched these diagnoses with those of three experts. Here are the results:

- Pathologists correctly diagnosed abnormal, pre-cancer cells about half the time, no better than a coin toss.
- Pathologists mistakenly found something suspicious in 13 percent of normal tissue.
- 13 percent of DCIS cases were misdiagnosed as less serious, while three percent were mistaken for invasive cancer.

Molecular profiling

While associated with a very high cancer-specific survival chance, ductal carcinoma in situ represents a group of diseases with various prognoses and needs for treatment. In the future, we should better understand who needs treatment (and who does not). Molecular profiling examines the genes and promises more tailored management for DCIS. Some factors that may influence DCIS prognosis include 1) p16 expression, 2) cyclooxygenase-2, and 3) Ki-67 proliferation index

The Oncotype DX test analyzes the activity of a group of genes in the DCIS to provide an individualized prediction of the 10-year risk of a future event (the return of DCIS or invasive cancer). This test can help some women with DCIS treated by surgery, with or without anti-estrogen therapy such as tamoxifen. In the USA, Medicare has established coverage for Oncotype DX for women with DCIS; coverage outside Medicare varies by insurance plan.

DCIS

How it works

The Oncotype DX test examines a sample of the DCIS that has already been removed during the original surgery. The test measures a group of cancer genes to see gauge their activity. The test result is reported as a score between 0 and 100, known as the DCIS Score results. A lower DCIS Score result means a lower chance that a tumor will come back in the same breast.

While the vast majority of patients with DCIS do not have an Oncotype DX Breast DCIS test, the score can help some women determine how aggressive to be with treatment (Radiation therapy? No radiation therapy?) One potential limitation of using the test is that the study that validated it defined cancer-free zones (margins) around the DCIS of at least 3 millimeters. The DCIS had to be 2.5 centimeters (2 inches) or smaller.

Depending on the recurrence score number, the DCIS has a low, intermediate, or high risk of recurrence. A low-risk score is less than 39, and a high-risk score is 55 or higher. A score of 39 to 54 is an intermediate risk. Here are the results during nearly ten years of follow-up:

In-breast DCIS recurrence

Low-risk score	5.4 percent
Intermediate-risk score	14.1 percent
High-risk score	13.7 percent

In-breast invasive disease recurrence

Low-risk score	8 percent
Intermediate-risk score	20.9 percent
High-risk score	15.5 percent

If you have DCIS, your doctor will recommend a treatment plan after surgery tailored to your specific recurrence risk for DCIS or invasive breast cancer, your personal preferences, and other factors. Your management plan may include radiation therapy, hormonal therapy, or neither.

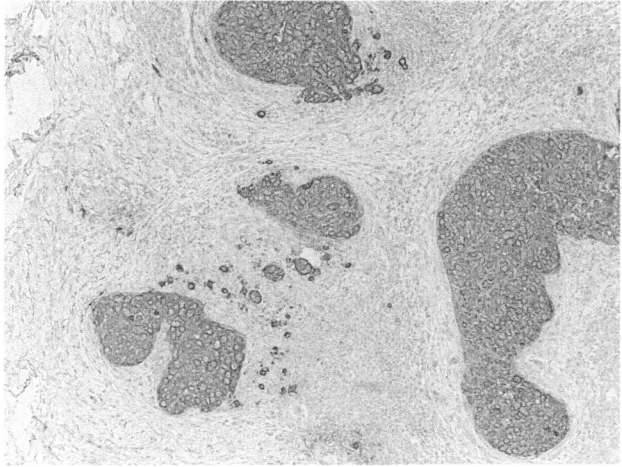

Microinvasion
A SMALL AMOUNT OF INVASIVE BREAST CANCER (1 millimeter or less)

Microinvasion describes a borderline difference between completely contained (with a duct) ductal carcinoma in situ (DCIS) and a minimally invasive ductal cancer. A very small amount of malignant cells are just beyond the duct lining, with this invasive component measuring less than one millimeter (1/25th of an inch). In cases with multiple foci of microinvasion (where no individual focus is larger than a millimeter), the pathologist should report the number of foci and range of sizes. We do not add the size of individual foci of microinvasion.

In the photomicrograph to the right, you can see abnormal cells stained to be brown. While most abnormal cells are confined to the ducts, small nests have escaped. Under the microscope, micro-invasive breast carcinoma tends to be associated with high-grade DCIS and comedo-type necrosis. There is some evidence that the risk of microinvasion increases with larger size DCIS lesions and multicentric (in several areas of the breast) ones.

LCIS (lobular carcinoma in situ)

Lobular means that the abnormal cells start growing in the lobules, the milk-producing glands at the end of breast ducts. Carcinoma begins in the skin or other tissues covering internal organs, such as breast tissue. In situ or "remaining in place" means that the abnormal growth remains inside the milk lobule and has not broken out into surrounding tissues. LCIS tends to affect more than one lobule.

Cancer?

Even though its name includes "carcinoma," LCIS is not a breast cancer. Rather, if you have LCIS, you have a higher risk for getting cancer in either breast in the future. Some experts prefer the descriptor lobular neoplasia (a collection of abnormal cells) *in situ*. Fortunately, we are a variety of means to reduce your risk of future cancer development in either breast.

Uncommon

Lobular carcinoma *in situ* (LCIS) seems uncommon, but we don't know how many people are affected. LCIS does not cause symptoms and usually does not appear on a mammogram. It tends to be found due to a breast biopsy performed for another reason. LCIS more common in premenopausal women, most commonly between the ages of 40 and 50. Less than 10 percent of women with LCIS have already gone through menopause. LCIS is extremely uncommon among men.

Aggressive variant: Pleomorphic

Surgery may be advised in certain circumstances. For example, surgery is often recommended for a specific LCIS called pleomorphic lobular carcinoma *in situ*. Pleomorphic LCIS has larger cells that demonstrate marked nuclear abnormality.

Suppose you have isolated pleomorphic LCIS on a biopsy. In that case, you have a high risk (about one in three) of upgrading to invasive cancer or ductal carcinoma *in situ* at the surgery (for example, a lumpectomy). Pleomorphic LCIS also has a greater risk of developing breast cancer than the more common classical type.

LOBULAR CARCINOMA IN SITU (LCIS)

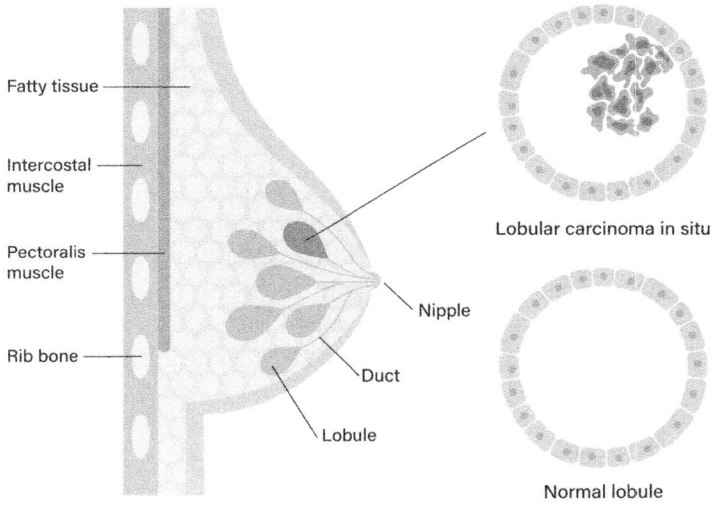

Fatty tissue

Intercostal muscle

Pectoralis muscle

Rib bone

Nipple

Duct

Lobule

Lobular carcinoma in situ

Normal lobule

LCIS

LCIS

Necrosis

Necrosis means that some of the LCIS cells have died. Pleomorphic means that the LCIS cells look more atypical under the microscope than in the usual case of LCIS. LCIS with either of these features (compared to LCIS without them) may be more aggressive (grow faster and be more likely to spread) and appears to be associated with an even higher risk of invasive cancer. LCIS with either of these features may be treated differently than most cases of LCIS.

DCIS versus LCIS

Cells of epithelial* lineage express adhesion protein molecules. These are calcium-dependent cell-to-cell adhesion proteins. One of these adhesion molecules is known as epithelial cadherin (E-cadherin). Loss of E-cadherin is a basic defect in invasive lobular carcinoma of the breast. Not surprisingly, the pre-invasive disease does not fully express it. Loss of E-cadherin can help distinguish LCIS (loss) from DCIS (no loss).

Microcalcifications

Calcifications may be associated with LCIS. Microcalcifications are mineral deposits that can be found in both non-cancerous and cancerous lesions. They can sometimes be seen both on mammograms and under the micro-scope. Because certain types of calcifications are in areas containing cancer, their presence on a mammogram may lead to a biopsy of the area. Then, following a biopsy, the pathologist looks at the tissue removed to be sure that it contains calcifications. Microcalcifications and calcifications matter when discovered in areas containing cancer. They are not important when found alone (without worrisome changes in the breast ducts or lobules).

---

*Epithelial tissues line the cavities and surfaces of structures throughout the body. Epithelial cells compose many glands.

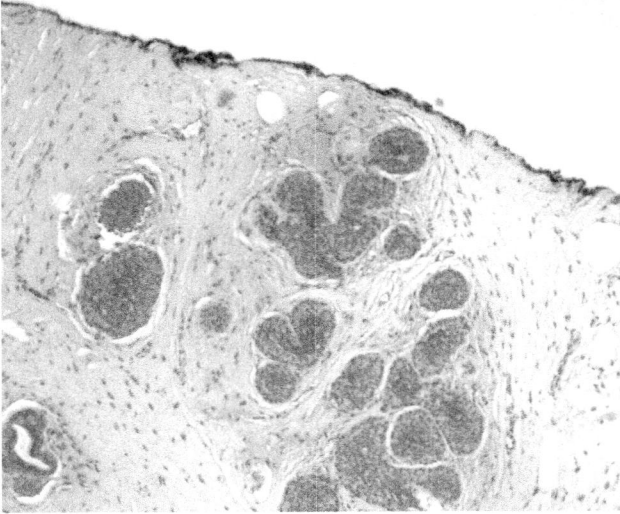

LCIS

Benign (not cancer)

Atypical hyperplasia (AH)

Hyperplasia describes an overgrowth (proliferation) of cells. It most often occurs inside the lobules or milk ducts. AH is a part of a multistep process that can lead to breast cancer. First, the cells increase in number (hyperplasia) but still look normal. Then, they can progress to become atypical: The cells stack on top of one another and begin to look abnormal. If the cells continue to change their appearance and multiply, they can evolve into non-invasive (in situ) carcinoma. With in situ carcinoma, the cells remain confined to the area where they started growing (the ducts or lobules). Ultimately, progression to invasive cancer can occur.

Types

There are two main kinds of hyperplasia—usual and atypical. Both increase breast cancer risk, though atypical hyperplasia does so to a greater degree. Special breast cancer screening and management recommendations exist for women with atypical hyperplasia (but not usual hyperplasia).

Atypical hyperplasia is not cancer but a cell abnormality that increases your chance of breast cancer in the future. It can be the ductal type (atypical ductal hyperplasia; ADH) or the lobular type (atypical lobular hyperplasia; ALH). We do not know what causes atypical hyperplasia.

Increased risk

While atypical ductal hyperplasia (ADH) and atypical lobular hyperplasia (ALH) are not cancers, when present, they can markedly increase the risk of the development of cancer in the breast in the future. Atypical hyperplasia is associated with a 30 percent chance of getting breast cancer over the ensuing 25 years.

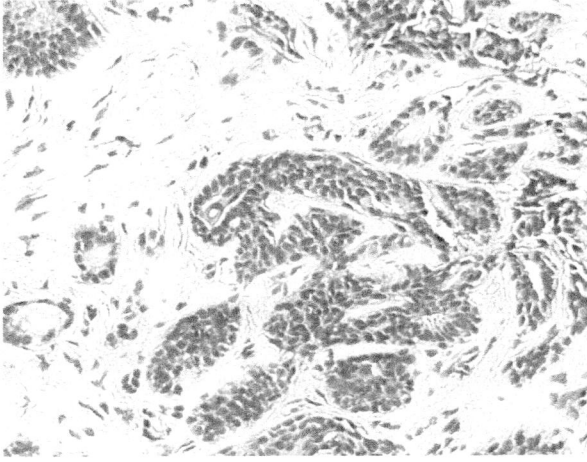

ADH

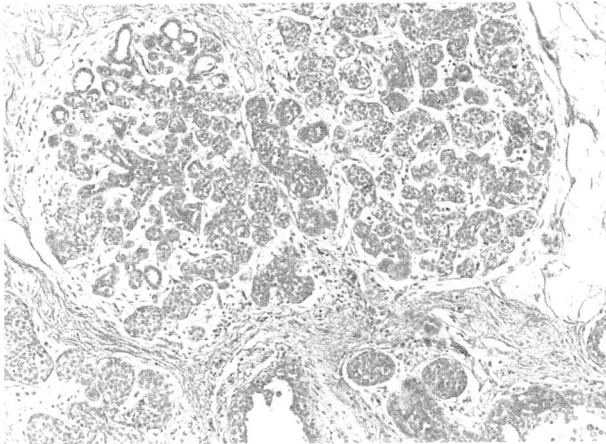

ALH

Benign (not cancer)

Simple cyst

A simple cyst is the most common cause of a palpable mass. Cysts are benign (not cancer) fluid-filled sacs. They are more common among premenopausal women and, in their pure form, do not increase the risk of breast cancer. Some cysts are palpable lumps in the breast, while others are not. If large enough, a cyst can cause pain. Breast ultrasound typically diagnoses cysts in women under 30 years old (non-invasive imaging that uses sound waves). For non-pregnant women over 30, clinicians may offer a mammogram, a breast ultrasound, or both.

Management

Simple (uncomplicated) cysts often do not need treatment, as most disappear over time. Half are gone within a year, and 70 percent within five years. However, if the cyst causes considerable pain, it may be aspirated (drained) with a very thin needle. We still need to get high-level evidence to suggest that diet change can decrease your probability of developing cysts.

> If ultrasound testing suggests that the abnormality is *not* a simple fluid-filled cavity, you will likely need tissue removed (biopsy) or even to see a surgeon.

Lipoma

Lipomas are benign fatty tumors that can appear almost anywhere in the body, including the breast. They are typically non-tender and may present as squishy non-tender lumps. When in doubt, a biopsy can confirm the diagnosis.

Other benign lumps in the breast include hamartomas, hemangiomas, hematomas, adenomyoeptheliomas, and neurofibromas. None of these conditions raises breast cancer risk, but they may need to be biopsied or removed to render a diagnosis.

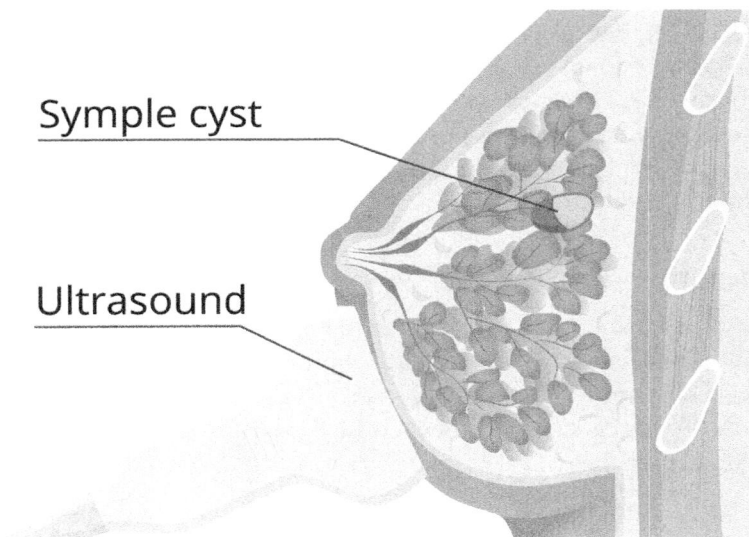

Symple cyst

Ultrasound

Benign (not cancer)

Fibroadenoma

Fibroadenomas are benign (not cancer) solid masses. Women are often between the ages of 15 to 35. Most fibroadenomas do not increase your risk of developing breast cancer. However, there is a slight increase in risk for those with a complex fibroadenoma, an associated proliferative disease, or a family history of breast cancer. Many recommend removing fibroadenomas, especially if they grow, cause discomfort, or change the breast shape. Sometimes, these tumors stop growing (or shrinking) in middle-aged or older adults without intervention. Suppose your doctors feel certain the masses are fibroadenomas (and not breast cancer) and are not painful. In that case, fibroadenomas are often left in place and carefully monitored to ensure they don't grow.

Radial scar

Radial scars (also known as complex sclerosing lesions) have a core of connective tissue fibers. Milk ducts and lobules grow out from this core. Radial scars may appear similar to breast cancer on a mammogram, but radial scars are *not* cancer. Treatment consists of removal. Some (but not all) studies suggest that radial scars may increase your risk of future breast cancer.

Adenosis (aggregate adenosis; adenosis tumor)

In adenosis, enlarged breast lobules contain more glands than usual. Biopsies of women with fibrocystic changes often show adenosis. This condition has many names, including aggregate adenosis, tumoral adenosis, or adenosis tumor. Even though some of these terms contain the term tumor, adenosis is not cancer.

Sclerosing adenosis is a special type in which the enlarged lobules are distorted by scar-like fibrous tissue. Some studies have associated sclerosing adenosis with a greater risk of developing breast cancer – about 1½ to 2 times the risk of women with no breast changes.

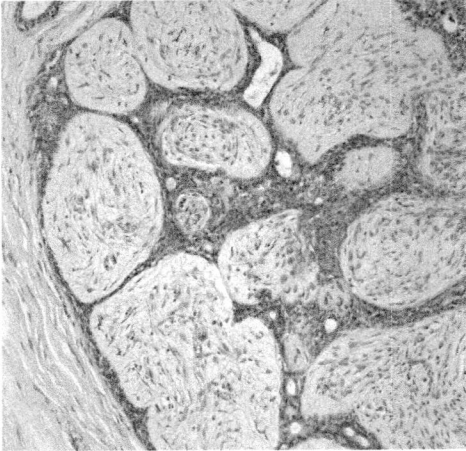

Fibroadenoma

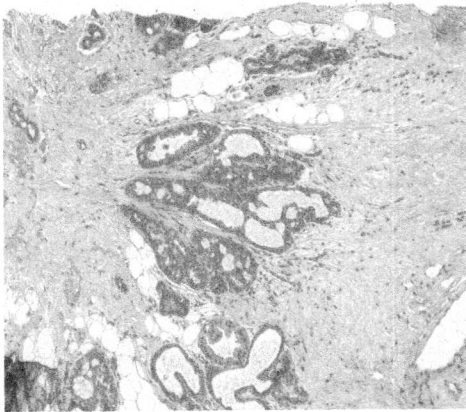

Radial scar

Benign (not cancer)

Phylloides

Phylloides tumors (full-OY-deez) are rare breast tumors that, like fibroadenomas, contain two types of breast tissue: stromal (connective) tissue and glandular (lobule and duct) tissue. They are most common in women in their 30s and 40s, but they may be found in women of any age.

Phylloides tumors are usually not true cancers, but in rare cases they may be. While up to one-third are classified as malignant based on how they look under the microscope, less than 5% of phylloides tumors overall are true cancers that spread to distant sites such as the lungs. Benign phylloides don't increase your future cancer risk. Malignant phylloides tumors are typically managed by removing them along with a wide margin of normal tissue (a margin), or by mastectomy (removing the entire breast) if needed. Close follow-up is required.

Intraductal papillomas

Intraductal papillomas are benign (not cancer) solid tumors that grow within the breast ducts. They are wart-like growths of gland tissue along with fibrous tissue and blood vessels. Solitary intraductal papillomas are a common cause of clear or bloody nipple discharge, especially when it comes from only one breast. Sometimes, they present as a small palpable lump behind or next to the nipple. They do not raise breast cancer risk unless there are other changes, such as atypical hyperplasia (AH).

Papillomas that are in small ducts in areas of the breast farther from the nipple may be multiple, and are less likely to cause nipple discharge. Papillomatosis is a type of hyperplasia in which there are very small areas of cell growth within the ducts, but they are not as distinct as papillomas. Finally, Papillomatosis is also linked to a slightly increased risk of breast cancer.

110

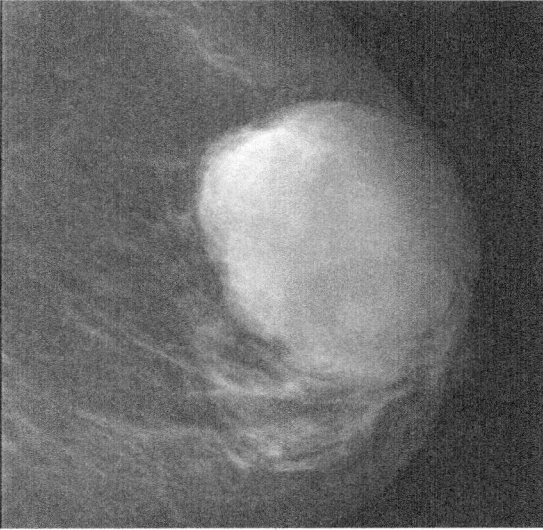

Phylloides
on a mammogram

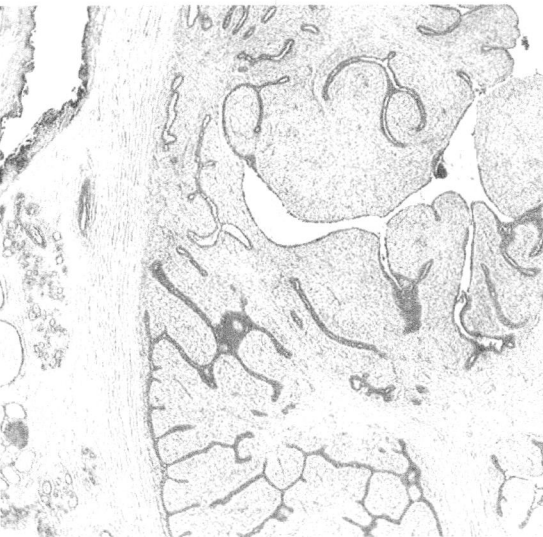

Phylloides
under the microscope

Fat necrosis and oil cysts

Here, breast injury damages breast tissue. Such injury may include radiation therapy directed at the breast or surgery. Scar tissue can be the result. Occasionally, scar tissue does not form in the usual way; instead, the fat cells die and release their contents. A sac-like collection of greasy fluid called an oil cyst can form.

This oil cyst may be able to be felt (it is palpable) and can be challenging to discern from true cancer by physical examination or mammograms. In this context, it is perhaps not surprising that your doctor may recommend a biopsy.

Mastitis

Mastitis is inflammation of the breast tissues. It results from a breast infection and may be seen in breastfeeding women, but it can happen in any woman. A break in the skin or an opening in the nipple can allow bacteria to enter the breast duct, allowing an infection to develop. Antibiotics often prove curative, but some women may need to remove pus (in an abscess).

Mastitis does *not* raise your breast cancer risk. However, because an aggressive form of breast cancer (inflammatory breast cancer) can mimic mastitis, it is important to consider a biopsy if your symptoms do not improve within a week or so.

Mastitis is managed with warm compresses, acetaminophen, ibuprofen, antibiotics, and breast massage. Vibration therapy may provide relief. Finally, a breast surgeon may be able to unclog ducts at the nipple surface and may use a thin needle to remove fluid (fine needle aspiration). Abscess management may include antibiotics, repeated aspiration, or even drainage through an open incision in the doctor's office or the operating room.

Duct ectasia

Mammary duct ectasia is common among women over 50. It occurs when a breast duct widens and its walls thicken, leading to a blockage and fluid build-up. A biopsy for a different reason may reveal it. Less commonly, you may experience a thick green or black discharge, with the nipple becoming tender, red, or pulled inward. A hard lump may develop because of the scar tissue.

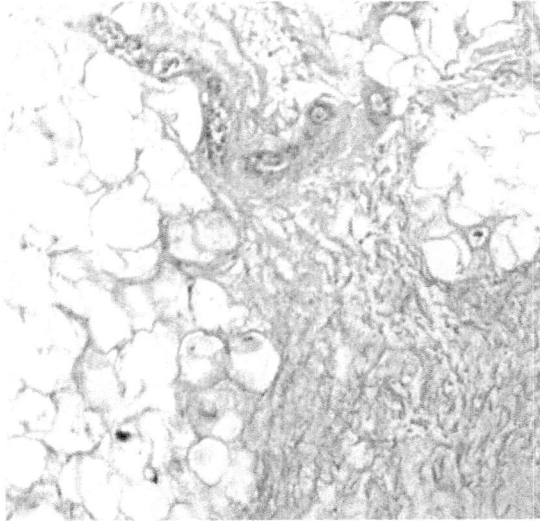

Fat necrosis

Benign (not cancer)

Duct ectasia sometimes improves without treatment or with warm compresses and antibiotics. The abnormal duct may be removed with surgery if symptoms do not resolve. Ectasia does not raise your risk of cancer.

PASH

Pseudoangiomatous stromal hyperplasia (PASH) is sometimes mistaken for cancer. Under the microscope, PASH has small slits in the tissues that look like blood vessels but aren't. Thus the name pseudo (false) angiomatous (blood vessels).

Alas, core needle biopsies with PASH may be mistaken for cancer; you may wish to consider getting a second opinion from an expert pathologist. PASH is typically found incidentally with other biopsies but sometimes presents as a palpable, non-tender thickening in the breast. PASH management is controversial. Those with enlarging masses or lesions with atypical features may consider an excision.

Hamartoma

Breast hamartomas are rare and benign tumors. The incidence of malignancy in normal breast tissue within the hamartoma is as low as one in a thousand.

They grow slowly, but in a disorganized fashion. These tumors can be soft and painless but may grow large. Obtaining a definitive diagnosis with a single imaging method can be challenging. A diagnosis may require complete excision. While cancer is rarely associated with hamartoma, an excision confirms it.

An excisional biopsy is usually needed to differentiate a hamartoma from other benign breast lesions (for example, fibroadenoma, lipoma, and cystosarcoma phyllodes.

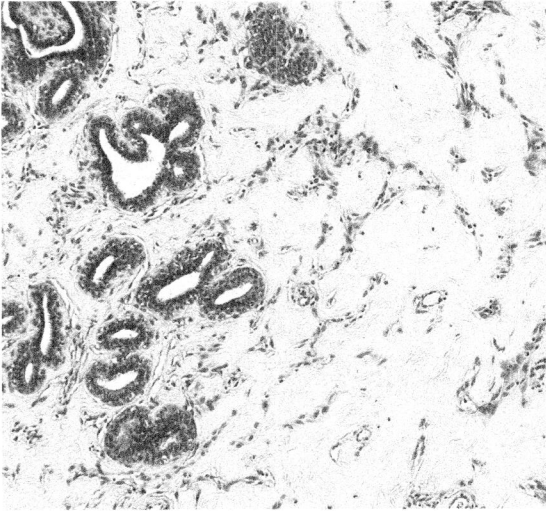

PASH

PATHOLOGY 2

INVASIVE

Invasive cancer

The analysis of the removed tissue can lead to several different reports. Some tests take longer than others, and the same laboratory may perform not all tests. Typically, you will hear some basic information in the first week after surgery, and all of the results are usually back within a few weeks. Your surgeon can let you know when the results are back, and if you don't hear from your doctor, give her a call.

There isn't just one face to breast cancer

Your doctor will order a series of tests on cancer and nearby tissues to create a "profile" of your breast cancer. Some of these tests may be performed after the initial biopsy, while others may be done after your lumpectomy or mastectomy. Your pathology report is important because it provides the information you and your doctor need to make the appropriate personalized management choices.
Management decisions depend on characteristics such as:

- The size and appearance of the cancer
- How quickly the cancer is growing
- Any signs of spread to nearby healthy tissues
- Whether hormones (estrogen, for example) or genetic mutations (such as overexpression of HER-2) — are factors in cancer's growth and development

What is cancer?

Cancer is a condition in which cells do not die at the normal rate. A tissue mass (tumor) can form as cell growth exceeds cell death. Breast cancer happens when cells in the breast divide and grow abnormally. Many (but not all) breast cancers grow slowly and are detected up to 10 to 15 years or more before we can feel it. Up to 75% of breast cancers begin in the milk ducts, while 10 to 15% begin in the lobules. The remainder starts in other breast tissues.

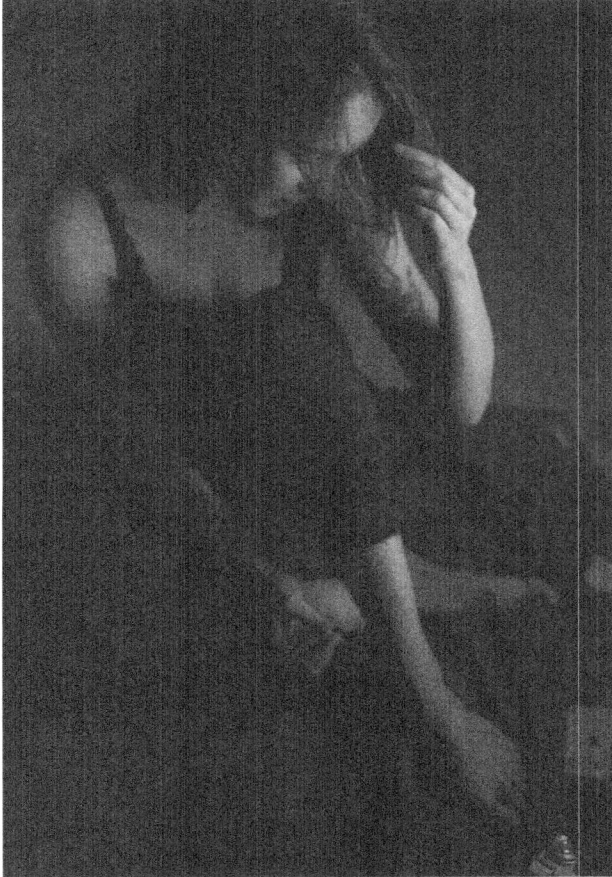

Invasive cancer

Invasive or non-invasive?

We may conveniently divide breast cancer into two categories: Invasive versus non-invasive breast cancer. The latter is also called carcinoma *in situ* (in SY-too). Only about 20 to 25% of breast cancer is non-invasive.

- **Ductal carcinoma *in situ* (DCIS)**
  A condition in which abnormal cells are confined to the milk ducts. In situ means "in place." With DCIS, the cancer cells stay within the milk ducts. Lobular carcinoma in situ is not true cancer (please see the previous chapter for info on LCIS).

- **Invasive breast cancer**
  Abnormal cells inside milk ducts have escaped through the duct wall into the nearby breast tissue. While most of the time, cancer does not spread to nodes or distant organs, invasive breast cancer can travel (through the bloodstream or lymphatic vessels) from the breast to other body parts.

The next section typically defines the removed tissue and, if cancer is present, provides information on features such as size, type, grade, hormone receptor status, and whether HER2/neu is over-expressed. If the surgeon removed lymph nodes, the pathology report should include the status of these nodes (are they involved with cancer or not).

Microscopic description

Here you will find what the pathologist saw and measured when she looked at the biopsy tissue under a microscope. The pathologist reports the tumor size in centimeters (cm) or millimeters (1 inch = 2.54 cm = 25.4 mm). The optimal way to measure tumor size is under a microscope. If the length and width of the biopsy containing cancer cells are measured, the longer of the two represents the tumor size.

DCIS

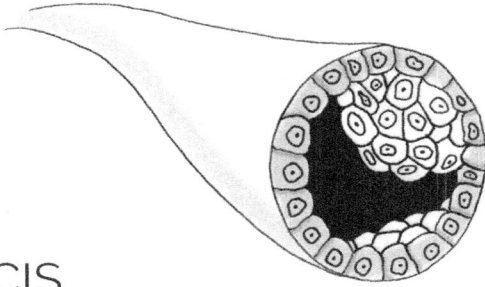

Invasive ductal

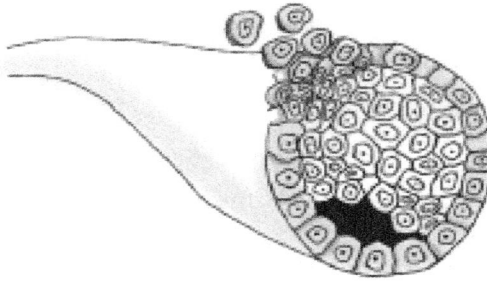

Invasive cancer

Types

Let's look at invasive breast cancer by subtype:

- Ductal   76 %
- Lobular   8 %
- Ductal/lobular   7 %
- Mucinous (colloid   2.4 %
- Tubular   1.5 %
- Medullary   1.2 %
- Papillary   1 %

Less common subtypes:

Paget disease of the breast (uncommon)

Abnormal cells are in the skin in or around the nipple. There may be an associated underlying mass in the breast.

Inflammatory breast cancer

This distinctive form of breast cancer is especially aggressive. Symptoms may include swelling and redness of the breast. Sometimes the skin has an orange peel-like appearance (peau d'orange).

Metaplastic breast cancer

This rare cancer can be hard to diagnose. These tumors tend to be larger and have a higher tumor grade.

Angiosarcoma

This cancer begins in cells that line blood or lymph vessels. This rare sometimes develops 5 to 10 years later (or more) as a complication of previous radiation treatments. Angiosarcoma can also occur in the arms of individuals who develop lymphedema as a result of lymph node surgery, radiation therapy, or both to manage breast cancer. Unfortunately, angiosarcomas tend to grow and spread quickly.

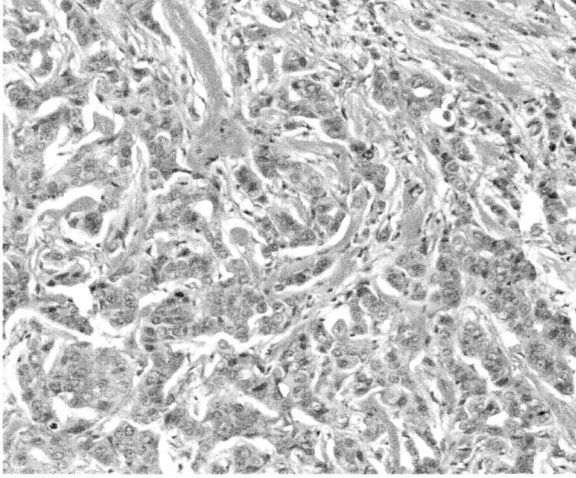

Ductal
(cords and nests of tumor cells)

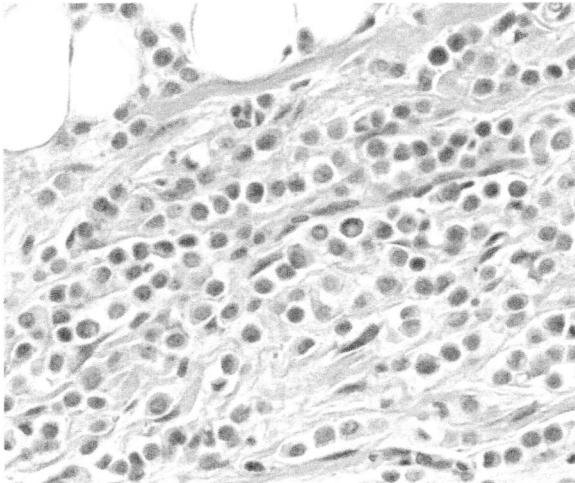

Lobular
Small cancer cells grow in a single file. LCIS is present in two-thirds of cases.

Invasive cancer

Paget's disease of the nipple

In 1874, Sir James Paget described 15 women with chronic nipple ulceration who all developed breast cancer within two years. While Paget believed the nipple changes were benign (not cancer), we subsequently discovered that the characteristic cells in the outer layer of the cells covering the nipple were indeed malignant. Please note that Paget's disease of the nipple a different entity than is Paget's disease of the bone.

Presentation

An underlying breast cancer (in situ or invasive) is present up to nearly 90 percent of the time, although there may or may not be an associated breast mass or mammogram abnormality. A palpable breast mass is associated with Paget's in about 50 percent of cases, with the mass often more than 2 cm from the nipple/areola. In 20 percent of cases, there is a mammogram abnormality but no palpable mass. A quarter will have no underlying mass or mammogram abnormality, but there is occult breast cancer. Finally, about 12 to 15 percent of cases are not associated with a palpable mass, mammogram abnormality, or cancer in the main breast tissue.

Skin biopsy

A doctor may use a nipple scraping to diagnose Paget's, but the diagnosis is more commonly made after a punch biopsy or wedging of the nipple. The hallmark of Paget's disease of the nipple is the presence of cancer cells (Paget cells) occurring singly or in small groups within the nipple's outer layer of cells. Sometimes, the cells can have a similar appearance to melanoma. More advanced testing (such as immunochemistry) may be done in cases with uncertainty about the diagnosis.

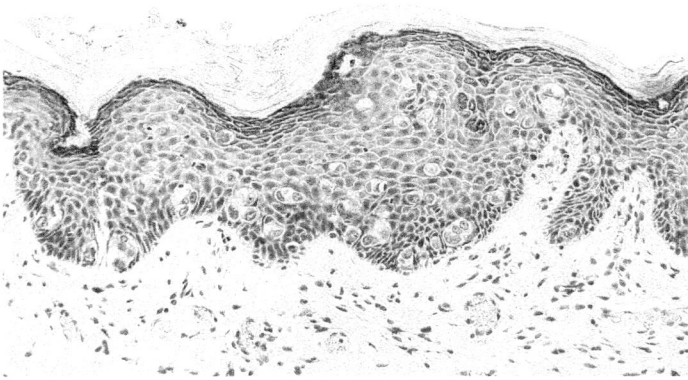

Paget's disease of the nipple
Paget cells are large cells with a clear halo

Invasive cancer

Types: Favorable

Certain breast cancers may have a better prognosis than "usual" infiltrating ductal carcinoma. Included among these cancers are:

- **Adenoid cystic**
  This rare cancer has an appearance similar to adenoid cystic cancers of the salivary glands. Spread to the axillary nodes is uncommon at about 5%.

- **Medullary carcinoma**
  More frequent in younger patients and among those with a BRCA-1 gene mutation.

- **Mucinous (colloid) carcinoma**
  Soft, gelatinous appearance grossly. The tumors tend to be well-circumscribed. There cell nests sitting in pools of mucus.

- **Papillary carcinoma**
  This rare is uncommon, accounting for less than 1-2% of invasive breast cancers. It is more common among women who have gone through menopause. This cancer typically has a well-defined border and small, finger-like projections.

- **Tubular carcinoma**
  Here, we see well-formed tubular or gland structures. About 75% of cases have associated DCIS (typically low-grade).

- **Low-grade adenosquamous carcinoma**
  A form of metaplastic carcinoma

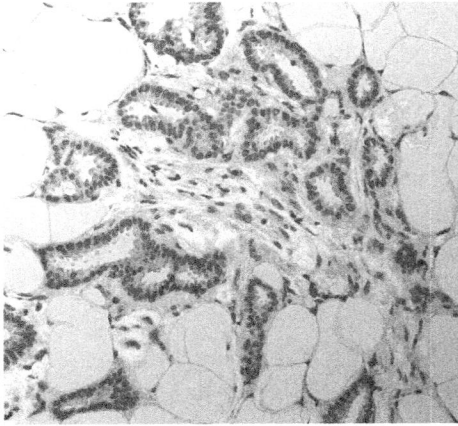

Tubular
Excellent prognosis

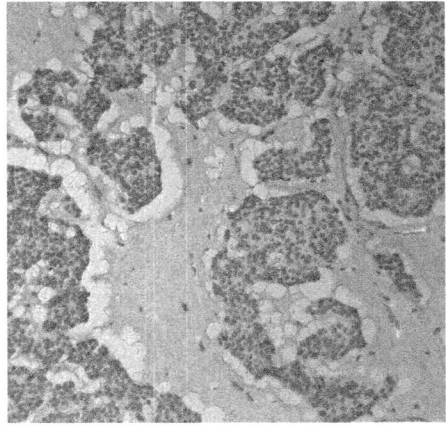

Mucinous
Cancer cells (red) floating
in pools of mucin (purple)

Types: Other

Other breast cancer subtypes have the same (or perhaps worse) prognosis as standard infiltrating carcinoma:

- **Micropapillary carcinoma**

  Invasive papillary carcinomas are rare, representing less than 1 to 2 percent of invasive breast cancers. These can be particularly aggressive, with a propensity for spread to regional nodes (even when small in size). An invasive papillary cancer typically has a well-defined boundary and is composed of small finger-like projections.

- **Metaplastic carcinoma**

  This subtype is rare, representing under 1 percent of all breast cancers. Like the more common invasive ductal carcinoma, metaplastic breast cancer starts in the breast's milk ducts and invades the tissues around the duct. Invasive ductal cancer cells, while abnormal, have some duct-like characteristics.

  Metaplastic tumors may have some breast cells but also contain cells that look like soft tissue and connective tissue of the breast. Metaplastic cancers can behave more aggressively than other breast cancer types. They are often (but not always) "triple negative," with no estrogen, progesterone, or HER2 receptors. Metaplastic tumors are often high-grade, larger (on average) than other types of breast cancer, and more likely to spread to nodes or distantly.

- **Tubulolobular carcinoma**

  Often misclassified as invasive carcinoma, tubulolobular carcinoma has invasive cancer exhibiting ductal and lobular characteristics. Cancer must have classic grade one features, intimately mixed tubular and linear architecture, and an overall infiltrative pattern of lobular cancer. Oddly, tubulolobular cancer is not tubular.

- **Mixed invasive ductal and lobular carcinoma**

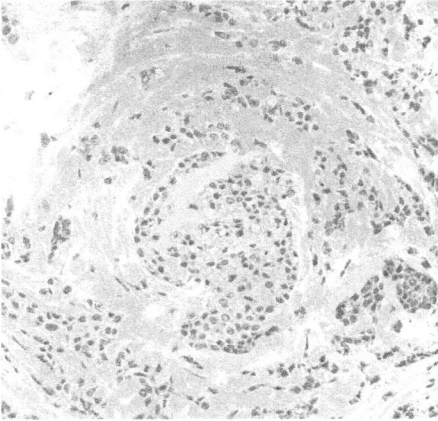

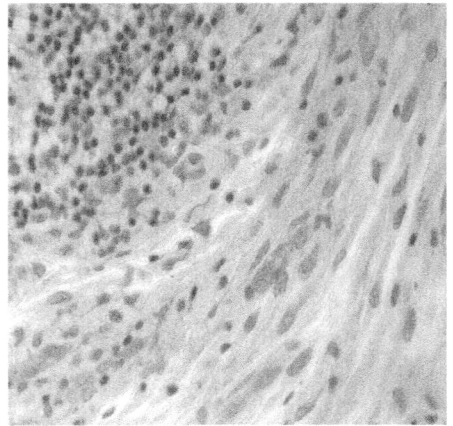

METAPLASTIC

Cancer is composed of breast cells and ones that look like soft tissue and connective tissue. These tumors are often bigger than other invasive breast cancers and the grade is usually high.

Invasive cancer

Grade

Tumor grade* describes cancer (seen under a microscope) based on how abnormal/aggressive the cells appear. Using a microscope, the pathologist examines the tissue removed from your body. She then decides if the cells are benign (not cancer) or malignant (cancer). Grade 1 (low grade) is the least aggressive, and grade 3 (high grade) is the most.

Nottingham grade

This system grades tumors based on tubule formation, nuclear grade, and mitotic rate. Each factor is assigned a score from 1 to 3 (1 is best). We then add the scores to get a total of 3 to 9, with nine being the most aggressive. In general, a lower grade means a better prognosis. Your care team will use the tumor grade and other factors (including stage, other cancer characteristics, general health, and personal preferences) to devise a systemic therapy plan tailored to you.

- Tubule formation
How close to normal do the breast (milk) duct structures appear?

- Nuclear grade
An evaluation of the size and shape of the cancer cell nucleus

- Mitotic rate (how fast is cancer growing?)
How many dividing cells are present in the microscope field?

Putting it all together

Total score 3 to 5: Low-grade (relatively non-aggressive); well-differentiated
Total score 6 or 7: Intermediate-grade; moderately differentiated
Total score 8 or 9: High grade (aggressive); poorly-differentiated

---

* Cancer grade is not the same as cancer stage. Cancer stage refers to the size and extent of cancer and whether cancer has spread.

Rate of cell growth

Your pathology report may have information about cell growth rate — what proportion of the cancer cells within the tumor is growing and dividing to form new cancer cells. A higher percentage points to a faster-growing, more aggressive cancer. Here are two tests that are sometimes used to determine the cell growth rate:

- *Ki-67*

This cell protein increases as cells prepare to divide and multiply. A staining process can measure the percentage of positive tumor cells for Ki-67. The more positive cells there are, the faster the growth rate. In breast cancer, a result of less than 10% is considered low, 10-20% intermediate, and high if greater than 20%.

- *S-phase*

This number tells you what percentage of cells in the sample are in the process of copying their genetic information (DNA). S-phase, short for the "synthesis phase," happens right before a cell divides into two new cells. A result of less than 6 percent is low, 6 to 10 percent intermediate, and more than 10 percent is considered high.

Experts don't agree on how to use the results of these tests when making management decisions. As a result, not all doctors order these tests routinely, so don't be alarmed if they are not in your pathology report.

Lymphvascular invasion (LVI)

Lymphovascular (angiolymphatic) invasion or LVI means that cancer cells are in the small lymph or blood vessels that drain lymph fluid and blood from your breast, ultimately into your circulation system.

Please note that lymphatic or vascular (blood) invasion differs from lymph node involvement. At the St. Gallen meeting in 2005, experts recognized LVI as a prognostic factor for survival for patients with no node involvement: Lymphvascular or angiolymphatic invasion appears to have prognosis implications only if you don't have lymph node involvement.

Margins

noun mar·gin \\'mär-jin\

a rim of normal breast tissue surrounding a suspicious area

A surgeon removes a rim of normal breast tissue (a margin) surrounding the suspicious area. The tumor with surrounding tissue is rolled in a special ink so that the outer edges, or margins, are visible under a microscope. A pathologist reports the margins:

> • **Positive margins** (ink on cancer or ductal carcinoma in situ) are associated with a two-fold increase in the risk of in-breast relapse compared to negative (clear) margins. Favorable biology, endocrine therapy, or a radiation boost do not significantly lower this higher risk.

> • **More widely clear margins** than no ink on the tumor do not significantly decrease the rate of in-breast recurrence. There is no evidence that more widely clear margins reduce recurrence for young patients, unfavorable biology, lobular cancers, or cancers with an extensive intraductal component. Finally, classic LCIS at the margin is not an indication for re-excision. The significance of pleomorphic LCIS at the margin remains uncertain.

The optimal cancer-free zone for a lumpectomy is controversial. In this context, an expert consensus panel considered a meta-analysis of 33 studies (with 28,162 patients) examining margin width and in-breast recurrence.

Researchers also looked at the results of randomized clinical trials, reproducibility of margin assessment, and current patterns of multi-modality care. They concluded that clear margins, no matter how small, as long as there is no ink on the cancer tumor, should be the standard for lumpectomy surgery. These guidelines apply to invasive cancer, Stages I and II managed with breast-conserving surgery followed by whole breast radiation therapy.

Margin width

The American Society for Radiation Oncology and the Society of Surgical Oncology concluded that **clear margins, no matter how small, as long as there is no ink on the cancer tumor, should be the standard for lumpectomy** surgery for *invasive* breast cancer. These guidelines apply Stages I and II cancer managed with breast-conserving surgery followed by whole breast radiation therapy.

Nodes

Lymph nodes are small tissue collections containing white blood cells (that fight infection). Nodes are part of the body's immune system and filter lymph fluid, which is made of fluid and waste products from body tissues. Nodes help fight infections, and nodal involvement with cancer influences breast cancer prognosis.

If breast cancer spreads, it most commonly goes first to regional lymph nodes:

- Axillary (underarm) nodes
- Supraclavicular (above the collarbone) nodes
- Internal mammary nodes (near the breastbone (the front center of the chest).

Sometimes cancer starts in the lymph nodes (lymphoma is an example) , but some others types of cancer (including breast cancer) can spread from one part of the body to another through lymph nodes and the lymphatic vessels.

Knowing if cancer has spread to your lymph nodes helps your care team determine the best management approach. Spread to regional lymph nodes can influence prognosis, systemic therapy choices (such as chemotherapy), and radiation therapy fields.

Checking the nodes

If the axillary lymph nodes are swollen, you may have a core needle biopsy (or fine needle aspiration). If cancer is in a node, more nodes are generally removed at the time of the main breast surgery.

For invasive breast cancer, even if the nodes are not known to be involved, they are usually checked for cancer. This node removal can be done through a sentinel node biopsy in which about one to three nodes are typically removed. Some patients have a more extensive axillary node dissection, which removes more lymph nodes.

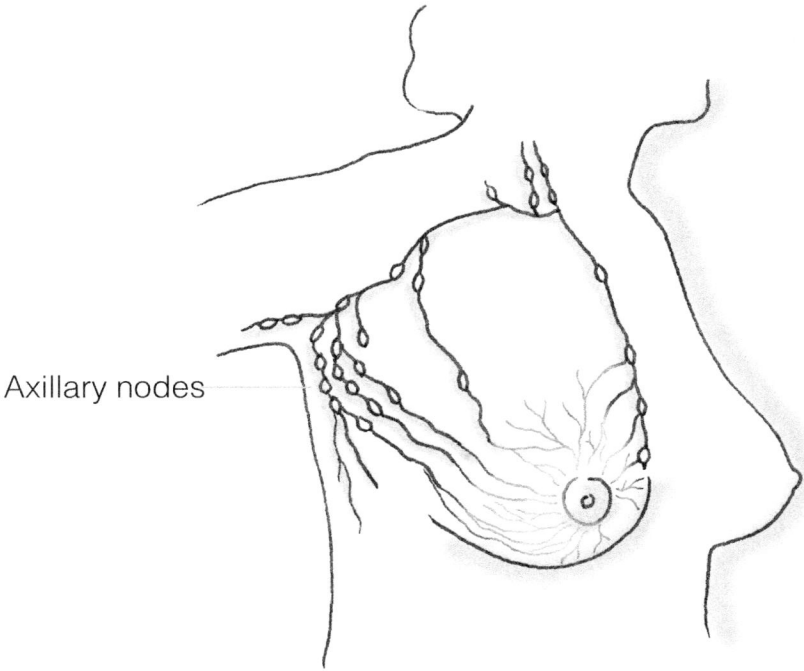

Axillary nodes

Number of nodes involved
is strongly associated with prognosis

Invasive cancer

Estrogen receptors (ER)

A pathologist checks your biopsy or surgical material to see if your breast cancer cells have receptors for the hormones estrogen and progesterone. Hormone receptors are proteins in and on breast cells that pick up hormone signals telling the cells to grow.

A cancer is estrogen receptor-positive (or ER+) if it has receptors for estrogen. This finding suggests that the cancer cells, like normal breast cells, receive signals from estrogen that promote their growth. The cancer is progesterone receptor-positive (PR+) if it has progesterone receptors; the cancer cells receive signals from progesterone that promote their growth. Just over two-thirds of breast cancers test positive for hormone receptors.

Why is ER/PR status important?

Hormone receptor status indicates whether your cancer will likely respond to endocrine (anti-hormonal) therapy. Endocrine therapy approaches include medications that either (1) lower the amount of estrogen in your body or (2) block estrogen from supporting the growth and function of breast cells. If the breast cancer cells have hormone receptors, these medications can stop their growth. If the cancer is hormone-receptor-negative (no receptors exist), hormonal therapy will not work. You and your doctor can then select other types of treatment.

ER/PR: Understanding your results

Your pathologist will check any invasive cancer for both estrogen and progesterone receptors. If your result is reported as "positive" or "negative," ask your doctor for a specific number. Different labs have varying cutoff points for calling a cancer hormone receptor-positive versus hormone receptor-negative. Even cancers with low numbers of hormone receptors may respond to hormonal therapy.

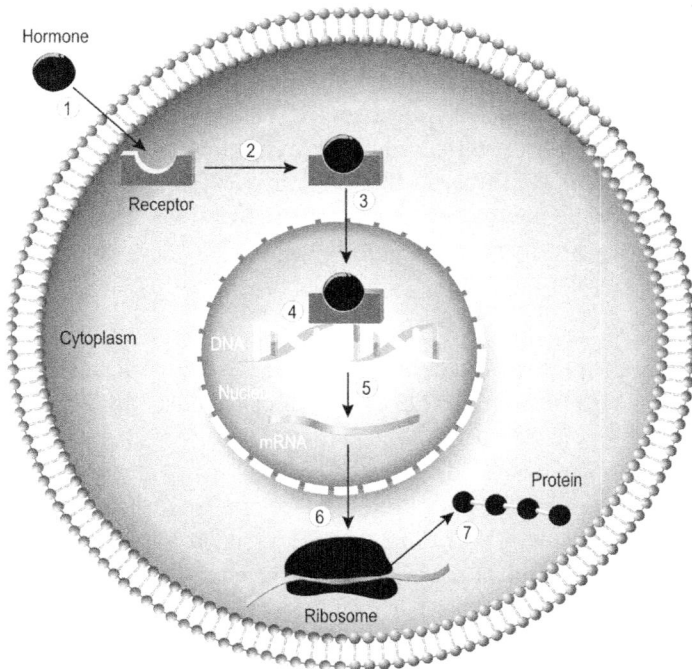

ESTROGEN hormone fuels the growth and division of some breast cancer cells

Invasive cancer

ER/PR

Estrogen and progesterone receptors are scored from 0 (no receptors) to 100 (all of your cancer cells appear to have receptors). A score of "0" generally means that hormonal therapy will not be helpful in treating the breast cancer. ER-low-positive (1 to 10 percent) may behave as if the estrogen receptors are negative. When the score is 0, the cancer is called hormone-receptor-negative. The alternative Allred system scores the ER from 0 to 8, the higher the better. Sometimes, a report will come back from the laboratory saying that the hormone status is "unknown." If you receive a result of "unknown," ask your doctor what this means, and ask what further steps should be taken to determine your hormone receptor status.

HER-2

Invasive breast cancers should be tested for HER2 (human epidermal growth factor receptor-2), a protein on the surface of cells charged with stimulating cell growth and repair. About 15 to 20 percent of patients have cells that have an excess of HER-2 genes inside the cell, leading to an extraordinary number of HER-2 receptors sticking out of the cell like antennae. These extra HER2 receptors receive a growth hormone, and then transmit a signal into the cell nucleus to make the cell more aggressive. Fortunately, we recently developed drugs that target the HER-2 pathway, dramatically improving the survival chance of patients with HER-2 overexpression. HER2 is reported for invasive breast cancer (but not typically for DCIS or LCIS). Two common tests:

- *Immunohistochemistry (IHC)*

  Detects the amount of HER2 protein on the surface of the cancer cells. IHC is often the first test done. If the IHC score is 0 or 1+, there is no HER-2 overexpression (HER-2 negative); if the score is 3+, there is overexpression (HER-2 positive); if the IHC score is 2+, the test is equivocal, and we move to FISH testing.

- *Fluorescence in situ hybridization (FISH) testing*

  Detects the number of HER2/neu genes in the cancer cell. DISH is typically scored as positive or negative for HER2 overexpression. If the answer is not clear, an IHC test may be done (please see above).

138

ER/PR

ER + / PR +	65%	Cancer cells have hormone receptors for estrogen and progesterone. These hormones support cancer growth.
ER + / PR -	13%	Estrogen (but not progesterone) may support the growth of cancer cells.
ER - / PR -	25%	Estrogen or progesterone does not feed cancer.
ER - / PR +	2%	Progesterone (but not estrogen) is likely to support cancer growth.

* the numbers do not sum to 100 because of rounding.

It is highly unusual for estrogen receptors to be negative for the following breast cancer subtypes:

- Low-grade invasive carcinomas of no special type (invasive ductal carcinoma)
- Lobular carcinomas (classic type)
- Pure tubular, mucinous, or cribriform carcinoma
- Encapsulated papillary and solid papillary carcinoma

On the other hand, it is highly unusual for estrogen receptors to be positive for the following breast cancer subtypes:

- Metaplastic carcinomas of all subtypes
- Adenoid cystic carcinomas and other salivary gland-like breast carcinomas
- Secretory carcinoma
- Carcinomas with apocrine differentiation

Invasive cancer

HER2

Breast cancer is not a single entity but rather a variety of diseases. Even breast cancers that appear similar under the microscope may have very different "personalities" or genetic fingerprints. HER2 overexpressing (HER2 positive) breast cancer is one subtype. Unfortunately, when cells are HER2-positive, they tend to be more aggressive.

HER2 function

HER2 is a normal gene; however, when amplified (too many), it causes cancer and is called an oncogene. Many scientists have postulated that oncogenes were related to growth factors. In the early 1980s, a Genentech scientist, a British protein chemist, and an Israeli protein expert proved that growth factors are related to cancer. They found an oncogene that was a mutated form of the epidermal growth factor (EGF) cell-surface receptor gene. This finding explained how an oncogene worked by linking the study of cell-growth signals and cancer.

HER2 positive

HER2 is a normal gene; however, when amplified (there are too many), it causes cancer and is called an oncogene. Many scientists had postulated that oncogenes were related to growth factors. In the early 1980s, a Genentech scientist, a British protein chemist, and an Israeli protein expert together proved that growth factors are related to cancer. They found an oncogene that was a mutated form of the epidermal growth factor (EGF) cell-surface receptor gene. By linking the study of cell-growth signals and cancer, this finding explained how an oncogene worked.

A healthy cell contains a normal quantity of approximately 20,000 HER2 proteins (or receptors) on the cell surface. Because of HER2 gene amplification, HER2-positive cancer cells have an abundance of HER2 receptors on the cell surface (approximately 2 million, or 100 times more than a healthy cell), leading to uncontrolled cancer cell growth. Up to 1 in 4 individuals with breast cancer are HER2-positive, a more aggressive form of the disease.

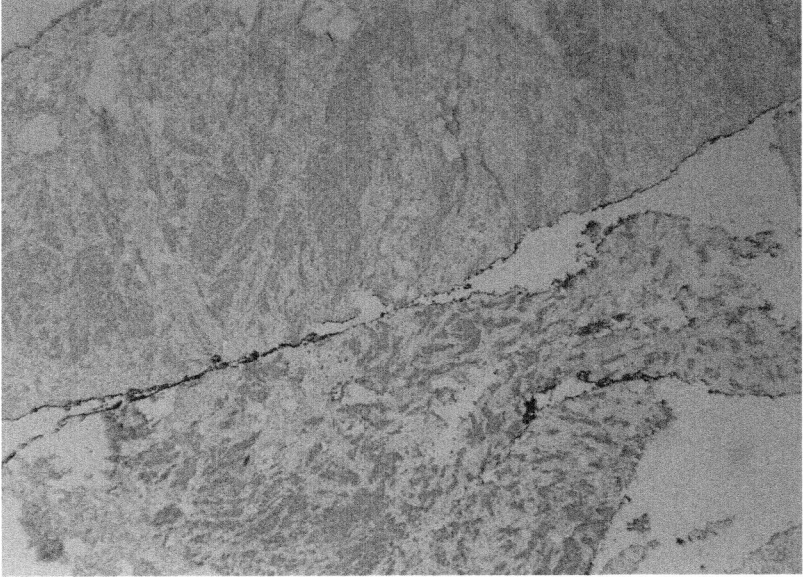

HER2

Some tumors are heterogeneous. The top part of the illustration
shows no overexpression of HER-2, while the bottom
part has overexpression (cells stain dark brown).

Invasive cancer

HER2

Dysregulation of ERBB2 (HER2) signaling in cancer involves an excess of signals that stimulate cancer cells to grow and spread.

1 *Amplify (genes)*

Up to 20 to 25% of individuals with breast cancer have cancer cells with too many copies of the HER2 gene. This overexpression results in an overabundance of HER-2 receptors (which stick out like antennae) on the cell surface.

2 *Dimerize*

The HER family sits on the cell surface. We have HER1 (EGFR), HER2 (ERBB2), HER3, and HER4. While each can bind (dimerize) to one of the others, HER2 is the preferred bonding partner. HER2 does not need an outside stimulant; it aids in activating a signal by binding with one of the other types of HER receptors. HER2 exists in an open conformation that makes it always ready to dimerize. HER2-containing dimers have increased signaling potency relative to dimers that do not contain HER2, as HER2 can decrease the disconnection rate from its dimerized partner.

3 *Send the signal*

A growth factor causes the dimerization of HER family receptors. It is as if the HER family members grab arms with another member if a growth hormone stimulates the first. Once the pair (known as an HER dimer) is created, the downstream signaling process begins. Signaling pathways include the so-called MAPK proliferation and the PI3K/Akt pro-survival pathways.

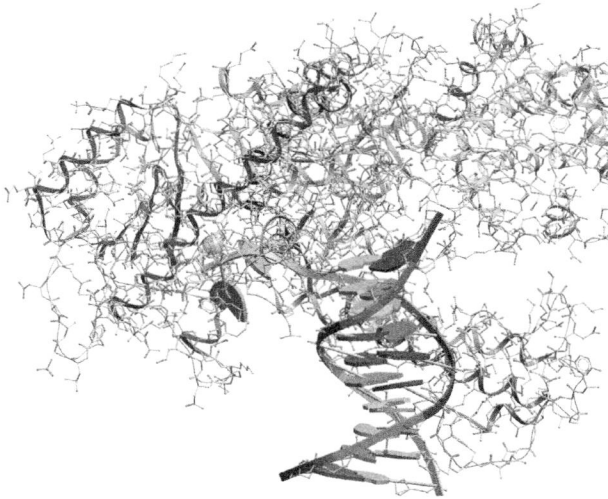

Signaling from HER2 can lead to the following:

· Increased/uncontrolled cell growth
· Decreased apoptosis (programmed cell suicide)
· Enhanced cancer cell movement
· Angiogenesis (formation of new blood vessels)

Invasive cancer

Molecular fingerprint

We may conveniently divide breast cancer into at least three subtypes based on the presence or absence of molecular markers for estrogen or progesterone receptors and human epidermal growth factor 2 (ERBB2):

- Hormone receptor (estrogen receptor and/or progesterone receptor positive) *and* HER2 (ERBB2) negative
- HER2 (ERBB2) positive
- Triple negative (estrogen- and/or progesterone-receptor negative)

There is an alternative classification system that divides breast cancer into at least four distinct molecular subtypes:

- Luminal A-like (best prognosis)
- Luminal B-like
- HER2-like
- Basal-like (triple negative/basal-like) (worst prognosis))

These same subtypes also appear in ductal carcinoma *in situ*. Breast cancers that do not fall into these subtypes are designated unclassified.

Okay, I know my cancer's ER, PR, HER2, and grade. Now what?

For invasive breast cancer, stage and cancer characteristics (such as estrogen receptor status (ER), HER2 status, and grade) influence management options and prognosis.

	ER or PR positive *and* ERBB2 -	ERBB2+ (HER2 +)	Triple-negative
What	One percent or more of cells positive for estrogen receptors (ER) or progesterone receptors (PR)	The cancer stains strongly for ERBB2 (3+) or FISH testing is HER2-positive.	The cancer is not positive for estrogen receptor, progesterone receptor, or ERBB2
How	Estrogen receptor activates cancer growth pathways	Oncogene ERBB2 overactive	Unknown (likely various ways)
Percent of breast cancer	70	15 to 20	15
Stage I: 5 year breast cancer survival	99 percent or more	94 percent or more	85 percent or more
Metastatic median survival	Four to five years	Five years	10-13 months

Invasive cancer

Genomic assay: Profiling your cancer

Each cell in your body contains about 25,000 to 35,000 genes. Genes carry the information that determines your traits, which you inherited from your parents. The DNA in a gene spells out specific instructions (like a recipe) for making proteins in the cell. Proteins are the building blocks for everything in your body.

A genomic assay uses a sample of your breast cancer tissue to analyze the activity of a group of genes. Genes contain the recipes for cell proteins needed to stay healthy and function normally. We can use information about your genes to predict your odds of breast cancer recurrence and whether chemotherapy should be a part of your treatment plan. Examples of genomic assays include:

- *Oncotype DX*

  Estimates the risk of recurrence of early-stage, hormone-receptor-positive breast cancer, as well as how likely it is that a woman diagnosed with this type of cancer will benefit from chemotherapy after surgery.

- *MammaPrint*

  Provides an estimate of recurrence risk for early-stage breast cancer-based on the level of expression of 70 genes associated with breast cancer recurrence. Breast cancer can be hormone-receptor-positive or hormone-receptor-negative.

- *EndoPredict*

  EndoPredict estimates the risk of distant recurrence of early-stage, hormone-receptor-positive, HER2-negative breast cancer that is either node-negative or has up to three positive lymph nodes.

Genomic assays

- *ProSigna (formerly PAM-50)*
  The Prosigna Breast Cancer Prognostic Gene Signature Assay estimates the risk of distant recurrence for postmenopausal women (within ten years of diagnosis of early-stage, hormone receptor-positive disease with up to three positive lymph nodes) after five years of hormonal therapy.

- *Breast Cancer Index*
  The Breast Cancer Index estimates the risk of node-negative, hormone receptor-positive breast cancer recurring for five to ten years after diagnosis and to predict the benefit of an additional five years of hormonal therapy.

These tests do a reasonably good job of estimating the risk of late distant recurrence for early-stage, hormone-receptor-positive, HER2-negative breast cancer.

Only the Oncotype DX test has strong evidence that it can predict how likely a woman diagnosed with this type of breast cancer will benefit from chemotherapy after surgery.

Please check to ensure your insurance covers these tests before one is ordered for you.

Ask

- **Where**

  Where is my cancer located in the breast? Has it spread to regional nodes or distant sites (metastasized)?

- **What**

  Can you explain my pathology report to me? What cancer type do I have? Is my breast cancer hormone receptor-positive or HER2-positive? What is my cancer grade? What does that mean for me?

- **Copies**

  Can I have a copy of my pathology report?

- **Second opinions**

  Most insurance plans will allow you to get a different opinion, as long as the second health care provider is a member of your health plan. It may be especially important to get a second opinion for rare types of breast cancer (for example, metaplastic breast cancer) and the low-grade type of ductal carcinoma in situ (DCIS). Sometimes that opinion is best obtained from an expert in pathology, reviewing the slides containing the material from your surgery.

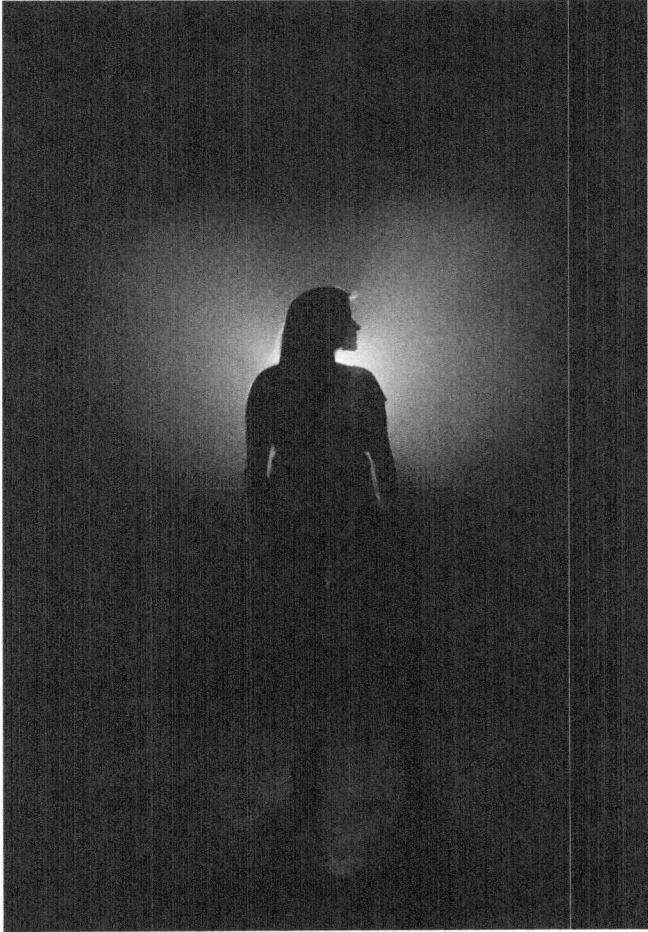

STAGE

CANCER EXTENT

Stage

Breast cancer stage describes the extent of cancer in the body. Your stage depends on whether the cancer is invasive or non-invasive, the tumor size, the number of nodes involved (if any), and whether the cancer has spread to distant body parts. Historically, we classified tumor stage using only these three measures. Beginning in 2018, the Tumor/Nodes/Metastases (TNM) added cancer cell features, including tumor grade, estrogen receptor, progesterone receptor, and HER2 status.

The stage is an important factor in determining prognosis and management. Staging provides a common language for healthcare team members to effectively communicate about a patient's cancer and collaborate on the best management courses. Understanding cancer's stage is also critical to identifying clinical trials that may be appropriate for particular patients.

Testing

Depending on the results of your physical exam and biopsy, your doctor may want you to have certain imaging tests such as a chest x-ray, mammograms of both breasts, bone scans, computed tomography (CT) scans, magnetic resonance imaging (MRI), or positron emission tomography (PET) scans. Blood tests may also be done to evaluate your overall health and can uncommonly indicate if cancer has spread to certain organs.

TNM (T is for Tumor, N is for Nodes, M is for Metastases)

We use a staging system that allows us to summarize the extent of cancer. The American Joint Committee on Cancer (AJCC) TNM system is the most commonly used system to describe breast cancer stages.

- **Clinical Stage**
Physical exams, biopsies, and imaging help define your clinical stage.

- **Pathologic stage**
Your pathologic stage uses information from the clinical stage. The pathologic stage adds in the findings from surgery (for example, for those having nodes removed, how many were involved, if any).

Staging

Metastases

Significant weight loss, unusual bone pain, a chronic cough, and shortness of breath can be symptoms of metastases.

Testing

Most patients who do *not* have concerning symptoms or abnormal blood tests do not need studies to check for distant spread. Selected patients may have:

- Blood tests to check for spread to the liver or bones
- X-ray/CT scans to test for spread to the chest, abdomen, and liver
- Bone scans to check for spread to the bones
- Positron emission tomography (PET) scan
- Brain MRI

Breast cancer stage combines cancer biology (ER, PR. HER2, and grade) with the geographic extent of disease. The latter includes the following:

- **T** (Tumor size)
- **N** (Lymph node status)
- **M** (Metastases)

The clinical stage is determined before any treatment; on the other hand, pathologic stage is determined

- Clinical stage is determined before surgery
- Pathologic stage is determined after surgery

Metastases

You may have tests to check for cancer spread to distant organs such as the bones, lungs, or liver). Although cancer starts in the breast, it can travel to other body parts through the lymph fluid or the blood. If your breast cancer has spread, the prognosis is poorer.

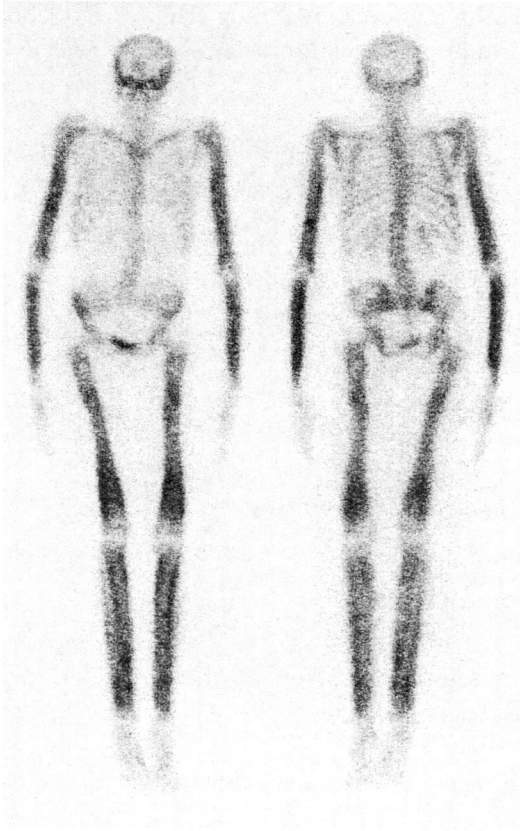

Metastasis
Cancer spreads to distant organs, such as the bones, lungs, or liver.

Staging

Comprehensive scans

Most patients who do not have concerning symptoms or abnormal blood tests do not need studies to check for distant spread (metastases). While we historically did routine body scans of patients, the National Comprehensive Cancer Network (NCCN) discontinued this recommendation in 1998. The most comprehensive testing is now typically reserved for patients with locally advanced disease (for example, very large tumors with cancer affecting several lymph nodes) or for patients whose physical symptoms may imply that breast cancer has spread elsewhere.

The American Society of Clinical Oncology (ASCO) offers a list of 10 things that physicians and patients should question. Included among them is this: Don't perform PET, CT, and radionuclide bone scans in staging early breast cancer at low risk for metastasis.

- Imaging with PET, CT, or radionuclide bone scans can be useful in staging specific cancer types. However, there is no evidence suggesting they improve the detection of metastases or survival for early breast cancer.

- In breast cancer, for example, there is a lack of evidence demonstrating a benefit for using PET, CT, or radionuclide bone scans in asymptomatic individuals with newly identified ductal carcinoma in situ (DCIS) or clinical stage I or II diseases.

- Unnecessary imaging can lead to harm through unnecessary invasive procedures, over-treatment, unnecessary radiation exposure, and misdiagnosis.

These are general guidelines, so please check with your physician to see if more extensive imaging is indicated for you as an individual based on your particular case characteristics.

Staging

New and improved system

In 2018, the American Joint Committee on Cancer (AJCC) updated the staging system for breast cancer. Stage incorporates the cancer amount (tumor size, spread to lymph nodes or distant sites). Now, the definitions of each stage vary depending on the cancer type. The cancer stage often correlates with outcomes, and management recommendations usually consider the disease stage.

Incorporating cancer cell biology

With an increasing understanding of tumor biology, it is clear that stage is not the only factor influencing prognosis. Tumor biology is very important, and may be more important than the stage in some cases. A small aggressive tumor may have a worse prognosis than a larger but slower-growing cancer.

Prognostic stage group

The 8th version of the AJCC staging system for breast cancer now considers tumor biology. Factors such as cell grade, estrogen receptor and HER2 status, grade, and (if performed) tumor genomic tests such as Oncotype DX are now incorporated into the clinical (before surgery) and pathological (after surgery) prognostic stage. Considering these biological factors means that the stage will have more meaningful prognostic information. Some larger tumors will now be considered stage I, and some smaller lesions will be upstaged based on their biology.

In a large validation study performed by researchers at the University of Texas MD Anderson Cancer Center, 31 percent of patients had upstaging, and 20 percent had downstaging. The updated prognostic stage performed better (predicting patient outcomes) than the standard anatomic stage. The pathologic prognostic stage does not apply to patients receiving neoadjuvant therapy. Many patients with triple-negative and HER2-positive breast cancer receive neoadjuvant chemotherapy.

Pathologic Prognostic Stage

TNM	Grade	HER2	ER	PR	Prognostic Group
Tis N0 M0	Any	Any	Any	Any	0
T1* N0 M0 T0 N1mi M0 T1* N1mi M0	G1	Any	Any	Any	IA
	G2 or G3	Positive	Any	Any	IA
		Negative	Positive	Any	IB
			Negative	Negative	IB
T0 N1** M0 T1* N1** M0 T2 N0 M0	G1	Positive	Positive	Positive	IA
				Negative	IB
			Negative	Positive	IB
				Negative	IIA
		Negative	Positive	Positive	IA
				Negative	IB
			Negative	Positive	IB
				Negative	IIA
	G2	Positive	Positive	Positive	IA
				Negative	IB
			Negative	Positive	IB
				Negative	IIA
		Negative	Positive	Positive	IA
				Negative	IIA
			Negative	Any	IIA
	G3	Positive	Positive	Positive	IA
				Negative	IIA
			Negative	Any	IIA
		Negative	Positive	Positive	IB
				Negative	IIA
			Negative	Any	IIA

Pathologic Prognostic Stage

TNM	Grade	HER2	ER	PR	Prognostic Group
T2 N1*** M0 T3 N0 M0	G1	Positive	Positive	Positive	IA
				Negative	IIB
			Negative	Any	IIB
		Negative	Positive	Positive	IA
				Negative	IIB
			Negative	Any	IIB
	G2	Positive	Positive	Positive	IB
				Negative	IIB
			Negative	Any	IIB
		Negative	Positive	Positive	IB
				Negative	IIB
			Negative	Any	IIB
	G3	Positive	Positive	Positive	IB
				Negative	IIB
			Negative	Any	IIB
		Negative	Positive	Positive	IIA
				Negative	IIB
			Negative	Positive	IIB
				Negative	IIIA
T0 N2 M0 T1* N2 M0 T2 N2 M0 T3 N1*** M0 T3 N2 M0	G1	Positive	Positive	Positive	IB
				Negative	IIIA
			Negative	Any	IIIA
		Negative	Positive	Positive	IB
				Negative	IIIA
			Negative	Any	IIIA
	G2	Positive	Positive	Positive	IB
				Negative	IIIA
			Negative	Any	IIIA

Pathologic Prognostic Stage

TNM	Grade	HER2	ER	PR	Prognostic Group
T0 N2 M0 T1 N2 M0 T1mi N2 M0 T2 N2 M0 T3 N1* M0 T3 N2 M0	G3	Positive	Positive	Positive	**IIA**
				Negative	**IIIA**
			Negative	Any	**IIIA**
		Negative	Positive	Positive	**IIB**
				Negative	**IIIA**
			Negative	Positive	**IIIA**
				Negative	**IIIC**
T4 N0 M0 T4 N1** M0 T4 N2 M0 Any T N3 M0	G1	Positive	Positive	Positive	**IIIA**
				Negative	**IIIB**
			Negative	Any	**IIIB**
		Negative	Positive	Positive	**IIIA**
				Negative	**IIIB**
			Negative	Any	**IIIB**
	G2	Positive	Positive	Positive	**IIIA**
				Negative	**IIIB**
			Negative	Any	**IIIB**
		Negative	Positive	Positive	**IIIA**
				Negative	**IIIB**
			Negative	Negative	**IIIC**
			Negative	Positive	**IIIB**
	G3	Positive	Any	Any	**IIIB**
		Negative			
Any T Any N M1	Any	Any	Any	Any	**IV**

* N1 does not include N1mi. T1, N1mi, M0 and T0, N1mi, M0 are included for prognostic staging with T1, N0, M0 cancers of the same prognostic factor status.

** N1 includes N1mi. T2, T3, and T4 cancers and N1mi are included for prognostic staging with T2, N1; T3, N1; and T4, N1, respectively.

Note: If performed, when OncoType DX score is less than 11 for T1-2, N0, M0 disease, if HER 2 negative, the Pathologic Prognostic Group is IA.

159

PROGNOSIS

DCIS and
Microinvasive carcinoma

DCIS

Survival

Researchers used the Surveillance, Epidemiology, and End Results (SEER) database to study women diagnosed with DCIS from 1988 to 2011. The study included 108,196 women. Researchers compared the subjects' risk of breast cancer death with women in the general population. The average age at diagnosis for women was nearly 54, and the average duration of follow-up was 7.5 years.

DCIS 10-year survival is 99%

The 10-year disease-specific survival probability following treatment for DCIS was 98.9%. By the 20-year mark, it dropped to 96.7%. The long-term death rate appeared to be higher for women who received a diagnosis before age 35 compared with older women (7.8 percent vs. 3.2 percent) and for black women compared with non-Hispanic white women (7 vs. 3 percent).

The authors note the finding of "greatest clinical importance" was that preventing an ipsilateral (on the same side of the body) invasive recurrence did not prevent death from breast cancer. Among all patients, the risk of same breast invasive recurrence at 20 years was 5.9 percent; the risk of invasive recurrence in the opposite was 6.2 percent.

Higher risk features

Your pathology report after a breast biopsy and after surgery discusses your DCIS features. You may never develop invasive breast cancer, even if you have several high-risk features. Higher risk features include:

- DCIS is in more than one area of your breast
- DCIS is high-grade
- DCIS margins are suboptimal (for example, involved)
- Young age: The US SEER database showed a 3.2% risk of breast cancer-related death for a patient with DCIS at age 35; however, for those under 35, the risk was 7.8 percent.

99%

That's the 10-year odds of surviving DCIS.
The 20-year cancer-specific survival is 96.7 percent.

DCIS

Local (in-breast) control

Local control

- Lumpectomy +/- radiation therapy

For women who had a lumpectomy, radiation therapy reduced the risk of developing an ipsilateral invasive recurrence (2.5 percent vs. 4.9 percent) but did not reduce breast cancer-specific death at ten years (0.8 percent vs. 0.9 percent), the results indicate.
- Mastectomy

Patients who had unilateral (single breast) mastectomy had a lower risk of ipsilateral invasive recurrence at ten years than patients who had lumpectomy (1.3 percent vs. 3.3 percent) but had a higher breast cancer-specific death rate (1.3 percent vs. 0.8 percent).

These data are from the US Surveillance, Epidemiology, and End Results (SEER) database. The bottom line? Adding radiation therapy to lumpectomy reduces the local recurrence risk by half but does not improve survival odds. A mastectomy yields a very low local recurrence rate at about one percent but has survival chances similar to a breast-preserving approach to management.

- Adding estrogen "blockers" to lumpectomy

Using drugs such as tamoxifen after lumpectomy and radiation therapy can reduce the risk of cancer in the opposite breast by about half and lower the same breast risk by about a third.

On the next page, we will turn to some of the individual studies (as well as meta-analyses or collections of studies) to get a better sense of the roles of radiation therapy, endocrine therapy, or both after breast-conserving surgery.

Radiation therapy (after lumpectomy)

High-level evidence for RT (in-breast control benefit)

A meta-analysis (an analysis of a collection of studies) of four large multicenter randomized trials confirmed the results of the individual trials: **Adding radiation therapy to breast-conserving surgery for DCIS significantly cuts the chances of a subsequent event in the same breast.** Rates of local failure at median follow-up intervals of approximately 13 to 17 years were 25% to 35% in the unirradiated arms compared with 10% to 20% in the irradiated arms. The National Surgical Adjuvant Breast and Bowel Project (NSABP) B-17 trial is illustrative:

- At a median follow-up of 17.25 years, compared with lumpectomy alone, radiation therapy lowered the chances of future invasive cancer in the same breast (crude local recurrence 20% versus 35%).
- Adding radiation therapy did *not* improve survival odds.

Are these studies relevant today? A contrarian view

Dr. Abram Recht of Harvard has an interesting take on whether the four first-generation randomized trials in DCIS are still relevant. So many aspects of patient evaluation and selection for breast-conserving therapy were different then than they are now; for example, there was much less use of magnification mammography, with resultant potential underestimation of the extent of DCIS. Pathologic evaluation was not standardized, and only limited sampling was performed, even with large specimens. Here is Dr. Recht's reply to the question of whether the studies noted above are valuable today:

They showed that RT substantially reduced local failure rates (but did not change the risk of metastases or breast cancer death). And no—even though life-threatening adverse effects of RT are rare, its ability to reduce the absolute risk of local recurrence is much smaller [than historically] for many (perhaps most) patients presenting today with ductal carcinoma in situ.

DCIS

Local (in-breast) control

Margins

A surgical margin is a cancer-free zone around the removed DCIS. Uninvolved margins lower the risk that the DCIS will return to the same place. Let's look at some of the available data.

- Meta-analysis (an analysis of a collection of studies)

In a meta-analysis of 4660 patients with DCIS treated with breast-conserving surgery and radiation, a surgical margin of under two millimeters (mm) appeared to be associated with increased rates of local recurrence compared with margins of two millimeters (mm) or more. There were no differences when comparing margins greater than 5 millimeters to margins of two millimeters.

Optimal margins for DCIS (and microinvasive carcinoma)

A multidisciplinary consensus panel used a meta-analysis of margin width and in-breast tumor recurrence from a systematic review of 20 studies, including 7883 patients and other published literature, as the evidence base for consensus.

This 2016 guideline (put out by three national cancer organizations in the USA) says that **two millimeters (about one-eight of an inch) clean margins should be the standard** for women diagnosed with ductal carcinoma in situ (DCIS) treated with lumpectomy and whole-breast radiation therapy.

Margins greater than two millimeters do not reduce the risk of cancer recurring in the breast in women with DCIS who are treated with lumpectomy *and* whole breast radiation therapy.

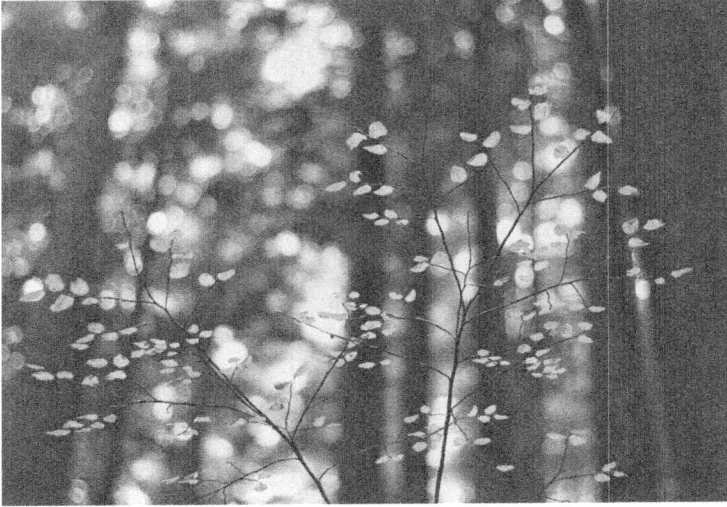

DCIS

Endocrine (anti-estrogen) therapy

Adding tamoxifen pills

Tamoxifen drops the risk of cancer events in both breasts. Let's look at the results of an important clinical trial that randomized women with DCIS (who had lumpectomy and radiation therapy) to the anti-estrogen pill tamoxifen for five years versus a placebo (a pill with no activity). Here are the results after a median follow-up of 13.6 years:

- Same breast risk reduction: Tamoxifen led to a 3.4% absolute reduction in ipsilateral (same) breast events.*

- Opposite breast risk reduction: Tamoxifen led to a 3.2% absolute reduction in contralateral (opposite) breast events.**

- Tamoxifen did *not* improve survival odds.

Other "anti-estrogen" pills

Researchers found that anastrozole (Arimidex) was better than tamoxifen at reducing recurrence risk among post-menopausal women diagnosed with hormone-receptor-positive DCIS.

---

* **Tamoxifen** led to a 10-year cumulative rate of 4.6% for invasive and 5.6% for non-invasive breast cancers in the ipsilateral (same) breast compared with 7.3% for invasive and 7.2% for non-invasive breast cancers in placebo-treated women.

**The cumulative 10-year frequency of invasive and non-invasive breast cancer in the contralateral (opposite) breast was 6.9% and 4.7% in the placebo and tamoxifen groups, respectively. The researchers discovered no differences in overall survival.

Tamoxifen versus anastrozole for DCIS

Here are the 10-year results for events in the same or opposite breast (Remember that we can only use anastrazole if you have already gone through menopause) for individuals who have DCIS:

- Anastrozole (Arimidex)
93.5% of the women had **no** recurrence

- Tamoxifen
89.2% of the women had **no** recurrence

Under 60?

Anastrozole appeared to be especially potent for post-menopausal women under 60 years of age:

- Anastrozole (Arimidex)
94.9% of the women had no recurrence

- Tamoxifen
88.2% of the women had no recurrence

For women older than 60, anastrozole (Arimidex) and tamoxifen were equally effective at reducing DCIS recurrence risk. The researchers said they didn't have a good explanation for why anastrozole and tamoxifen offered equal benefits to women older than 60 (as opposed to the post-menopausal women under 60, for whom anastrozole provided more benefits than tamoxifen).

DCIS

Into the future: HER2 and prognosis

Her2 overexpression may predict an increased risk of local (in-breast) recurrence. Radiation therapy reduces local failure rates for HER2-positive DCIS. Here are the results (with a median follow-up of 7.6 years) from the European Institute of Oncology, in which roughly a third of patients with DCIS had HER2 overexpression:

> The adjusted risk of a DCIS breast cancer recurrence was higher in the HER2-positive group than in the HER2-negative group by a factor of 1.59. This study did not support the premise that HER2-overexpression in primary DCIS is important for tumor progression toward invasive breast cancer.

HER2 testing is not routine for DCIS

While we do not routinely test DCIS for HER2, there is an ongoing trial (NSABP B-43) randomizing patients to adding the anti-HER2 drug Herceptin (trastuzumab) or not to conventional surgery and radiation therapy of patients whose DCIS over-expresses HER2.

High-risk DCIS treated with breast-conserving surgery, and radiation therapy has a low risk of local recurrence. Adding a costly drug such as trastuzumab (Herceptin) to reduce this small risk further is unlikely to be cost-effective. It could be considered over-treatment of a non-fatal disease that is sufficiently managed with current approaches.

DCIS

Into the future: Genomics

Oncotype DX DCIS is a 12-panel gene test with a scoring system that categorizes ductal carcinoma *in situ* as low, intermediate, or high risk for local recurrence over the ten years following treatment with breast-conserving surgery alone. A large population-based study presented at the 2014 San Antonio Breast Cancer Symposium validated this gene test in a diverse population of women with DCIS.

Should you have Oncotype DX testing for DCIS?

This test needs further study and is not yet part of standard practice. However, if you and your doctor agree that the test is appropriate, you will likely want to find out if your insurance covers the test. During surgery, your doctor will remove and preserve a small amount of the tumor. The pathologist will send the tumor sections to Genomic Health to generate a DCIS Score™ result. The DCIS Score results tell the likelihood or possibility of DCIS returning in the same breast as either a DCIS tumor or as an invasive breast cancer tumor:

Risk group	Local recurrence
Low	13%
Intermediate	**28%**
High	**33%**

Oncotype DX produces the DCIS Score™ result between 0 and 100. Women with lower DCIS Score results have a lower risk of their DCIS returning as DCIS or as an invasive tumor. A higher DCIS Score result means a greater chance of the DCIS returning. While promising, this test needs additional study is not yet part of standard care.

171

Microinvasion

Prognosis: Excellent

Microinvasive breast carcinoma is an invasive carcinoma of the breast with no invasive focus measuring more than 1 millimeter. It is often associated with ductal carcinoma in situ (DCIS); some refer to it as DCIS with microinvasion. It represents less than one percent of all cancers. For microinvasive carcinoma, however, taking out a sentinel node from the underarm area is typically recommended.

Microinvasive carcinoma prognosis is excellent, with 5-year survival chances ranging from 97 to 100%. A Yale (USA) series with a median follow-up of 8.5 years showed no difference in the recurrence rate or 5-year survival odds when comparing patients with microinvasion versus pure DCIS.

In-breast recurrence

The local recurrence risk following breast-conserving- or mastectomy-is small. Researchers from the Harvard-affiliated Brigham & Women's Hospital/Dana-Farber Cancer Institute have reported their experience. Here is the 5-year local recurrence rate following breast-conserving management:

	Local recurrence
Breast-conserving management	4.2 percent

* Close (2 mm or less) or involved (as opposed to negative or clear) surgical margins increased the risk of an in-breast recurrence after breast-conserving management or mastectomy by a whopping factor of 8.8 times. On the other hand, HER-2 overexpression did not appear to be associated with recurrence.

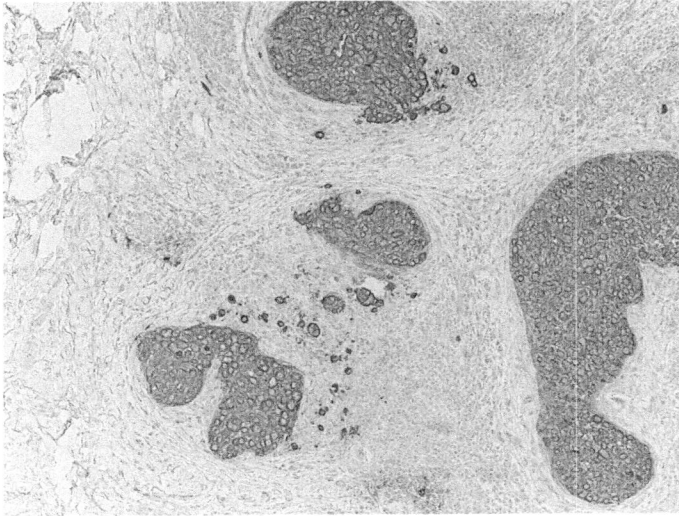

Microinvasive

PROGNOSIS

Invasive cancer;
Inflammatory cancer

Invasive cancer

Prognosis

Some factors are both prognostic and predictive. Suppose you have a newly diagnosed breast cancer that has not spread to distant sites such as the bones, liver, lungs, or brain. In that case, your healthcare providers will typically use clinical factors to help determine your prognosis (chances of survival, for example). These prognosticators include:

- Age
- Race
- Extent of cancer (stage)
- Tissue markers (for example, whether your cancer over-expresses HER2 or if it is positive for estrogen receptors and progesterone receptors (ER and PR))
- Gene expression profiles

Age

Both very young and advanced age is associated with a worse breast cancer prognosis. For very young women, breast cancer is generally more biologically aggressive. However, the relationship between age and prognosis is complex, as breast cancer subtype appears to play a role: Researchers found the age of 40 or younger to be associated with a 2.1-times increase in breast cancer mortality among those with luminal A type*, and a 1.4-fold increase among those with luminal B types. Age was of only borderline significance for those with "triple negative" (ER/PR/HER2 negative) breast cancer and did not matter for those with the human epidermal growth factor receptor 2 (HER2 positive or overexpressing) subtype.

---

* ER+ and/or PR+ ; HER2-negative, low Ki-67 (generally tumor grade 1-2)

prog-nos-tik

A *prognostic factor* provides information on clinical outcomes,

at the time of diagnosis, independent of therapy.

pre-dik-tiv

A *predictive factor* provides information on the likelihood of

a response to a given therapy.

Age (continued)

One study of the relationship between age and prognosis found that women under 35 have a lower probability of surviving five years or longer than women ages 35 to 69. Younger patients often have more advanced-stage disease and are more likely to have cancer cells that are hormone receptor negative (ER/PR negative). This worse prognosis is even though the women in the very young group tend to receive more aggressive treatment, suggesting more aggressive cancer biology among the younger patients.

Patients at the other end of the age spectrum also fare less well. Patients over the age of 65 have a higher breast cancer-specific mortality. This worse outcome is thought attributable to the fact that these older women tend to have more advanced-stage disease, co-morbidities (other health problems that can threaten their lives), and may be treated less aggressively.

Race

There are significant racial disparities in breast cancer outcomes. African-American women have a higher breast cancer mortality than other races: Breast cancer-specific mortality per 100,000 people was 32 for African-Americans and 22 for whites in 2007.

While the reasons for this lower breast cancer-specific survival among African-Americans are not entirely understood, the available data suggests several potential explanations:

- Lower rates of breast cancer screening
- Significantly longer delays to the start of treatment
- Lower rates of primary care visits
- A higher chance of having the biologically aggressive basal-like subtype of breast cancer

In a recent study, researchers used a sophisticated statistical method to determine the contributions of screening and tumor biology (with a focus on estrogen receptor status). To explain the declining breast cancer mortality rates among American women over the last four decades, using data from the Surveillance, Epidemiology, and End Results (SEER) Program, the investigators concluded that most of this survival benefit could not be attributed to cancer size and receptor status, leaving treatment as the major factor.

In an elegant editorial, Elkin and Hudis offer that these trends mask well-documented disparities in breast cancer survival linked to racial/ethnic identity. Ju-Hyun Park and colleagues offer the cumulative 5-year disease-specific survival (DSS) by age and race, using data from the Surveillance, Epidemiology, and End Results database (2005-2010):

Under 50, local only	Five-year DSS
African-American	94.9
White, non-Hispanic	98.1

50-59, local-only disease	
African-American	96.5
White, non-Hispanic	98

70+, local-only disease	
African-American	92.5
White, non-Hispanic	95.8

Under 50, regional disease	Five- year DSS
African-American	82.3
White, non-Hispanic	93.4

50-59, regional disease	
African-American	81.1
White, non-Hispanic	92.2

70+, regional disease	
African-American	76.6
White, non-Hispanic	81.5

* at presentation

Age (continued)

Under 50, distant	Five-year DSS
African-American	35.4
White, non-Hispanic	54.2

50-59, distant metastases	
African-American	32.3
White, non-Hispanic	44.6

70+, distant metastases	
African-American	17.8
White, non-Hispanic	31.7

Why? Fewer estrogen-driven cancers to target

Dr. Lisa Newman adds that breast cancer mortality rates for black and white American women did not begin to separate until around 1983 when mortality rates began declining for white women. She challenges that it cannot be coincidental that tamoxifen (our first targeted treatment for breast cancer) became widely available approximately five years before these race-based mortality differences began to emerge.

The prevalence of estrogen receptor-negative breast cancer is two-fold higher for black compared to white American patients: Availability of tamoxifen treatment has led to a favorable shift towards improved breast cancer survival. However, this outcome benefit is less evident among black patients, for whom fewer tumors are amenable to treatments targeting estrogen.

Fewer HER-2 over-expressing cancers to target

Additional advances in the systemic treatment of breast cancer have targeted human epidermal growth factor receptor 2 (HER2)-over-expressing cancers with anti-HER2 drugs such as Herceptin. The incidence of the so-called triple-negative (ER/PR/HER2 negative) breast cancer subtype is three times as high among blacks as it is for whites. This finding means that this new, exciting class of medicine is less likely to apply to black women.

Means of detection

Those with breast cancer found by a screening mammogram have a better prognosis than those found on physical exam. Screening mammogram-detected breast cancers tend to be smaller and less likely to have spread to regional lymph nodes.

Multifocal or multicentric cancer

Multifocal breast cancer means more than one cancer within the same breast quadrant; multicentric disease is in multiple separate quadrants. It is controversial whether multifocality or multicentricity influences prognosis.

Stage

In general, stage (extent of cancer) is a prognostic factor for survival. Breast cancer stage is based on tumor size, whether and how many lymph nodes are involved with cancer, and whether metastases (distant spread) are present.

Tumor size

The maximum diameter of primary cancer in the breast is prognostic. While we correlate size with the number of axillary nodes involved with cancer, both size and node status are prognostic. Here are the US Surveillance, Epidemiology, and End Results (SEER) program results

Size	Survival chances
2 cm or less	91%
2 to 5 cm	80%
More than 5 cm	**63%**

These numbers don't necessarily reflect your survival chances as an individual. There is variability in age, the number of nodes involved with cancer, grade (how aggressive the cancer cells appear), different measures of proliferation, and other factors.

Lymph node involvement

The number of axillary nodes involved with cancer is a strong prognosticator. For those without metastatic cancer, the five-year survival rate for women with localized (that is, breast only) cancer is approximately 96%. For those with one to three nodes involved, survival is 86%. Finally, for those with four or more nodes involved, the survival is 66%.

Micrometastases (under 2 mm of tumor spread to axillary nodes) are associated with a worse prognosis than no spread. A meta-analysis of 58 studies showed this increase by a factor of 1.44. On the other hand, patients who are treated appropriately aggressively at MD. Anderson Cancer Center (USA) appeared to have no increased risk compared to those with no nodal involvement. However, as the authors remarked, chemotherapy was administered to a greater proportion of stage IB patients than stage IA patients (70.5% versus 26.9%).

Isolated tumor cells (ITCs) in regional nodes do *not* affect prognosis or treatment.

Metastases (spread to distant organs)

The presence of distant metastases is a negative prognosticator. Later in this chapter, we will provide more information about metastases and prognosis.

Grade

Tumor grade incorporates cancer cell features such as the percentage of tubule formation, the aggressiveness of the nuclei (nuclear pleomorphism), and the rate of cell division (mitoses). While the grade is prognostic, interobserver ratings are too frequently in disagreement.

Lymphovascular (angiolymphatic) invasion

Tumors associated with lymphovascular invasion (cancer cells in a small blood or lymph vessels within the breast) may be associated with a higher chance of local or distant relapse. This association appears to be especially true when the cancer grade is high.

One study suggests that lymphovascular invasion is associated with other poor prognosticators and may not be an independent risk factor. In addition, endocrine therapy may diminish its value as a poor prognosticator.

Hormone receptors

Estrogen receptor status is a prognostic factor. ER-positive tumors tend to be linked to better survival chances than tumors with few or no estrogen receptors: Five-year survival is about 10 percent better for women with ER-positive breast cancer. However, after five years, this survival difference begins to decrease and, over time, may even disappear. As ER-negative breast cancers tend to recur earlier than ER-positive, ten-year survival odds may not differ.

Those with estrogen receptor scores of one to 10 percent are considered to have ER-low-positive cancers. There is limited data about the use of endocrine therapy (such as tamoxifen or the aromatase inhibitors for this group.

HER2-enriched

Her2 overexpression is associated with a poorer prognosis, especially for patients without chemotherapy and drugs targeting HER2. For those with appropriately aggressive management incorporating these drugs, HER2 overexpression may be especially valuable as a predictive factor for the efficacy of anti-HER2 drugs such as trastuzumab (Herceptin), pertuzumab (Perjeta), and others.

Tumor-Infiltrating lymphocytes in triple-negative breast cancer

The immune system appears to affect breast cancer prognosis. Recently, tumor-infiltrating lymphocytes (TILs) have been evaluated in randomized trials using contemporary chemotherapy; these studies have confirmed that TILs are most frequently found in highly proliferative tumors (triple-negative [ER/PR/HER2-negative] and HER2-positive). The presence of TILs at diagnosis is associated with a better pathologic response to neoadjuvant therapy as well as disease-free (DFS) and overall survival (OS) after adjuvant chemotherapy in certain subtypes. The BIG 02-98 trial showed TILs at diagnosis associated with outcomes among patients with triple-negative breast cancer who receive chemotherapy.

Gene profiles

Gene expression profiling measures thousands of genes' activity (expression) in a breast cancer cell. Studies examining gene expression show several breast cancer subtypes that differ in prognosis. Several genes are associated with estrogen receptor expression, HER2 expression, and proliferation. There is also a cluster of genes known as the basal cluster.

Gene expression profiles

Unlock information unique to you

Your breast cancer biology is unique. Identifying the most effective and tailored management strategies for you is based on factors such as age, tumor size, and grade, whether cancer has spread to regional lymph nodes, your hormone receptors, and whether your tumor over-expresses HER-2. Now, we can factor in more hidden breast cancer biology, giving your care team more information to personalize your breast cancer management.

Examining the patterns of various genes (gene expression profiling) can provide prognostic and predictive information for patients with early breast cancer. Information provided in 2016 suggests that such testing may also be prognostic for patients with more advanced Stage IV disease. The table to the right shows three tests (examining different sets of genes), including The Oncotype DX®, MammaPrint®, and the Prosignia test.

Oncotype DX*

The 21-gene recurrence score (RS) is among the most validated prognostic assays. It is indicated for women with estrogen receptor-positive, node-negative breast cancer. (Selected patients with node involvement may have the test, but we have less validation in that clinical setting.) The test can help determine the prognosis for patients recommended to proceed with at least a five-year course of endocrine therapy. Here's the company's take: :

> The Oncotype DX breast cancer test examines a sample of your breast cancer (obtained, for example, from cancer removed at your surgery). The test measures a group of breast cancer genes in this sample to see how active they are (also known as how they are expressed). The test result is reported as a number between 0 and 100, known as the Recurrence Score® result. A lower score means cancer has a lower chance of returning, and a higher score means a higher chance of cancer returning over the next nine years.

* Endorsed by the American Society of Clinical Oncology and two expert panels (National Comprehensive Cancer Network; St. Gallen International Expert Consensus).

Gene Expression Profile Tests

Assay	Who
OncoType DX	• Stage I, II, or IIIA • Hormone (estrogen) receptor-positive • No more than three nodes involved • You and your care team are making decisions about chemotherapy
MammaPrint	• Tumor size no larger than 5 cm (or if larger, can be surgically removed) • Hormone (estrogen) receptor-positive and will be treated with endocrine therapy • HER2-negative • 0 to 3 lymph nodes involved.
Prosigna	• Stage I or stage II and node-negative *or* stage II with one to three positive nodes • Hormone receptor-positive • Endocrine therapy alone planned after surgery
EndoPredict	• Stage I or stage II invasive breast cancer • Maximum 3 nodes involved • You and your doctor are making decisions about chemotherapy

Oncotype: Would you benefit from chemotherapy?

The Oncotype DX® score also provides information regarding the potential benefit of adding chemotherapy to endocrine therapy. Most (51 percent) will have a low recurrence score, while 27 percent have a high recurrence score (over 30). Finally, 22 percent of patients fall into the intermediate risk group. Those with T1b, N0 tumors that is low-grade and not associated with lymphovascular invasion should be treated with endocrine therapy alone.

Validation of Recurrence Score (RS)

The National Surgical Adjuvant Breast and Bowel Project (NSABP) B-14 trial validated the recurrence score (RS). This study examined the benefit of tamoxifen for hormone receptor-positive, node-negative breast cancer.

  • Chemotherapy improves the odds for the high-risk group.

  • RS may predict both locoregional and distant recurrence. RS can identify patients whose prognosis is so favorable that the benefit of chemotherapy is likely to be quite low.

Premenopausal women with hormone receptor-positive, HER2-negative with pT1-3 (over 5 mm), pN0 tumors should strongly consider Oncotype DX testing.

Premenopausal women with no nodes involved: Usual recommendations

RS 26 to 100	Chemotherapy and endocrine therapy
RS 16 to 25	There may be a small chemotherapy benefit, but it is unclear if the benefit is due to chemotherapy or the ovarian suppression caused by chemotherapy. Many consider chemotherapy plus endocrine therapy versus ovarian suppression plus endocrine therapy.
RS 15 or less	Chemotherapy unlikely to add much benefit; endocrine therapy is usually recommended.

Premenopausal women with 1 to 3 nodes involved

RS 25 or less	There may be a small chemotherapy benefit, but it is unclear if the benefit is due to chemotherapy or the ovarian suppression caused by chemotherapy. Many consider chemotherapy plus endocrine therapy versus ovarian suppression plus endocrine therapy.
RS 26-100	Substantial potential benefits from adding chemotherapy to endocrine therapy.

Postmenopausal women

RS 26 or higher An aggressive program including both endocrine therapy and chemotherapy is usually recommended.

RS 25 or lower Endocrine therapy (without chemotherapy)

For postmenopausal women with four or more involved nodes measuring more than two millimeters), chemotherapy followed by endocrine therapy is supported by high-level evidence.

MammaPrint

The MammaPrint 70-gene breast cancer recurrence assay may help you to answer some of the most important clinical questions for management:

- What is your risk for recurrence?
- Are you a candidate to avoid chemotherapy?
- What is the optimal treatment for you as an individual?

MammaPrint is based on the Amsterdam 70-gene prognostic profile. Unlike the Oncotype DX assay, MammaPrint can determine the prognosis in patients with breast cancer regardless of hormone receptor status and for patients with HER2-positive breast cancer.

Cancer spread

The development of metastatic disease has seven critical steps. First, there is the growth and proliferation of the primary tumor, followed by the growth of blood vessels into the primary tumor (angiogenesis). The third step is a local invasion. The cancer cells insert themselves into the blood system, a process known as intravasation. After drifting into the bloodstream, the cells must exit (extravasation). The last step is the adaptation of the cancer cell to the new microenvironment. The process can then begin anew.

MammaPrint analyzes all seven genomic steps of the metastatic cascade. The test provides a numerical index with a range of -1 to +1, allowing for the placement of the patient into one of two categories: Low risk (can safely withhold chemotherapy) and high risk. The next box illustrates outcomes associated with the risk group, as determined by MammaPrint.

	Cancer recurrence (by ten years)
• MammaPrint, Low risk	10%
• MammaPrint, High risk	29%

These percentages assume you do not have endocrine therapy or chemo-therapy. Researchers based the selection of the 70 predictor genes on analyses of tumors from patients under 55 years of age with node-negative cancer. No published studies show if adjuvant therapy modification based on this test would improve disease-free or overall survival. While the test seems promising, the major guideline groups in the USA need to include the MammaPrint test in management pathways.

MINDACT

A large randomized trial (Microarray in Node-Negative and 1 to 3 Positive Lymph Node Disease May Avoid Chemotherapy [MINDACT]) evaluated the clinical utility of MammaPrint. While not designed to predict a benefit (or not) from chemotherapy, it showed that patients with a high risk based on clinical factors but with a low MammoPrint score had a favorable distant metastasis-free survival chance of more than 92 percent. (The study was not sufficiently powered to exclude a potential small benefit from chemotherapy.)

Prosigna Breast Cancer Prognostic Gene Signature Assay

This assay (formerly called the PAM50 test) analyzes the activity of certain genes in early-stage hormone receptor-positive breast cancer. The test may eventually be used to help make treatments decisions based on the risk of distant relapse (metastases) for postmenopausal women within ten years of diagnosis of early hormone-receptor-positive disease with up to three positive lymph nodes after five years of endocrine ("anti-estrogen") therapy treatment.

The Prosignia Assay proved effective in an analysis of 1,478 postmenopausal women who participated in the Austrian Breast Cancer Study Group 8 (ABC-SG-8) trial. Among all patients, the estimated 10-year distant relapse-free survival rates were approximately 97%, 91%, and 80% in the low, intermediate, and high-risk groups based on the risk of recurrence (ROR) score. These results were seen whether the axillary nodes were involved or not involved.

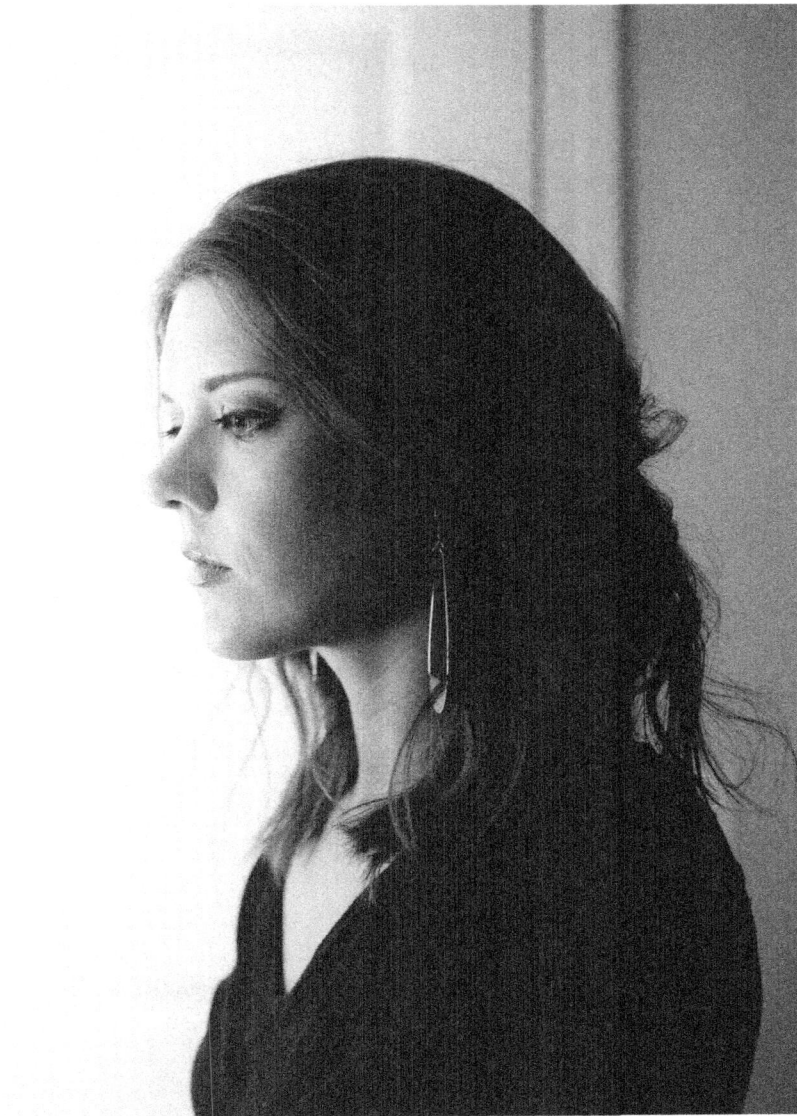

There are few data regarding the role of gene expression assays for those with four or more involved axillary nodes. Decisions to administer chemotherapy for this group should be based on clinical factors.

Other gene expression tests

Other genomic tests include the Rotterdam 76-gene signature assay, Genomic Grade Index (GGI), Breast Cancer Index (BCI), IHC4, EndoPredict, etc.

Proliferation markers (Ki-67; p53)

Here are some measures of how rapidly the cancer cells are dividing:

Disseminated tumor cells (DTCs)

Overt metastases (cancer spread to distant organs) represent a late event in the natural history of breast cancer. In contrast, the presence of breast cancer cells in the bone marrow can be detected much earlier and likely play an important role in the development of overtly metastatic disease. The data is not yet sufficiently compelling to warrant routine testing for disseminated tumor cells.

Circulating tumor cells (CTCs)

While not a routine test, newly diagnosed patients with circulating tumor (cancer) cells in their blood appear to have a poorer prognosis. This association has been demonstrated among patients at high-risk for recurrence who received chemotherapy. Two prospective studies are demonstrative:

> • Among patients with Stages I to III breast cancer, the presence of one or more CTCs was associated with a 4.6 times increase in the risk of disease progression and a four times increase in the risk of death.

> • In a separate study, the presence of CTCs led to a 2.2 times increased risk of death. Those with five or more CTCs per 30 milliliters of blood had a 3.6 times increased risk of death. In addition, those with persistent CTCs after chemotherapy had 1.16 times higher risk of death.

Other

Ki-67 is a protein associated with cell proliferation. The American Society of Clinical Oncology (ASCO) tumor marker expert panel cautions against its use as a prognostic factor. Twenty to 30 percent of breast cancers have p53 (also known as TP53) tumor suppressor gene mutations. The data regarding the implications of p53 gene mutation remain inconclusive.

Survival by cancer extent

Stage

The cancer stage at diagnosis determines management options and is strongly related to projected survival length. In general, if the cancer is found only in the part of the body where it started, it is localized. If it has spread to nearby lymph nodes, the stage is regional. Finally, the stage is advanced if there are metastases to organs such as the bones, lungs, liver, or brain.

The earlier breast cancer is discovered, the better the chances of surviving more than five years after diagnosis. For breast cancer, about 61% of patients are diagnosed with local-only cancer. The United States SEER analysis (www.seer.cancer.gov) shows relative survival probabilities are as follows:

Disease extent	5-year survival
Local	99 percent
Regional	86 percent
Distant	29 percent

Relative survival statistics compare the survival of patients diagnosed with cancer with the survival of people in the general population who are the same age, race, and sex and who have not been diagnosed with cancer. Because survival statistics are based on large groups of people, they cannot be used to predict exactly what will happen to you as an individual patient.

Cancer-Specific Survival

Adding risk profile to pathologic stage

Here are MD Anderson (USA) analysis results: Researchers determined cancer-specific survival by adding the risk profile (estrogen receptors, HER2 status, and grade) to the TNM pathologic stage. Using these prognostic groups has greatly improved our ability to provide a good estimate of prognosis. First, determine your risk profile (add your points to get a total of 0 to 3)

	0 points	1 point
Grade	Grade 1/2	Grade 3
Estrogen receptors	ER-positive	ER-negative
HER2 status	HER2 positive	HER2 negative

Look up your pathologic (after surgery) stage using the tables from the previous chapter on Stage. Finally, plug your status into the table to the right.

Contemporary outcomes

We now have reliable data showing us what proportion of women with breast cancer will develop metastases. Researchers performed a massive meta-analysis of more than 400 studies performed worldwide. They presented their results at the Advanced Breast Cancer Sixth International Consensus Conference: Abstract OR91 on October 15, 2021.

After evaluating tens of thousands of women, the meta-analysis discovered that the overall metastasis risk is between 6 percent and 22 percent. Younger women have a higher risk in general.

By cancer biology, luminal B cancers have a 4.2 to 35.5 percent risk of metastasis. Those with luminal A-type (for example, strongly estrogen- and progesterone receptor positive, HER2 negative, and lower grade) cancers had a risk ranging from 2.3 percent to 11.8 percent.

Putting It All Together

Stage	Risk profile	5 year disease-specific survival
IA / IB	0	100%
	1	99.4%
	2	98.8%
	3	96.6%
IIA	0	100%
	1	99.4%
	2	97.5%
	3	91%
IIB	0	100%
	1	96.9%
	2	92.9%
	3	91.5%
IIIA / IIIB	0	100%
	1	98.3%
	2	92.2%
	3	68.6%
IIIC	0	*
	1	92.2%
	2	80.8%
	3	33.3%

Calculate Take your stage and add the risk profile from the previous page. Use this table to calculate 5 year breast cancer specific survival odds. Remember that these numbers don't tell you the value of a particular treatment (for example chemotherapy), and may include many patients who received such treatment.

* Insufficient data

Neoadjuvant

HER-2 overexpressing cancers

Neoadjuvant therapy uses drugs (for example, chemotherapy) before surgery. Neoadjuvant treatment isn't routinely used to treat early-stage breast cancer but may be offered if the cancer is large, locally advanced, or aggressive.

Response is associated with survival

One way to check the effectiveness of neoadjuvant treatment is by looking at the tissue removed during surgery to see if any active cancer cells are present. If there are no active cancer cells, we call it a pathologic complete response. Those with a complete pathologic response to neoadjuvant treatment are less likely to have a recurrence, as compared to women who don't have a complete pathologic response. The German Taxol Epirubicin Cyclophosphamide Herceptin Neoadjuvant (TECHNO) trial used chemotherapy and trastuzumab (Herceptin) for patients whose cancer had overexpression of HER-2. Researchers found that 39% of patients had a pathologic complete response. Here are the results with a three-year follow-up:

	Pathologic complete response	
	Yes	**No**
Disease-free survival	88%	71%
Overall survival	96%	85%

There are no differences in breast cancer recurrence rates or overall survival when comparing systemic therapy before (neoadjuvant) or after (adjuvant) surgery. That's the conclusion of a so-called meta-analysis that combined the results of eight individual studies.

Neoadjuvant chemotherapy and locoregional recurrence

Researchers analyzed 12 clinical trials on neoadjuvant chemotherapy that involved nearly 12,000 people. Of these, 61% had primary cancers measuring 2 to 5 cm, and 47% had involvement of regional nodes. Here are five-year results:

	Locoregional Relapse
Surgery type	
Lumpectomy	8%
Mastectomy	10%
Breast cancer type	
Grade 1-2, hormone receptor +, Her2 -	4%
Grade 3, hormone receptor +, Her2 -	9%
Hormone receptor - , HER2 +	15%
Hormone receptor +, HER2 +	10%
Hormone receptor -, HER2 - (triple negative)	12%
Response type	
Pathologic complete response	5.5%
• Lumpectomy	6%
• Mastectomy	4%
No pathologic complete response	7%
• Lumpectomy	6%
• Mastectomy	8%
Radiation therapy (after surgery)	
Pathologic complete response	
• Lumpectomy	4%
• Mastectomy	2%
No pathologic complete response	
• Lumpectomy	8%
• Mastectomy	6.5%

Nodes: Micrometastases

Basics

Evaluation of axillary (underarm) lymph nodes for the presence of cancer is an important part of breast cancer staging. To assess these nodes, a surgeon performs either an axillary lymph dissection (many nodes are surgically removed and evaluated) or a less extensive procedure known as a sentinel node biopsy.

A sentinel node biopsy is a means of evaluating whether cancer has spread to nodes in your axilla. The procedure is typically done at the time of your surgery. It represents an innovative and thorough method of evaluating the sentinel node to ensure that no regional spread of cancer was missed. Whereas around three sections per axillary node were typically examined in the pre-sentinel node biopsy era, the sentinel node is now more thoroughly examined. This change has led to the more frequent identification of micro-metastatic (that is, 2 millimeters or less in size) disease in nodes.

Micrometastases to nodes - Prognosis

Among women with early breast cancer, micrometastases in the axillary nodes may lead to a higher risk of recurrence than those without node involvement. A study of 3,369 patients discovered:

	Recurrence-free survival (5 years)
No node involvement	87%
Isolated tumor cells	89%
Micro-metastases	80%
Macro-metastases	80%

These numbers refer to relapse-free survival. **In terms of overall survival, there were no differences when comparing those with *micrometastases* (or isolated tumor cells) with women with cancer-free nodes.**

Nodes: Isolated tumor cells

Isolated Tumor Cells - Not Clinically Significant

Isolated tumor cells (ITCs) are small clusters of cells not greater than 0.2 mm, or cancer cells not exceeding 200 in number in a single lymph node cross-section (as seen under a microscope). The discovery of isolated tumor cells in lymphatics can result from cancer cell displacement by the surgeon. Many (but not all) studies suggest that ITCs are *not clinically significant*.

Triple Negative Breast Cancer: Role for TILs?

Breast cancers negative for estrogen receptors, progesterone receptors, and HER2 are colloquially known as "triple negative" breast cancers (TNBC). Emerging evidence suggests an association between the number of immune cells attacking cancer and prognosis.

Researchers at Peter MacCallum Cancer Centre, University of Melbourne, Australia, demonstrated the strong predictive value of so-called stromal tumor-infiltrating lymphocytes (TILs; immune system cells) for outcomes in patients with early-stage triple-negative breast cancer (TNBC) who receive adjuvant chemotherapy. More study is needed to validate this provocative observation.

Locoregional relapse

re·lapse [rē´laps], local

The breast cancer comes back in the same breast (after lumpectomy) or chest wall (after mastectomy) region.

Patients with local or regional recurrence only may be conveniently divided into three groups, including those who initially had:

- Mastectomy
- Mastectomy plus radiation therapy
- Breast-conserving therapy

Let's look at the prognosis after a local recurrence. Analysis of a combined database of patients from the European Organization for the Research and Treatment of Cancer (EORTC) 10801 and Danish Breast Cancer Cooperative Group 82TM trials provide data.

The research compared breast-conserving therapy with mastectomy in patients with stage I and stage II disease. The 133 (approximately 8%) patients with a local recurrence as an initial event were equally divided between those who had undergone mastectomy and those who had received breast-conserving therapy as initial treatment for breast cancer. Of those in the former group, 51 (76%) were able to undergo radiation therapy with or without surgery as a treatment for local disease recurrence.

Does initial local treatment type affect prognosis?

No differences in survival emerged between patients receiving treatment for recurrence after initial treatment with mastectomy or breast-conserving therapy. Approximately 50% of both groups were alive at 10-year follow-up.

How much risk does a locoregional recurrence add?

The Early Breast Cancer Trialists' Collaborative Group (Oxford Overview) offers this striking observation: For every six patients with a local recurrence (in-

The Early Breast Cancer Trialists' Collaborative Group (Oxford Overview) offers this striking observation: For every six patients with a local recurrence (in-breast after lumpectomy or chest wall after mastectomy) by the ten-year mark, there will be one additional death from breast cancer by the 15-year mark.

Local recurrence

The risk for a local (in the region of the breast or chest wall) decreases as event-free survival lengthens, at least according to an analysis of a large database from the Netherlands. The study also suggested that recurrence risk varies substantially by cancer subtype. Fortunately, the risk of a local recurrence as the first event within five years of diagnosis was low, at three percent. The risk appears highest for those with so-called triple-negative cancer (estrogen receptor, progesterone receptor, HER2 negative) and lowest for those with ER-positive, PR-positive, and HER2-negative breast cancer.

We typically express prognosis as a five-year or 10-year probability of event-free survival. Various studies have shown the five-year local recurrence rate for breast cancer is around three percent, but what is the rate if you are out from diagnosis for two years and have not had a recurrence? Here's what Dutch investigators discovered (numbers given with the assumption that there have been no breast events to that particular time point):

	At diagnosis	1 year	2 years	3 years	4 years
ER+, PR+, HER2 -	2.2%	2%	1.5%	1%	0.6%
ER+, PR -, HER2 -	2.4%	2%	1.4%	0.9%	0.5%
ER+, HER2 +	2.8%	2.2%	1.5%	1%	0.4%
ER -, HER2 +	4.7%	3.4%	2%	0.7%	0.2%
ER -, PR -, HER2 -	6.8%	4.6%	2.7%	1.6%	1.1%

Locoregional relapse

Relapse after breast-conserving management

After breast-conserving surgery (lumpectomy) followed by whole-breast radiation therapy (WBRT), breast cancer can recur locally, regionally, or at distant metastatic sites. A local recurrence is defined as the reappearance of cancer in the ipsilateral preserved breast. In contrast, a regional recurrence denotes a tumor involving the regional lymph nodes, usually ipsilateral axillary or supraclavicular, less commonly infraclavicular or internal mammary. The term locoregional recurrence indicates a recurrence in either the breast or regional nodes.

Locoregional control after recurrence
Many patients with an isolated locoregional recurrence will survive at least ten years. For women who have an in-breast recurrence managed with a mastectomy, modern series show a broad range of future locoregional control:

	Future locoregional control
• Mastectomy after *invasive* first relapse	48%
• Mastectomy after *non-invasive* relapse	100%

Interval to recurrence
Contemporary studies indicate that 10-year survival rates range from 39 to 80 percent. There are many prognostic factors, with invasive recurrences having a worse prognosis (compared to non-invasive). In addition, a short disease-free interval between initial breast-conserving management and local recurrence is a poor prognostic factor. In one study, the rates of distant disease were 92, 53, and 22 percent when the interval from primary treatment was less than two, two to five, and longer than five years, respectively.

200

Interval to locoregional relapse

Prognostic factors for patients experiencing a local or regional relapse include the disease-free interval from initial diagnosis and the location and volume of the recurrence (please see the next pages). Here are outcomes from one series from the Mallinckrodt Institute of Radiology (USA), based on the interval from diagnosis until locoregional recurrence:

	Survival (5 year)
Two years or less	35 percent
More than two years	50 percent

Results in the modern era

British Columbia (Canada) researchers explored the impact of local or regional recurrence on survival in breast cancer in the modern era. They conducted a retrospective study of patients with stages I, II, or III disease treated with surgery who experienced a subsequent locoregional relapse. 10 year survival varied by breast cancer biology:

	10 year survival	Median survival
Luminal A	65 percent	Not reached
Luminal B	27 percent	4.8 years
Her2-positive	44 percent	7.3 years
Triple-negative	24 percent	3.1 years

Locoregional relapse

Regional relapse

Recurrences in regional lymph nodes in the axillary (underarm area) or paraclavicular (around the collarbone) regions are relatively uncommon. Regional lymph node recurrence after breast conservation therapy may be salvaged but is associated with a high rate of either simultaneous or subsequent distant metastases and poor overall prognosis. A study from the University of Pennsylvania examining 10-year outcomes following regional recurrence is illustrative:

	Disease-specific survival
Regional (nodes) only relapse	44%
Local *and* regional relapse	40%
Regional *and* distant relapse	12%*

* If the regional and distant relapses are simultaneous, the median survival drops to 1.1 years. This outcome compares to 5.2 years if the distant metastases are after the regional recurrence.

Locoregional relapse

Supraclavicular relapse

There is a range of findings regarding outcomes for patients with an isolated supraclavicular (above the collarbone) recurrence. Let's look at the largest series. The Danish Breast Cancer Cooperative Group looked at 305 patients with a supraclavicular relapse (but without a distant spread of cancer). Patients initially had either mastectomy or breast-conserving surgery, and 23 percent received radiation therapy.

	Progression-free survival
Supraclavicular only relapse	**15 percent (five years)** Combination salvage therapy and low cancer grade were associated with to longer progression-free survival.

Locoregional management included the removal of at least the measurable tumor (19 percent) or curative radiation therapy (33 percent), with only 10 percent having combined surgery and radiation therapy. Overall, 26% had combined locoregional and systemic (endocrine or chemotherapy) therapy, while 49% had systemic therapy only, and 25 percent had locoregional treatment alone.

Locoregional relapse

Chemotherapy?

Chemotherapy ups survival odds

The CALOR trial examined outcomes following a complete resection for patients with an isolated (no distant spread of cancer) locoregional recurrence. The individual doctor selected the chemotherapy type; multiple drugs for at least four courses were recommended) versus no chemotherapy. After a median follow-up of 4.9 years, here is the overall disease-free survival:

	Disease-free survival	Survival
Chemotherapy	69 percent	88%
No chemotherapy	57 percent	76%

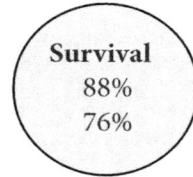

Chemotherapy may benefit ER-negative most

Chemotherapy appeared to be significantly more effective for women with the estrogen-receptor-negative disease. The authors concluded that adjuvant chemotherapy should be recommended for patients with completely resected locoregional breast cancer recurrence, especially if the recurrence is estrogen-receptor negative.

Chemotherapy downsides

Of the 81 patients who got chemotherapy, 12 (15 percent) had serious side events. The most common events were neutropenia (very low white blood cell level), febrile neutropenia, and intestinal infection.

Cigarettes

Prognosis

Smoking before and after breast cancer is associated with increased mortality from breast cancer and other conditions, including respiratory and cardiovascular disease.

Researchers in the Collaborative Breast Cancer and Women's Longevity Study followed women for a median of 12 years following diagnosis. Researchers found that:

- Women who smoked a year before their breast cancer diagnosis were 1.25 times more likely to die of breast cancer than never-smokers.

- Breast cancer mortality was highest among long-term smokers, heavy smokers, or former smokers who quit less than five years before being diagnosed.

- One in 10 study participants who did not quit smoking following their diagnosis were 1.72 times more likely to die of breast cancer than the never smokers or those who quit smoking following their cancer diagnosis. Women who quit had about a third lower mortality from breast cancer and a more than halving risk of death from respiratory cancer.

According to lead author Michael Passarelli, Ph.D., these results should motivate smoking women diagnosed with breast cancer to quit smoking. "Our study shows the consequences facing both active and former smokers with a history of breast cancer," he said in an associated press release, adding, "Smoking cessation programs should be considered part of cancer therapy."

Breast density

Tamoxifen

Tamoxifen (and the aromatase inhibitors such as anastrozole, exemestane, and letrozole) is highly effective in treating estrogen receptor (ER) –positive breast cancer. Tamoxifen treatment for five years reduces 10-year recurrence risk and 15-year breast cancer mortality by nearly one-third (event rate ratio, 0.70).

Tamoxifen and breast density
Breast density is a measure of how the breasts appear on mammograms. Breast density compares the breast and connective tissue area to the fat area. Breast and connective tissue are denser than fat, a difference seen on a mammogram.

- High breast density means greater breast and connective tissue than fat.
- Low breast density means greater fat than breast and connective tissue.

Women with the highest levels of percent density (75% or higher) have a four- to six-fold increased risk of developing breast cancer compared with women with the lowest percentage (25% or less) when adjusted for confounding factors. A decrease in density may be a-needed predictor of a favorable response to the selective estrogen receptor modulator tamoxifen.

Women whose mammographic density declined in the unaffected breast after initiation of tamoxifen therapy appear to have a lower risk of recurrence or death from breast cancer. That's the conclusion of four retrospective analyses. The magnitude of the observed benefit associated with a decline (approximately 10%) in breast density was remarkably similar among the studies. Furthermore, the ability of tamoxifen to lower mammographic density may increase mammogram effectiveness among some women.

Inflammatory

Prognosis

With appropriately aggressive treatment, up to 62 percent of those with inflammatory breast cancer (IBC) will live at least five years, and 41 to 47 percent will have no signs of breast cancer ten years after diagnosis. While these rates are not nearly as high as for other types of breast cancer, new treatments continue to improve survival.

Inflammatory, non-metastatic: Median survival 57 months

Let's look at survival differently: Median survival is the length of time for half of the patients in a group to have died. By definition, half of the patients in that group are still alive. The US Surveillance, Epidemiology, and End Results (SEER) database shows that the median survival for non-metastatic inflammatory breast cancer is 57 months.

Survival rates improving

With modern treatment, the survival rate has improved significantly. An analysis from the Surveillance, Epidemiology, and End Results database demonstrated 20-year cancer-specific survival of 20 versus 9 percent for patients with invasive breast cancer treated in 1995 compared with 1975. Despite these improvements, the survival rate for patients with IBC remains significantly worse compared with women with non-inflammatory, locally advanced breast cancer. For Stage IV IBC, the median survival drops to 21 months.

Poor prognostic features

Poor prognostic features include triple-negative receptor status, hormone receptor-positive/human epidermal growth factor receptor 2 (HER2)-negative status, four or more involved lymph nodes before therapy, and lack of response to neoadjuvant chemotherapy. HER2-positive inflammatory breast cancer may have an equivalent or marginally better prognosis than HER2-negative disease, unlike non-inflammatory breast cancer.

Race; older patients

Black women

Black women appeared nearly six times more likely (than white women) to develop distant metastases after a breast cancer diagnosis. Even after Blanter and colleagues at Mt. Sinai Hospital (New York City) researchers adjusted for disease stage and patient age, this finding held.

The reason for this disparity needs to be clarified. Contributing factors may include surveillance, treatment differences, or follow-up.

Over 70

Can we use endocrine (anti-estrogen) therapy in place of surgery? A meta-analysis compared primary surgery with primary endocrine therapy using tamoxifen in women more than 70 years of age. Here are their findings:

- No significant difference in *survival* between the two treatments;
- Patients receiving surgery had a superior progression-free survival (nearly half as likely to progress after surgery).

The CALGB 9343 clinical trial looked at lumpectomy with or without irradiation in women age 70 years or older with early breast cancer. All had estrogen receptor-positive breast cancer treated by lumpectomy and were randomly assigned to receive tamoxifen plus radiation therapy or tamoxifen alone. Here are the ten-year results:

In-breast control was 98 percent in the radiation therapy-containing group and 90 percent in the tamoxifen alone group. The study found no difference in overall survival, distant disease-free survival, or breast preservation.

6x

Black women are 5.75 times more likely to develop a distant cancer spread than white women.

Summary

Prognostic factors

• **Prognostic factors** provide information on outcomes independent of treatment. In contrast, **predictive factors** provide information on the likelihood of a response to a given treatment. Some factors are both prognostic and predictive.

• **Stage (extent of cancer at diagnosis)** is a critical determinant of prognosis.

• **Lymphvascular (angiolymphatic) space invasion** (LVI) is a risk factor for local recurrence after breast-conserving management.

• **Both very younger and very old age** at diagnosis are associated with worse prognoses.

• **African-American women** (as a group) have a worse prognosis than white and Asian women (even after controlling for disease characteristics at diagnosis).

• **Genomic assays** allow for the simultaneous measurement of thousands of genes and have led to the identification of biology-based prognostic profiles in clinical use today. These assays incorporate important gene clusters relating to estrogen receptor expression (the luminal cluster), HER2 expression, proliferation, and the basal gene cluster. Breast cancer subtypes differ in prognosis.

• **Local or regional recurrence prognostic factors** include the site of recurrence, volume of disease, and interval from original diagnosis to the time of recurrence.

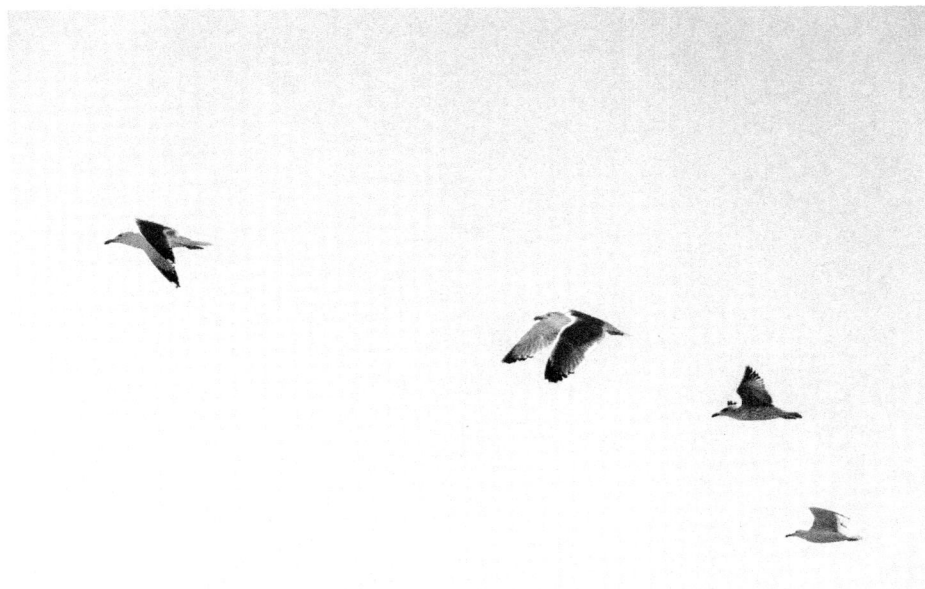

PROGNOSIS

Metastases

Metastases

Prognostic factors

According to the US National Cancer Institute SEER database, stage IV breast cancer has an overall 5-year survival probability of 30 percent. While patients with metastatic breast cancer cannot typically be cured, we have recently had meaningful improvements in survival. That said, there is great variability among patients, and in this chapter, we will look at some of the variables that may influence your prognosis.

Prognostic versus predictive factors

Prognostic factors provide information (at the time of diagnosis or various times during the patient's course with metastatic cancer) on projected clinical outcomes. Note that prognostic factors are independent of therapy. In contrast, predictive factors provide information on the likelihood of a response to a given treatment. Some factors are both prognostic and predictive.

Prognostic factors

- **Relapse-free interval (RFS):** A relapse-free survival of two years or more is more favorable than a shorter time to relapse.

- **Location of metastases:** Those with metastases involving the chest wall or bones have a more prolonged progression-free survival on average, as compared with patients who have liver, lung, or brain metastases.

- **Hormone receptors:** Those with positive estrogen and progesterone receptors (ER+/PR+) have a significantly longer survival length (on average) than those with single hormone receptor-positive tumors (ER+/PR- or ER-/PR+).

- **HER2 overexpression** (at least, in the era before we had targeted therapies such as trastuzumab (Herceptin)).

• **Triple negative** type of cancer (ER/PR/HER2 negative) is linked to a worse prognosis than cancers with other combinations of these markers.

• **Other:** Weight loss, poor performance status, or elevated blood levels of lactic dehydrogenase (LDH) can affect prognosis.

• **Circulating tumor cells (CTCs):** Patients with elevated CTCs (5 or more cancer cells in 7.5 milliliters) appear to have a worse prognosis.

The Southwest Oncology Group (SWOG) 0500 trial examined chemotherapy patients. Patients with no baseline elevation of CTCs had a median survival of 35 months. This outcome was compared to 23 months for those who had elevated CTCs at baseline (but had a decline in CTCs after their first cycle of chemotherapy). The median survival was 13 months for those with persistently elevated CTCs.

While the available data points to prognostic value for CTCs, their role in patient surveillance remains controversial and is not routinely used to determine patient management in the USA.

• **Next-generation sequencing of breast tumors**

Understanding the molecular drivers of cancer progression is an area of active clinical investigation to identify specific genetic abnormalities. While several tests are commercially available, these are only sometimes used. It is unclear whether these tests are prognostic or how much they will allow for effective individualization of treatment.

Metastases

Prognostic factors

ER, PR, and HER2

Investigators at the Department of Pathology at the Academic Medical Center in Amsterdam used tissue from 263 patients with metastatic breast cancer and stained the samples for a host of markers. These included ER, PR, HER2, EGFR (epidermal growth factor receptor), CK5/6, CK14, E-cadherin, TP53, and Ki-67. The tumors were then classified by molecular subtype, incorporating factors such as estrogen and progesterone receptor status, HER2, and Ki-67 (a measure of cancer cell growth rate). Here are the results:

Patients developed metastasis by 30 months (on average)

The average time to the development of metastases was 30 months. For those who developed metastases, more than three-quarters did so within 5 years of treatment of the primary breast tumor. Data showed that women with hormone-negative disease developed distant metastases earlier than women with other subtypes. Using tissue microarrays, the authors found that the median survival varied according to breast cancer subtype. About 76% of patients who developed metastasis did so within the first five years of initial diagnosis.

	Median survival
ER-negative, HER2 negative	27 months
HER2 positive	52 months
ER-positive, HER2 negative, Ki-67 high	76 months
ER-positive, HER2 negative, Ki-67 low	79 months

The most common site of distant metastasis is the bone (71%), followed by the liver (55%), and then the lung (31%). Visceral (internal organs such as the liver and lungs) metastases occurred in 77% of patients. For those who developed distant spread, there appear to be differences by cancer subtype:

216

	Visceral	Bone
ER-negative, HER2 negative	81%	55%
HER2 positive	77%	70%
ER-negative, HER2 negative, Ki-67 high	76%	88%
ER-positive, HER2 negative, Ki-67 low	77%	73%

While there is currently no cure for metastatic breast cancer, treatment can meaningfully extend life while helping maintain quality of life. There are also clinical trials available that offer hope.

ER, PR, and HER2

As a general rule, there should be an attempt to biopsy recurrent cancer. This allows for a re-check of estrogen receptors (ER), progesterone receptors (PR), and human epidermal growth factor receptor 2 (HER2). The receptor status can change: 1) The original tumor ER and PR differ from the recurrent tumor ER and PR about 13 percent and 30 percent of the time, respectively; 2) the HER2 differs from 3 to 5 percent of the time. The ER, PR, and HER2 status can predict response to various treatments.

Tumor markers

Tumor markers include CA 15-3 and CA 27.29. Assays can determine levels of circulating MUC-1, a protein in the bloodstream. CA 15-3 and CA 27.29 levels may be used to monitor the disease status of patients having treatment for metastatic breast cancer. While prognostic, serum tumor markers are not predictive of treatment outcomes and don't help with treatment selection.

Elevations in tumor markers are occasionally "false positives" or spurious. Indeed, up to 20 percent of patients treated with systemic therapy may have a temporary increase during the first month or two after treatment starts. Some individuals with abnormal liver function can have a falsely elevated marker level, and those with a vitamin B12 deficiency and megaloblastic anemia (as well as those with thalassemia or sickle cell disease) may have CA 15-3 levels that are elevated.

Metastases

Brain

Risk

Breast cancer is the second (behind lung cancer) most common cancer associated with brain metastases in the USA. The breast cancer subtype appears to be associated with an individual's probability of developing brain metastases. Among a group of 1434 higher-risk women managed with breast-conserving therapy plus chemotherapy, brain metastases developed in 2.5 percent. Here are the numbers at the ten-year mark:

Luminal A	0.1 percent
Luminal B	3.3 percent
Luminal-HER2	3.2 percent
HER2	3.7 percent
ER/PR/HER2 negative	**7.4 percent**

Patients with ER/PR/HER2 negative ("triple negative") have an increased risk of brain metastases as the initial site of metastases compared to other breast cancer subtypes. In one study, the odds of developing brain metastases by the 5-year mark were three percent for Stage I, five percent for Stage II, and 10 percent for Stage III, respectively.

Prognosis

The Radiation Therapy Oncology Group (RTOG) used a sophisticated analysis to show the prognosis for patients with breast cancer who develop metastases to the brain. A score (graded prognostic assessment, or GPA) is created based on performance status, breast cancer subtype, and age.

Calculating survival

Step #1: Calculate score

	0	0.5	1	1.5	2	TOTAL
KPS	50 or less	60	70-80	90-100	-	
Subtype	ER/PR/ HER2 -	-	ER/PR+, HER2 -	HER2 +	ER/PR/ HER2 +	
Age	60+	Under 60	-	-	-	
					Sum	

Step #2: Find median* survival (months)

Score 0-1	3.4 months
Score 1.5-2	7.7 months
Score 2.5-3	15.1 months
Score 3.5-4	25.3 months

---

* Karnofsky Performance Status: 100 = no complaints; 90 = minor symptoms; 80 = normal activity with effort; 70 = cares for self, but unable to carry on normal activity or do active work; 60 = requires considerable assistance but able to care for most of the personal needs; 50 = requires considerable assistance and frequent medical care; 40 = disabled, requiring special care and assistance
** Half of the patients in this group will live past the median survival.

Summary

Metastases and prognosis

- Stage IV breast cancer is associated with an overall 5-year survival probability of 22%. However, the prognosis for an *individual* is challenging to estimate, as a host of factors can play a role.

- **Relapse-free interval (RFS): A** relapse-free interval of two years or more is more favorable than a shorter time to relapse.

- **Location:** The most common site of distant metastasis is the bone (71%), followed by the liver (55%), and then the lung (31%). On average, those with metastases involving the chest wall or bones have a more prolonged progression-free survival compared to patients with liver, lung, or brain metastases.

- **Hormone receptors:** Those with positive estrogen and progesterone receptors (ER+/PR+) have a significantly longer survival length (on average) than those with single hormone receptor-positive tumors (ER+/PR- or ER-/PR+).

- **HER2 overexpression** (at least, in the era before we had targeted therapies such as trastuzumab (Herceptin)).

- **Triple negative type of cancer** (ER/PR/HER2 negative) is linked to a worse prognosis than cancers with other combinations of these markers.

- **Other:** Weight loss, poor performance status, or elevated blood levels of lactic dehydrogenase (LDH) can affect prognosis.

Metastases

Brain: Leptomeningeal spread

Leptomeningeal

The meninges are the three membranes that envelop the brain and spinal cord. Leptomeningeal (lep-toh-men-IN-jee-ul) carcinomatosis is an unusual complication of cancer in which the disease spreads to the membranes (meninges) surrounding the brain and spinal cord. Symptoms may be divided into three groups:

- Brain involvement: Headaches (may be associated with nausea, vomiting, and light-headedness), significant fatigue, behavioral changes, gait disturbances, and memory problems
- Cranial nerve involvement: Impaired or double vision, hearing loss, sensory deficits, vertigo, and others
- Spinal root involvement: Neck stiffness and pain

Prognosis

One series of 68 women with metastatic breast cancer who had cancer spread to the leptomeninges had a median survival of four months, with a one-year survival chance of 13 percent. Variables linked to survival length included:

- Conversion to no cancer cells in the spinal fluid.
- The absence of systemic metastases (for example, to the liver, bone, or lung).
- Combined modality management (chemotherapy and radiation therapy, for example).

MANAGEMENT

DCIS

DCIS

Overview

Basics

Ductal carcinoma in situ (DCIS) is non-invasive. However, abnormal cells sometimes evolve to become invasive cancer over time. If DCIS is left untreated, approximately 40 to 50 percent of DCIS cases may progress to invasive breast cancer. The diagnosis of DCIS increased dramatically following the introduction of screening mammograms and now represents up to a quarter of all newly diagnosed breast cancer. In this chapter, we will review the management of DCIS.

Work-up

1) History and physical exam; 2) diagnostic mammograms of both breasts; 3) a review of the biopsy by a pathologist, and 4) determination of whether the DCIS has estrogen receptors (ER-positive or ER-negative). Individuals at high risk for hereditary breast cancer should strongly consider genetic counseling.

Management

- Breast-conserving surgery ("lumpectomy") + radiation therapy

- Breast removal (mastectomy)

- Breast-conserving surgery

"Anti-estrogen" therapy such as tamoxifen pills (for pre- or post-menopausal women) or an aromatase inhibitor (for women who are after menopause) may be advised for those with estrogen-receptor positive DCIS. Follow-up is then history and physical exam every 6 to 12 months for five years, then annually. Mammograms are done every 12 months (and 6 to 12 months after radiation therapy).

DCIS

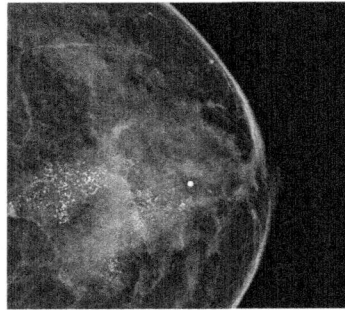

Imaging

Mammograms

A screening mammogram is the primary imaging tool for the early detection of breast cancer. Researchers developed a prototype mammography unit in 1965. A technologist typically obtains two views of the breast; one from the top-down and the other from the side-to-side of the breast. A single view can miss 11 to 25 percent of cancers. A newer form of mammograms is known as tomosynthesis or "3-D" mammograms. A large study found that the addition of tomosynthesis to digital mammography resulted in a decrease in recall rates and an increase in cancer detection rates.

We use screening mammograms for those with no clinical symptoms or findings on exam. On the other hand, a diagnostic mammogram is for patients who present with breast symptoms or have an abnormal clinical exam. The diagnostic mammogram is supervised by a radiologist, with images obtained to evaluate a specific abnormality. A spot compression view may be added, using focal compression to the area of interest in the breast using a small compression paddle. Magnification spot compression view can better characterize the shape and size of calcifications or better characterize a mass.

Roughly 90 percent of women with DCIS have microcalcifications on mammography. DCIS accounts for 80 percent of breast cancer among those who present with calcifications on screening mammography. However, tomosynthesis did *not* improve detection rates for DCIS.

Ultrasound

Ultrasound uses sound waves to follow up on an abnormal mammogram. Ultrasound can provide more information about masses or asymmetry and may distinguish a solid mass from a non-cancerous cyst. Ultrasound does not emit radiation.

DCIS

Imaging

MRI

Magnetic resonance imaging as a screening tool for women at average risk is controversial. While its use for DCIS remains unclear, the test may help to determine the extent of DCIS and to identify disease that is scattered in the breast (multicentric DCIS) or find cancer in the opposite (contralateral) breast. Many centers do not use MRI for DCIS: While MRI is quite good at finding DCIS, it has a high risk of false alarms (false positives).

Should everyone with ductal carcinoma in situ have a breast MRI? About one-third of surgeons in the United States will order an MRI for women with DCIS. Yet routine MRI before or after surgery in women with DCIS may not be a sound clinical strategy: It does not appear to improve long-term outcomes. Researchers at Memorial Sloan Kettering Cancer Center (New York City) identified 2321 women who had undergone lumpectomy for DCIS between 1997 and 2010. Of these patients, 596 received an MRI either before or immediately after surgery, and 1725 did not.

After eight years, local recurrence rates were not significantly different between the MRI and no MRI groups (14.6 vs. 10.2 percent). Even after controlling for nine patient variables (including age, menopausal status, family history, and use of radiation or endocrine therapy), there was no significant difference in the risk of local recurrence. This multivariable analysis is important because women undergoing MRI typically have a higher risk profile.

Finally, contralateral (the other) breast cancer rates in the MRI and no MRI groups were the same: Contralateral breast cancer rates in the MRI and no MRI groups were the same at five years (3.5% versus 3.5%) and similar at eight years (3.5% versus 5.1%). This observation does not mean that no patient with DCIS should have an MRI; we need high-level evidence to advocate for its routine use for patients with ductal carcinoma in situ.

DCIS

Biopsy types

Core needle biopsy

A core tissue sampling can evaluate most abnormalities. We usually prefer this approach to alternatives, such as removing the lesion (excisional biopsy). The core biopsy is done with image guidance.

Wire localization excisional biopsy

For those who are not candidates for non-surgical approaches (such as a core biopsy) to establish the diagnosis, an alternative is a so-called wire localization excisional biopsy. This technique involves the placement of a very thin wire. This approach allows your surgeon to localize the tissue that needs removal. A radiologist places the wire (typically in the radiology department of a hospital or surgery center where your breast biopsy ("lumpectomy') is to be performed).

You are awake for the placement of the very fine wire, but the radiologist injects a local anesthetic to numb the breast before placement. You may experience a sting from the anesthetic needle, but most patients feel much more comfortable as the anesthetic begins to act. The radiology technologist obtains images of your breast. A radiologist then inserts a very fine needle to target the breast abnormality. The aim is to rest the needle's tip at the abnormality's location. A slender wire is threaded down through the needle, and the needle is then removed (with the wire left in place). Feeling pressure or a pulling sensation during the wire placement is not unusual.

What entities could be mistaken for DCIS? Atypical ductal hyperplasia (ADH), microinvasive carcinoma, and lobular carcinoma in situ (LCIS) all can look like DCIS. The odds that a seemingly pure DCIS on a core needle biopsy will be associated with invasive cancer at surgery is about 25 percent.

DCIS

Paget disease of the nipple

Paget disease of the breast (also known as Paget disease of the nipple and mammary Paget disease) is a rare type of cancer involving the skin of the nipple and often the darker circle of skin around it (areola). Most people with Paget disease of the breast also have one or more tumors inside the same breast. A biopsy of the nipple abnormality is required to diagnose Paget disease of the breast. Several types of biopsy are available:

Less commonly, the surgeon may remove the entire nipple. A pathologist then examines the cells under a microscope to make a diagnosis. It is not uncommon for individuals with Paget disease of the nipple to simultaneously have different cancer in the same breast. Thus the imaging and physical exam are critical. As many as 50 percent of patients with Paget disease of the nipple may have an underlying palpable mass in the breast.

Here are some the features for which the pathologist looks to make the diagnosis of Paget disease: 1) intraepithelial (within the layer of cells that forms the surface or lining the nipple) population of large, atypical (Paget) cells; 2) large nuclei, with prominent nucleoli (small dense spherical structures in the nucleus of a cell during interphase part of the cell life cycle); 3) an underlying *in situ* or invasive breast carcinoma is commonly present.

Here are some of the features for which the pathologist looks to make the diagnosis of Paget disease:

- Intraepithelial (within the layer of cells that forms the surface or lining the nipple) population of large, atypical (Paget) cells.

- Large nuclei, with prominent nucleoli (small dense spherical structures in the nucleus of a cell during the interphase part of the cell life cycle).

- An underlying *in situ* or invasive breast carcinoma is commonly present.

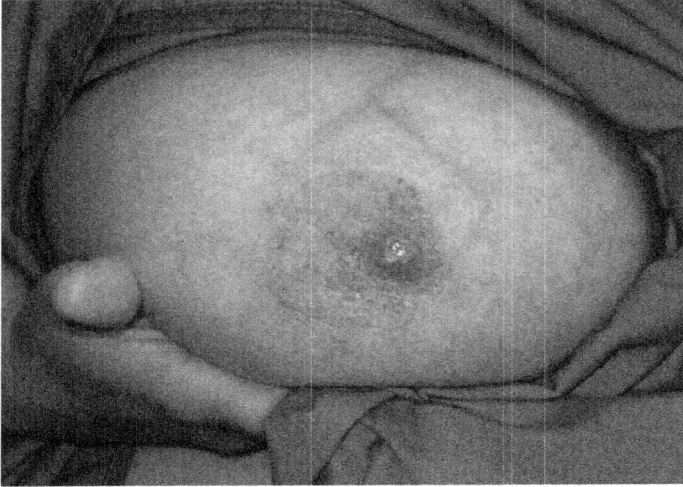

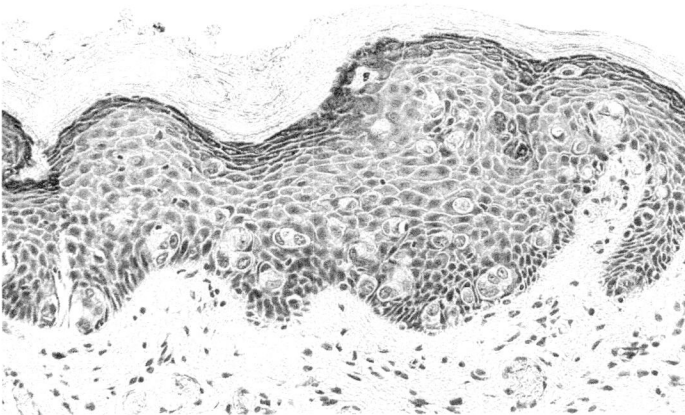

DCIS

Management

Goals

The term ductal carcinoma in situ (DCIS) of the breast refers to various diseases with various potential behaviors. All DCIS types have this in common: They are confined to the breast ducts and, in their pure form, cannot spread or threaten your life. In situ means "remaining in place." Our management goal is to prevent the development of invasive breast cancer. Potential tools include surgery, radiation therapy, and anti-estrogen (endocrine) therapy.

Surgery

We begin with surgery. Women with DCIS may have local (breast) treatment with a mastectomy or a breast-conserving approach. Breast-conserving management consists of a lumpectomy (wide excision; partial mastectomy), typically followed by radiation therapy. Let's look at these approaches:

Mastectomy versus lumpectomy

Both are reasonable options for most women with small-volume DCIS confined to a single breast area. If you meet the criteria for a lumpectomy, the surgery choice is personal. A mastectomy is excellent for long-term disease-specific survival (and local control). Still, mastectomy may be an overly aggressive surgery for most women with DCIS. While a lumpectomy is generally better tolerated, there is a higher chance of a local (in-breast) recurrence with a breast-conserving approach.

The 20-year odds of surviving are similar (about 97% overall) when comparing mastectomy with lumpectomy-based approaches. However, there is a higher local recurrence rate (for example, 3.3 percent versus 1.3 percent in one series) with breast-conserving management.

Criteria for breast-conserving surgery

Breast-conserving management for DCIS results in a low rate of in-breast recurrence with a favorable side effect profile. Still, mastectomy is a reasonable alternative approach for many women. You must meet certain criteria to be an optimal candidate for breast-conserving management.

> • *Limited*
>
> The DCIS should be limited to one quadrant or section of the breast. A mastectomy is generally recommended for those with multicentric disease (DCIS in breast locations far apart from one another). The finding of multiple lesions close to one another does not necessarily mean you cannot have breast-conserving surgery.
>
> • *Reasonable cosmetic outcome*
> A resection would yield a cosmetic outcome acceptable to you.
>
> • *Margins*
> A reasonable cancer-free zone (clear or negative margins) around the DCIS can be achieved. Margin status is an important factor for achieving local (in-breast) control. Re-resections may be done in an effort to obtain negative margins in those desiring breast-conserving management. Patients in whom adequate margins cannot be achieved with breast-conservation surgery should have a mastectomy.

Mastectomy

A mastectomy is usually the preferred management approach if you do not meet these criteria. Mastectomy is curative for over 98 percent of patients with DCIS. Some women who have a mastectomy for the breast with the DCIS will elect to remove the other breast as a risk-reducing maneuver (prophylactic contralateral mastectomy). I am unaware of an associated survival benefit for doing so, however. Other women use endocrine therapy (such as tamoxifen or aromatase inhibitor pills) as a risk-reducing maneuver.

While axillary node removal is not indicated for most women with DCIS, those having a mastectomy may benefit from a so-called sentinel lymph node biopsy (removal). After a total mastectomy, the lymphatic drainage is permanently changed, rendering it impossible to perform an accurate sentinel node biopsy if we discover you have invasive cancer in the removed breast tissue.

DCIS

Treatment

Margins

The margin width (distance between the edge of the DCIS and the nearest inked margin) reflects the completeness of surgical removal of the DCIS. Margins are an important predictor of local recurrence. This observation is especially true for those who opt to avoid radiation therapy. We characterize the margins as follows:

> • *Negative ("clean," "not involved," or "clear")*
> The margins don't contain cancer cells: There is only normal tissue at the edges of the tissue removed from the breast. No additional DCIS surgery is typically needed.

> • *Positive ("involved") margins*
> The margins contain cancer cells. Additional surgery is usually recommended to get clear margins. On occasion, it is impossible to get clear margins due to location (for example, if it is at the chest wall).

> • *Close margins*
> DCIS approaches but doesn't touch the edge of the breast tissue removed. More surgery may or may not be needed.

The excised breast tissue may be X-rayed ("specimen radiograph") to ensure your surgeon has removed the DCIS. These X-rays may be especially useful when microcalcifications are found on a mammogram and are related to cancer. Depending on the X-ray results, your surgeon may need to remove additional tissue (immediate re-excision). After surgery, selected patients may have a mammogram of the affected breast if there is any concern that the disease (calcifications) is left behind. Mammograms can be particularly valuable if the calcifications are extensive before surgery, approach the edge of the surgical specimen, or the surgical margins need to be completely clear.

Clear margins are important for local control

For women with ductal carcinoma in situ (DCIS) treated with breast-conserving surgery, margin status is recognized as one of the most important predictors of local recurrence, regardless of whether radiation therapy is given after surgery. A recent meta-analysis (an analysis of a collection of studies) showed:

- *Positive (involved) margins:* In-breast relapse is 2.25 times higher

- *Negative (uninvolved) margins:* In-breast relapse is lower with margins larger than 10 mm, compared to a negative margin larger than 2 mm

Let's look in graphic form at the predicted probabilities of an in-breast recurrence, stratified by margin threshold and treatment:

	Positive	Margin threshold			
		0 mm	2 mm	5 mm	10 mm
Lumpectomy + RT	**20%**	10%	9%	11%	**4%**
Lumpectomy alone	**35%**	20%	17%	20%	**9%**

There has been a lack of consensus about what constitutes an optimal cancer-free or "negative" margin for ductal carcinoma in situ, and as a result, about one in three DCIS surgeries are currently repeated. After evaluating a new meta-analysis (collection of studies), a consensus panel concluded that 2 millimeters (mm) are optimal: Wider margins were not associated with a lower in-breast recurrence rate, and margins less than this led to a higher probability of an in-breast recurrence.

⚠️ **Clear surgical margins** should be obtained for DCIS patients after breast-conserving surgery, regardless of whether radiation therapy is to be given. Within cosmetic constraints, surgeons should attempt to achieve negative margins as wide as reasonably achievable in their first attempt.

DCIS

Treatment

Radiation therapy (RT)

Breast-conserving surgery ("lumpectomy") with the achievement of clear margins is commonly followed by radiation therapy. Patients at very low risk may opt to decline radiation therapy, as may those with other medical problems or limited life expectancy. RT reduces the risk of local invasive and non-invasive recurrences. Randomized trials have shown radiation therapy applied after surgery reduces the risk of an in-breast tumor recurrence by 50 percent or more, compared with excision alone. Let's look at one of the best studies comparing radiation therapy versus surgery with no radiation therapy (15-year results):

National Surgical Breast and Bowel Project (NSABP) Trial B-17

	RT	No RT
• In-breast *invasive* recurrence	9%	**19%**
• Survival	83%	84%

Radiation therapy reduces recurrence risk by half

A systematic review of radiation therapy after surgery for DCIS included four randomized controlled trials involving 3925 women. Radiation therapy reduced the risk of in-breast recurrence by half. All subgroups (margin status, age, and grade) benefited from the addition of radiation therapy.

Nine women required treatment with radiotherapy to prevent one in-breast recurrence. Deaths from vascular disease, lung toxicity, and second cancers were low and not significantly higher for women who received radiation therapy. The authors concluded that radiation therapy was beneficial for all clinically relevant subgroups.

Radiation therapy or no RT: Long-term results

The SweDCIS (Swedish Ductal Carcinoma in Situ) trial was set up in 1987 to study the value of radiation therapy (RT) after breast-conserving surgery for breast ductal carcinoma *in situ* (DCIS). Here are the findings at the 20-year follow-up mark:

- Breast cancer–specific death
  Radiation therapy had no effect.

- Overall survival
  Radiation therapy had no effect.

- Half of the recurrences were in situ, and half were invasive cancer.

- Younger women had a relatively higher risk of local relapse.

- **Radiation therapy reduced the risk of in situ recurrences for all age groups,** whereas radiation therapy reduced the chances of an invasive local recurrence only for women 52 or older.

What you need to know

The Swedish researchers concluded that 20-year follow-up results support radiation therapy (after lumpectomy). Long-term results have been presented for three similar studies randomly assigning patients to radiation therapy or not after breast-conserving surgery for primary ductal carcinoma in situ. These studies found that radiation therapy led to an absolute reduced risk of in-breast recurrence of 10% after 15 years. The effect appears similar for in situ and invasive breast events. No effect on breast cancer survival was reported in any of the studies: Radiation therapy improves local (in-breast) control but has no effects on survival odds.

Into the future: Gene expression testing

Gene expression analyses (testing some of the genes of your removed DCIS) represent an attempt to move beyond historical clinical and pathology characteristics to stratify DCIS by risk. Can we find a group of patients with a low enough rate of local recurrence with wide excision alone that radiation therapy might confer little benefit? Genomic tests such as Oncotype DX and DCISionRT others suggest the answer may be yes.

DCIS

Treatment

Radiation therapy (RT)

Not all women who have had a lumpectomy for DCIS need radiation therapy. Still, RT can meaningfully lower the risk of an in-breast recurrence: The goal is to kill any DCIS cells left in the breast after breast-preserving surgery (Radiation therapy is rarely used after a mastectomy for DCIS). However, radiation therapy does not improve your odds of long-term survival. If radiation therapy is being considered, you will be referred to a radiation oncologist. The first step is a consultation, a meeting in which you will review the pros and cons of RT, alternatives to it, and logistics.

Am I a candidate for radiation therapy?

Some women with DCIS are not candidates for radiation therapy. For example, being pregnant or having certain health conditions can increase radiation therapy risks. The latter includes active scleroderma or lupus. Unfortunately, these disorders can cause harm to normal tissue during and after radiation therapy. In addition, if you have had radiation therapy to the same breast (or the same general region of the chest area), you may not be a candidate for breast radiation therapy.

Simulation for external beam radiation therapy

If you opt for radiation therapy, you must have a treatment planning session (simulation). Here, the radiation oncology physician and a simulation therapist map out the target. Typically, you have a CT scan of your breast region, with no contrast administered by vein or mouth. The most common treatment position is on your back (supine) on a hard flat table, arms overhead. Many patients appreciate some support placed behind their knees. During the planning session, the radiation simulation therapist will likely put small marks (about the size of a pinhead) on your skin, as these can help optimize targeting for each daily radiation treatment. The marks are commonly permanent tattoos.

Radiation treatment planning: Special considerations for left side

If radiation hits your heart, you may be injured. Typically, we use tangential fields, with the patient having arms over the head and the heart not receiving a significant dose. If your treatment targets the left breast, you may be asked to hold your breath (for short periods) during the planning session. This approach is one way to minimize radiation exposure to the heart: Deep inspirations typically cause the heart to fall backward out of the radiation field. Some cannot hold their breath consistently for the required time, and many radiation therapy centers don't have the necessary technology.

Each daily (Monday through Friday) radiation therapy session lasts about 20 minutes. A treatment course usually ranges from one to 7 weeks, most commonly three to four. The radiation schedule varies from person to person, depending on factors such as margin status, life expectancy, and body habitus.

Radiation dose: To boost or not to boost

Radiation therapy is most commonly delivered to the whole breast, for example, over approximately 3 or 5 weeks. After the whole breast treatment, you may receive a supplemental dose of radiation targeting the area of the "lumpectomy." This extra dose is called a "boost" and typically aims at a small volume. Most patients get their boost dose with a special form of external radiation called electrons. For example, we can regulate the depth of the radiation beam penetrance with electrons by choosing a particular energy. A radiation "boost" to the tumor bed (the area from which the surgeon removed the DCIS) can yield a small but statistically significant reduction in in-breast recurrence after a lumpectomy for ductal carcinoma in situ, retrospective study from the USA, Canada, and France has shown.

Women with DCIS who received the extra radiation therapy or boost had a 15-year in-breast control rate of 91.6% compared with 88% for those who had lumpectomy and radiation therapy but no boost to the tumor bed.

Partial breast radiation therapy

Whole breast radiation therapy is a category 1 recommendation of the National Comprehensive Cancer Network (meaning consensus based on high-level evidence). Highly selected individuals may be candidates for no RT versus more recently introduced radiation therapy techniques that target only the partial breast. These approaches include brachytherapy (MammoSite® is a well-known example) and external beam radiation therapy. For accelerated partial breast irradiation (APBI), the DCIS should have been detected by a screening mammogram, not high-grade, 2.5 centimeters or less, and with margins more than three millimeters.

DCIS

Management

Into the future: Genomic testing for DCIS

The Oncotype DX DCIS test examines the DCIS removed during your initial surgery. The Oncotype DX DCIS test analyzes the activity of 12 genes. Then it estimates a woman's recurrence risk of DCIS (ductal carcinoma in situ) or the risk of a new invasive cancer developing in the same breast, as well as how likely she is to benefit from radiation therapy after DCIS surgery.

The DCIS Score is between 0 and 100 and is represented in two graphs. One graph shows the chances of any breast event (either DCIS or invasive breast cancer), while the other. A lower DCIS Score result means there is a lower chance that this will occur, and a higher score means a higher chance of this. The other graph represents the chances of the tumor returning to the same breast as invasive breast cancer. A lower score means there is a lower chance that this will occur, and a higher score means a higher chance of this.

The DCIS Score results can help guide personalized management decisions. Because everyone's DCIS is unique, a DCIS Score may help facilitate creating a treatment approach tailored to you. Here are the local recurrence rates in a study validating the Oncotype DX test at a median follow-up of 9.6 years:

- Low-risk score: 13 percent
- Intermediate risk score: 28 percent
- High-risk score: 33 percent

Additional validation is needed before we can routinely use this test. Those with an Oncotype DX for DCIS should discuss balancing the recurrence reduction associated with radiation therapy and its risks.

DCISionRT is another risk assessment test for women with DCIS. It evaluates a patient's individual biology along with other risk factors and predicts the 10-year risk of a DCIS or invasive breast cancer recurrence in that same breast. It also predicts radiation therapy benefit.

DCIS: Management with endocrine therapy

Tamoxifen (for five years)

Tamoxifen is an "anti-estrogen" pill. The NSABP B-24 randomized trial showed tamoxifen could reduce the probability of future events in the breast treated for DCIS and in the opposite (contralateral) breast among women with DCIS who undergo lumpectomy followed by radiation therapy. There are clear benefits if the DCIS is estrogen receptor-positive (ER +).

The NSABP B-24 trial was a randomized clinical trial that randomized women with DCIS to either lumpectomy and radiation versus the same treatment followed by the anti-estrogen pill tamoxifen (taken for five years). The study showed the following at 17-year follow-up:

- Tamoxifen lowered the risk of future invasive or non-invasive cancer in either breast. The risk of invasive cancer dropped by 6 per 1000 to 19 per 1000, or about one-third (relative risk 0.68);

- Tamoxifen benefit appeared limited to women with estrogen receptor-positive DCIS.

The United Kingdom Coordinating Committee on Cancer Research study found:

- Tamoxifen did not lower the risk of invasive cancer in the same breast but did lower the risk of invasive cancer in the opposite breast. The researchers did not provide absolute reduction numbers.

- Tamoxifen lowered the risk of DCIS recurrence in the same breast.

- Tamoxifen did not lower the risk of DCIS in the opposite breast.

The standard dose of tamoxifen is 20 mg/day for five years. Low-dose tamoxifen (five milligram/day for three years) is an option if a patient is symptomatic on the 20 milligram dose or if patient is unwilling or unable to take standard-dose tamoxifen.

Meta-analysis (putting the studies together)

- Tamoxifen lowers the risk of a future ipsilateral (same) invasive breast cancer by about one-fifth (relative risk 0.79).
- Tamoxifen lowers the risk of a future contralateral (other breast) event risk by nearly half (relative risk 0.57).

Aromatase inhibitor (AI) pills better than tamoxifen

Treatment of **post-menopausal** women with DCIS with the aromatase inhibitor anastrozole resulted in higher breast cancer–free survival rates than standard treatment with tamoxifen. The NSABP B-35/SWOG-35 study randomized 3,104 post-menopausal women with hormone receptor–positive DCIS to either daily 20 mg tamoxifen or one mg anastrozole for five years. All patients had a lumpectomy and radiation therapy before starting their 5-year regimen of "anti-estrogen" pills. Here are the results with a median follow-up of 8.6 years:

- The estimated percentage of patients with a 10-year breast cancer-free interval was 89.1 in the tamoxifen group and 93.1 percent in the anastrazole group. Moreover, anastrazole resulted in further improvement in breast cancer-free interval in those under age 60.
- Anastrozole appeared to reduce the diagnosis of a second primary breast cancer in the opposite breast more than tamoxifen, but this trend was not statistically significant. There were no survival differences when comparing the tamoxifen with anastrazole.

For those with ER-positive DCIS, tamoxifen or an aromatase inhibitor anastrozole can reduce the future event probability in either breast. Premenopausal women have tamoxifen as a potential treatment tool. Postmenopausal with ER-positive DCIS may consider tamoxifen or an aromatase inhibitor (AI).

Systemic therapy for local recurrence

For patients who have had appropriate management of the breast (in which cancer recurred), consideration is given to systemic therapy to surgery for those with estrogen receptor-positive disease, especially if the recurrence is invasive. For some, this may mean anti-estrogen approaches such as tamoxifen or an aromatase inhibitor pill (for example, if the invasive cancer is estrogen receptor-positive). Selected patients with a higher-risk disease may receive chemotherapy, and those whose invasive recurrence is positive for HER2 (human epidermal growth factor receptor-2) should receive a HER2-directed drug such as trastuzumab (Herceptin).

Recurrence

With appropriate management, the **prognosis for patients with DCIS is excellent.** An analysis of over 100,000 patients with DCIS enrolled in a national database in the USA found the 20-year disease-specific survival to approach 97%. The risk of in-breast recurrence at 20 years was 5.9 percent, and the risk of other breast invasive cancer was 6.2 percent. In this review, predictors of higher risk for death from breast cancer included young age at diagnosis (those under 35 had a 2.16 times increase in risk), high-grade (risk increased by 1.88 times), and black ethnicity (2.55 fold increase in risk).

Approximately one-half of all local recurrences are invasive, regardless of the initial treatment approach. Management hinges on the extent of the disease, location, and prior surgical approach (mastectomy versus lumpectomy). For patients with an invasive local recurrence after management for DCIS, consideration may be given to staging studies to check for the distant spread of cancer. There should also be a check on the recurrence of the disease for estrogen/progesterone receptor and HER2 statuses.

Original treatment	Management for local recurrence
Lumpectomy + RT*	Mastectomy
Lumpectomy with no RT*	Repeat lumpectomy + radiation therapy *or* mastectomy
Mastectomy	Excision of recurrence in mastectomy flap, then *consider* RT*

* RT = Radiation therapy

DCIS: Controversies

• *Is DCIS cancer?*

Is ductal carcinoma in situ cancer? When I think of cancer, I imagine a disease that, left untreated, eventually leads to death. Yet, this does not seem inevitable for DCIS. While DCIS can become invasive and spread to distant sites, the United States SEER large database suggests a long-term disease-specific survival probability of approximately 97%. Breast cancer encompasses a variety of abnormalities and has a great range of aggressiveness and destructive potential. If you have DCIS, you may need some treatment (but not chemotherapy). I think the term cancer is not entirely appropriate for DCIS, and I look forward to introducing more appropriate terminology.

• *Are you sure it's DCIS?*

DCIS is a part of a continuum from hyperplasia (too many cells, but normal-appearing) to atypical hyperplasia (somewhat abnormal-appearing cells) to DCIS to invasive cancer. Differentiating atypical ductal hyperplasia (ADH) from lower-grade DCIS can be remarkably challenging. Some consider getting a second opinion from an outside pathologist if you have low-grade ductal carcinoma in situ.

• *Do we overtreat DCIS?*

As our understanding of DCIS has evolved, management has become complex and controversial. Who needs radiation therapy? RT for DCIS is *not* associated with a survival advantage. What about endocrine therapy, such as tamoxifen or aromatase inhibitors? Most patients do not, but we cannot answer these questions accurately. And what constitutes an adequate surgical margin? The most benign-appearing forms of DCIS (including low-grade DCIS without necrosis estrogen receptor-positive) may never cause clinically meaningful disease, even if untreated. Alternatively, more aggressive forms of DCIS would progress to become invasive. How do we select who needs more aggressive treatment?

Current data are insufficient to support the use of HER2-directed therapy in DCIS. The American Society of Clinical Oncology/College of Pathologists guidelines do not support HER2 testing of DCIS.

DCIS

Follow-up

Risk does not plateau

For women with low-risk DCIS who opt for breast-conserving surgery without radiation therapy, the risk of a local recurrence of DCIS or invasive cancer increases steadily over the ensuing 12 years. There appears to be no plateau in risk, a prospective, non-randomized study suggests.

A team of researchers determined the 12-year risk of a local (in the same breast) recurrence among women who opted for lumpectomy without radiation therapy. The surgical margins had to be at least 3 millimeters. Tamoxifen (not randomly assigned) was given to 30 percent of the patients. The local (in-breast) recurrence rate did not appear to plateau over time. This observation highlights the importance of appropriately aggressive follow-up. Fortunately, for DCIS, the follow-up is fairly simple:

NCCN Guidelines

The National Comprehensive Cancer Network (NCCN) is a group of 32 top cancer centers in the USA. Here is what the NCCN recommends for follow-up for ductal carcinoma *in situ:*

- *History and physical exam* every six to 12 months for five years, then annually

- *Mammogram* every 12 months (first mammogram 6–12 months after breast conservation management). Patients who have had a mastectomy (with or without reconstruction) do *not* need imaging of the affected side but should have annual mammograms for the opposite breast (if present).

Summary

DCIS

• **Excellent outcomes**

The 20-year disease-specific survival odds approach 97%.

• **Improving recurrence rates**

The management of ductal carcinoma *in situ* in the USA keeps improving. The 5-year recurrence rate dropped from 13.6% to 6.6% when comparing lumpectomy-based results in the 1978 to 1998 period with 1999 to 2010.

• **Local therapy**

Surgery goes first (lumpectomy versus mastectomy). Then strong consideration should be given to radiation therapy for those who have had breast-conserving surgery (no radiation therapy is an alternative approach). Those who have a mastectomy may consider breast reconstruction. Reconstruction can be immediate or delayed.

• **Clear margins are important**

The local recurrence rate (even with radiation therapy) is as high as 20% if the margins are involved.

• **Systemic therapy**

Risk reduction therapy (such as tamoxifen (or an aromatase inhibitor for postmenopausal women)) for five years should be considered for patients managed with lumpectomy for estrogen receptor-positive DCIS. Those who do not tolerate tamoxifen at the standard dose of 20 milligrams daily may try five milligrams daily for three years. There should also be counseling regarding risk reduction strategies for the opposite breast.

• **Gene testing**

Those at high risk for hereditary breast cancer should have genetic counseling.

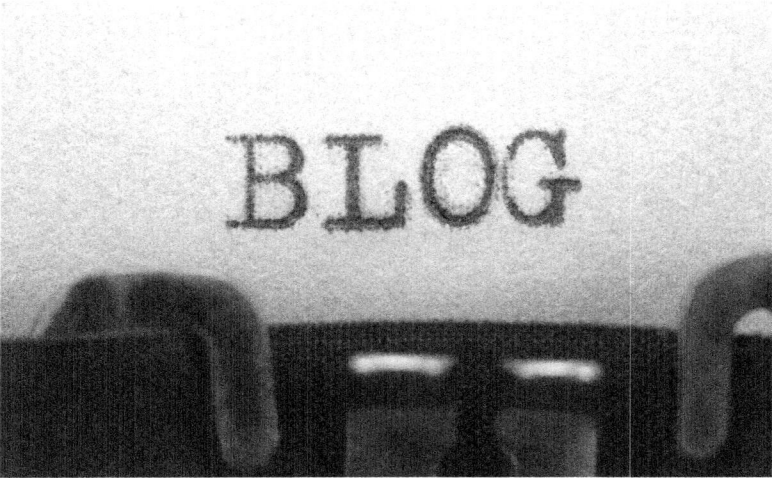

www.newcancerinfo.com

MANAGEMENT

Invasive cancer:
Surgery and radiation

Invasive

Management: Basics

Early versus locally advanced

Let's begin by explaining what we mean by "early" invasive breast cancer. I think of early breast cancer as stage I and IIA disease, with a subset of patients with stage IIB, also fitting into the category. In the United States, most patients will present with no evidence of distant spread (metastases). On the other hand, Locally advanced breast cancer includes a subset of patients with clinical stage IIB disease (T3, N0) and patients with stage III disease.

IA	T1, N0, M0
IB	T0-T1, N1mi, M0
IIA	T0-T2; N0-1; M0
IIB	T2-3; N0-1; M0

Distant spread (metastasis)

Approximately 5 percent of patients will have simultaneous metastatic disease identified at initial presentation. For more details on the meaning of T, N, and M, please go to chapter 6 (breast cancer staging).

Invasive

Management: Initial evaluation

A breast cancer diagnosis is based on clinical examination in combination with imaging and confirmed by pathological assessment such as a biopsy (tissue sampling). Clinical examination includes palpation of the breasts and regional lymph nodes and an assessment for distant metastases (bones, liver, and lungs; a neurological examination is required if there are concerning symptoms).

Guidelines

The National Comprehensive Cancer Network (www.nccn.org) offers recommendations for the initial workup of patients with early breast cancer.

- History and physical exam
- Diagnostic bilateral mammograms
- Pathology review (include Ki-67 test if considering abemaciclib after surgery).
- Determination of tumor estrogen receptor (ER), progesterone receptor (PR) status, and HER-2.
- Genetic counseling if you are at high-risk for hereditary breast cancer or have triple-negative breast cancer
- Pregnancy test in all patients with childbearing potential
- Breast MRI (optional). MRI may be useful for characterizing axillary or internal mammary nodal disease.

Cancer spread (metastasis)

Routine systemic staging is not indicated for non-metastatic cancer in the absence of systemic symptoms. Approximately 5 percent of patients will present with cancer spread (metastasis) to distant sites such as the bones, liver, lungs, or brain. If metastases are present, the disease is Stage IV breast cancer.

Invasive

Management: Genetic counseling

Hereditary breast cancer means that breast cancer runs in your family, and could be caused by an inherited change in your genes. About five to 10 percent of breast cancers are hereditary. You may have a higher risk for hereditary breast cancer if breast cancer runs in your family. The US Centers for Disease Control offers that genetic testing is usually recommended if you have:

You have breast cancer plus any of the following:	• A strong family health history of breast and ovarian cancer
	• A moderate family health history of breast and ovarian cancer and are of Ashkenazi Jewish or Eastern European ancestry
	• A personal history of breast cancer and meet certain criteria (related to age of diagnosis, type of cancer, presence of certain other cancers or cancer in both breasts, ancestry, and family health history)
	• A personal history of ovarian, fallopian tube, or primary peritoneal cancer
	• A known BRCA1, BRCA2, or other inherited mutation in your family
You have a personal history of **ovarian cancer**	

Other criteria include a personal or family history of at least three of these:

- Breast, pancreas, prostate (Gleason score 7+), diffuse stomach (gastric), colon, endometrial, thyroid, or kidney cancer, melanoma, sarcoma, adrenocortical carcinoma, brain tumors, or leukemia

- Skin problems consistent with Cowden syndrome

- Macrocephaly, hamartomatous polyps of the gastrointestinal tract

---

* bilateral disease or at least two separate cancers in the same breast

BRCA

Breast cancer genes (basics)

Patients at high risk for having hereditary (inherited) breast cancer should receive **genetic counseling.** Approximately five to 10 percent of breast cancer patients have an inherited genetic mutation related to their cancer. The most common gene mutations (mistakes) associated with breast cancer are in tumor suppression genes BRCA1 and BRCA2 (BReast CAncer genes #1 and #2). You may recall that the actress Angelina Jolie had a BRCA mutation.

Breast cancer risk

About 12 percent of women in the general population will develop breast cancer during their lives. By contrast, 72 percent of women who inherit a harmful BRCA1 mutation and around 69 percent of women who inherit a harmful BRCA2 mutation will develop breast cancer by 80 years of age. In addition, breast cancer incidence rise in early adulthood until 30 to 40 years for BRCA1 carriers and until 40 to 50 years for BRCA2 carriers, after which it plateaus at 20 to 30 per 1000 person-years until at least age 80. BRCA1 carriers are more likely to develop triple-negative breast cancer, an especially aggressive disease.

Ovarian cancer risk

About 1.3 percent of women in the general population will develop ovarian cancer sometime during their lives. By contrast, 44 percent of women who inherit a harmful BRCA1 mutation (and 17 percent of women who inherit a harmful BRCA2 mutation) will develop ovarian cancer by age 70.

BRCA mutations increase risk of other cancers, too

The incidence may increase for cancer of the opposite breast, colon (BRCA1; amount uncertain), male prostate cancer (BRCA2 may increase risk five- to 9 fold; the magnitude of increase for BRCA1 carriers is not well-understood), and pancreas cancer (BRCA1 unclear; BRCA2 five percent, compared to 1.5 percent in the general population). We are learning about the risk of stomach and biliary cancer (BRCA2), skin or uveal (eye) melanoma for those with BRCA2 mutations, fallopian tube cancer (lifetime risk about 0.6 percent), uterine papillary serous carcinoma, and others.

Invasive

Genes

While BRCA mutations are involved in most hereditary breast cancer, other gene mutations can also lead to inherited breast cancers. Mutations in these other genes do not increase the breast cancer risk as much as BRCA.

- **ATM.** This gene helps to fix damaged DNA. Alternatively, ATM can help kill the cell if the cell cannot repair the damage. Inheriting two abnormal copies of ATM causes the disease ataxia-telangiectasia. Inheriting one abnormal ATM gene copy raises breast cancer risk in some families.

- **PALB2.** The PALB2 gene signals the creation of a protein that interacts with a protein created by the BRCA2 gene. PALB2 mutations can raise breast cancer risk.

- **TP53.** This gene helps stop cell growth when there is damaged DNA. TP53 gene mutations are associated with **Li-Fraumeni syndrome**, a condition linked to a higher risk of breast cancer. Individuals also have a higher risk of other cancers, including leukemia, sarcomas (cancer of the bones or connective tissue), and the brain.

- **CHEK2.** This gene helps with DNA repair. Mutations in CHEK2 are associated with a higher breast cancer risk.

- **CDH1.** Inherited mutations of CDH1 raise hereditary diffuse gastric (stomach) cancer risk. Women with CDH1 gene mutations also have a higher chance of developing invasive lobular cancer.

- **PTEN.** The PTEN gene is important for cell growth regulation. Inherited mutations can cause **Cowden syndrome**, a rare condition that raises the risk of cancer and benign (non-cancer) breast tumors. Those with a PTEN mutation also have a higher chance of developing growths in the digestive tract, thyroid, ovaries, and uterus.

Genes

- **STK11.** Defects in this gene can lead to **Peutz-Jeghers syndrome**. Those with the disorder have pigmented spots on their lips and their mouths, abnormal growths (polyps) in the digestive and urinary tracts, and a higher risk of cancer, including breast cancer.

Are you concerned about your risk because of a personal or family history of breast (or other) cancer? Please talk with your doctor or other appropriate healthcare professional. Often, you will use one of several risk assessment tools first.

Regardless of the mathematical model used. A healthcare team member may suggest that you speak with a genetic counselor. This expert can review your personal and family history to assess your probability of having a family cancer syndrome.

How genetic testing is done

A genetic test may use blood or saliva samples. Alternatively, you may swab material from inside your cheek. The samples then go to a lab for analysis.

Testing may target one (or a few) specific mutations; however, more comprehensive testing can look for many different BRCA (and other) gene mutations. Please remember that genetic testing is not perfect - the tests don't always provide clarity for some individuals. A genetic counselor or other experts can guide you through interpretation. Genetic results may come back as:

- **Positive for a mutation.** This finding may affect your breast cancer management options. In addition, there may be steps you can take to lower your risk of breast (and other) cancers.

- **Negative for the mutation(s) tested for**. While this result doesn't guarantee that you're not at increased risk, it provides some reassurance.

- **Inconclusive.** The test cannot say for sure if you have a gene mutation.

- **Variant of unknown significance (VUS).** The test discovered a gene change (variant), but we do not understand if this VUS affects your risk.

Invasive

Management: Overview

Surgery

In general, surgery is the first step (after the initial work-up just described) for patients with early invasive (infiltrating) breast cancer. There are two major types of surgery:

- Mastectomy (breast removal)
- Lumpectomy

These surgeries generally remove one or more axillary (underarm) lymph nodes.

After surgery

Following surgery, your care team may offer treatment from one of these categories:

- Systemic therapy
  Examples include chemotherapy, targeted drugs such as trastuzumab (Herceptin), "anti-estrogen" therapy such as tamoxifen pills
- Additional local (breast region) therapy
  Radiation therapy (RT)

Many patients confuse local and systemic therapies. In general, decisions about one have little to do with decisions about the other. We assess the risk of locoregional recurrence in the chest wall and nodes following a mastectomy. We also assess the risk of a locoregional recurrence in the breast or regional nodes following a lumpectomy to make appropriate recommendations regarding additional (adjuvant) therapies.

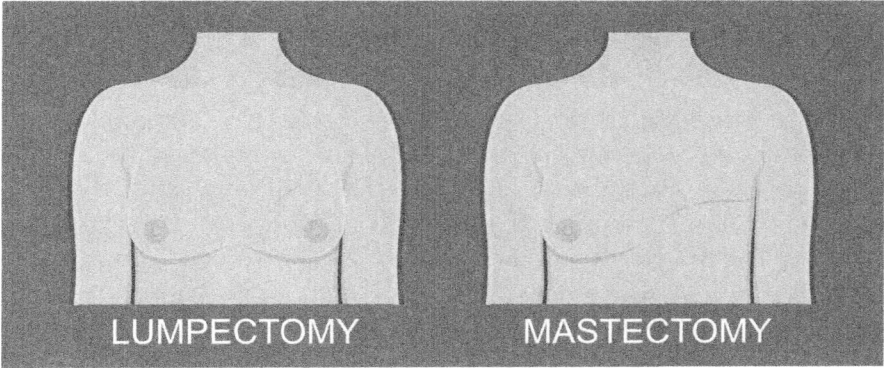

LUMPECTOMY

MASTECTOMY

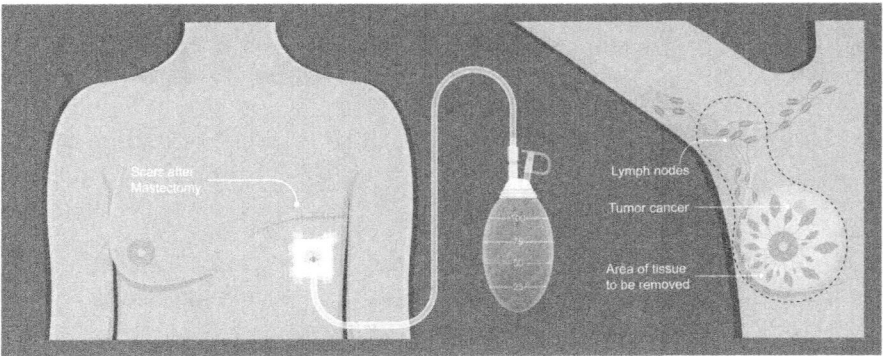

Scars after
Mastectomy

Lymph nodes

Tumor cancer

Area of tissue
to be removed

Invasive

Management: Breast

Surgery: Lumpectomy or mastectomy?

Breast-conserving local management generally consists of a lumpectomy and removal of one (or more) underarm nodes, followed by radiation therapy. The goal is to provide a survival probability equivalent to that associated with a mastectomy while providing a high probability of permanently retaining the breast. Six prospective, randomized trials have compared breast-conserving management with mastectomy for appropriately selected patients. Long-term survival shows equivalence in survival probability. More recently, with better systemic therapies, there are hints that breast-conserving management may even be associated with better survival in some cases.

Are you a candidate to keep your breast?

While breast-conserving management yields survival chances equivalent to those associated with breast removal, there are some caveats. Here are some of the conditions that would lead us to recommend a mastectomy:

- A large tumor relative to your breast size*
- Multicentric (cancer in multiple areas of your breast) or multifocal*
- Persistently (after multiple attempts to clear them) diffusely involved margins
- You are not able to receive radiation therapy (pregnancy; active connective tissue disease involving the skin, especially lupus and scleroderma; prior radiation therapy to the same area)

---

* **Neoadjuvant therapy:** Selected individuals may be candidates for systemic therapy such as chemotherapy (to try to shrink cancer) *before* surgery.

** Cancer in multiple areas close to one another; selected patients may be candidates for breast conservation if your surgeon can use a single incision to remove cancer with acceptable margins and cosmetic outcome.

Lumpectomy v. Mastectomy
Survival odds are the same

| Study* | No. | Stage | F/U* | Survival (overall) | |
				Mastec-tomy	Lumpectomy + radiation
NSABP	**1,851**	**I-II**	**21 yrs**	**47%**	**46%**
EORTC	868	I-II	22 yrs	45%	39%
Denmark	731	I-III	20 yrs	58%	51%
Milan	701	I	20 yrs	58%	59%
NCI	237	I-II	26 yrs	44%	38%
France	179	I	22 yrs	52%	60%

For appropriately selected patients, there are no differences in survival odds when comparing breast-conserving approaches with mastectomy-based ones: A meta-analysis (study of studies) concludes that appropriately selected patients who choose breast-conserving surgery (with radiation therapy) have the same odds of long-term survival as those who select a mastectomy-based treatment.

The chance of cancer returning in the breast (local recurrence) is slightly higher with lumpectomy/radiation therapy than with mastectomy. For appropriately selected patients, however, the risk of cancer spreading to other organs (distant metastasis) is the same for a lumpectomy followed by radiation therapy as it is for mastectomy.

---

* National Surgical Adjuvant Breast and Bowel Project B-06 (USA)
  European Organization for the Research and Treatment of Cancer
  National Cancer Institute (USA)
  Arriagada (France)

** F/U = follow-up (years)

Invasive

Management: Breast

Most patients who are candidates for either breast-conserving surgery or a mastectomy prefer the less invasive, breast-conserving management approach. How can you select which surgery is appropriate for you?

- *Do I want to keep my breast?*

If deemed an appropriate candidate, you may wish to consider lumpectomy followed by radiation therapy.

- *Am I anxious about cancer coming back in the breast?*

If breast removal would significantly reduce your anxiety about an in-breast recurrence (and if you understand that even after a mastectomy, cancer sometimes comes back on the chest wall), you may wish to consider a mastectomy. While there are no long-term differences in your odds of survival, there is a higher risk of a local recurrence after a lumpectomy.

- *Are you okay with receiving radiation therapy?*

RT courses vary in length but are often composed of 15-minute appointments, Monday through Friday, for 3 to 7 weeks. Most patients having a mastectomy for early breast cancer do not need radiation therapy unless the lymph nodes are involved or the margins are under a millimeter.

- *Does having a mastectomy mean I won't need chemotherapy?*

No. I think breast (and node) and body management are separate issues. Your medical oncologist will recommend chemotherapy based on your risk for distant recurrence and breast cancer-related death. The breast surgery type doesn't influence this calculation. Please consider the breast/nodes and body system as two spaces we address separately.

- *My tumor is fairly large. Must I have a mastectomy?*

Selected patients with large tumors (relative to their breast size) may attempt breast-conserving management using systemic therapy (such as chemotherapy) before surgery. We call the use of treatments such as chemotherapy before surgery neoadjuvant.

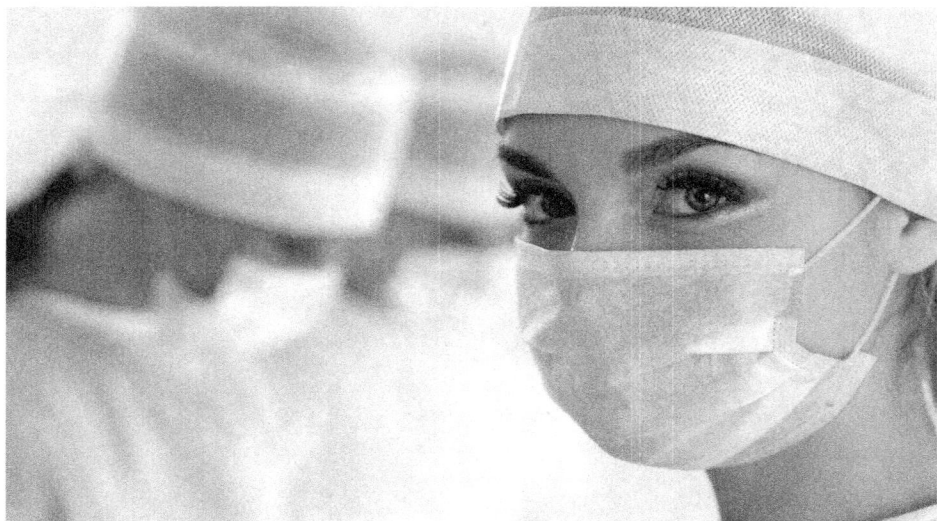

Surgery: Logistics

Preoperative (before surgery)

If your cancer cannot be felt or seen, you will need a procedure before surgery to mark the target tumor using imaging such as a mammogram. A care provider may also draw marks (using a felt-tip marker, for example) on your breast that show where the surgeon should make an incision.

You go to the anesthesia room, where a nurse inserts an intravenous (IV) line into your hand or arm, taping it into place. While selected patients may have a lumpectomy with local numbing anesthesia, most have general anesthesia. General anesthesia is standard if you will also have lymph nodes removed.

A lumpectomy surgery usually lasts about 30 to 45 minutes. Your surgeon will likely use an electric scalpel that uses heat to reduce bleeding. The scar is often (but not always) curved, following your breast's natural curves. The tumor is removed, along with a small surrounding rim of normal-appearing breast tissue. With a lumpectomy, most patients do not need a drain placed in the breast or axilla, At the end of the operation, your surgeon will stitch the incision closed and cover the wound.

259

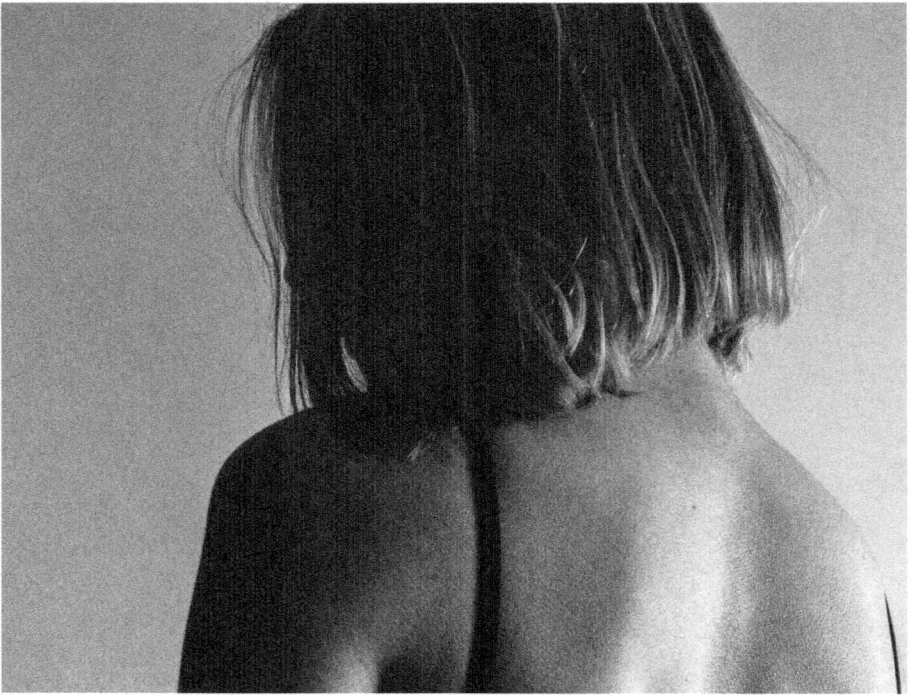

After mastectomy: Reconstruction

Breast reconstruction should be available to those women undergoing mastectomy. Immediate reconstruction for many women can make the prospect of losing a breast easier to accept. Still, not all patients are candidates for immediate reconstruction: Some are advised against immediate reconstruction for cancer reasons, especially in the case of locally advanced breast cancer, such as inflammatory carcinoma. Some women may decline or defer reconstruction because of personal preference.

Autologous tissue-based techniques generally tolerate post-operative radiation therapy (RT) well. Implant-based reconstruction can result in an unfavorable aesthetic outcome following post-operative RT. Skin-sparing mastectomy allows for the conservation of a skin envelope for use in breast reconstruction. If your care team recommends post-mastectomy radiotherapy (PMRT), a plastic surgeon typically places a temporary implant before radiation therapy for those desiring an implant-based reconstruction.

Invasive

A special note for those with a BRCA mutation

Many women with a harmful BRCA1 or BRCA2 mutation who develop breast cancer in one breast choose a bilateral (double) mastectomy, even if they would otherwise be candidates for breast-conserving surgery.

And the ovaries, too?

We do not have very effective tools for ovarian cancer screening. You may also wish to consider removing your ovaries and fallopian tubes in a bilateral salpingo-oophorectomy (BSO) procedure, depending on where you are in your life and whether you wish to have biological children. Some women choose to delay the procedure until age 40 to 45. I recommend a referral to a gynecologic oncologist to discuss this surgery. The surgery appears to reduce the risk of ovarian cancer among BRCA mutation carriers and decrease the risk of dying of the disease.

Other risk-reducing surgery?

Risk-reducing removal of the ovaries and fallopian tubes is the procedure of choice, with the removal of the uterus (hysterectomy) not routinely recommended. I am unaware of national guidelines pointing to the taking of the uterus, even though there may be a small increase in the incidence of uterus cancer among BRCA mutation carriers. There is controversy about removing only the fallopian tubes for those who want to keep their ovaries for some time. We do not have high-level evidence from clinical trials to support this limited approach.

Hormone replacement (HRT)

Before using HRT to manage menopausal symptoms in BRCA carriers who have had a risk-reducing removal of their ovaries and fallopian tubes, there should be a shared decision-making process, including counseling about non-hormonal options and our lack of high-level evidence regarding hormone replacement therapy for carriers of BRCA mutations. Similarly, we lack high-level evidence regarding vaginal estrogen therapy for carriers.

Invasive

Management: Care after surgery

A care team member will move you to the recovery room, where care providers monitor your heart rate, blood pressure, and temperature. Most patients with a lumpectomy outpatient surgery (they don't stay in the hospital overnight). As you recover at home, you may need to:

• **Take pain medication**
Many patients have the prescription filled on their way home). While you may or may not need pain medicine, it is wise to have it available.

• **Take care of a bandage.**
Your surgeon or valued care team member should give you instructions. The surgeon will occasionally ask you to wait to remove it until your first follow-up visit when she removes the bandage (dressing).

• **Stitches and staples**
Stitches (sutures) are typically used and dissolve over time. It is not rare to see the end of the stitch (suture) sticking out of the incision like a whisker. If this is the case, your surgeon can remove it. Staples are not common, but if used, the doctor removes them during your first postoperative follow-up visit.

• **Consider good support, such as a sports bra.**
This approach may reduce movement that can cause pain. Many with larger breasts prefer to sleep on the side that has not been operated upon, sometimes with the healing breast supported by a pillow.

• **Consider sponge baths until your doctor removes your drains or stitches (sutures)**
Sponge baths may prove refreshing until your doctor gives you the okay for showers or baths.

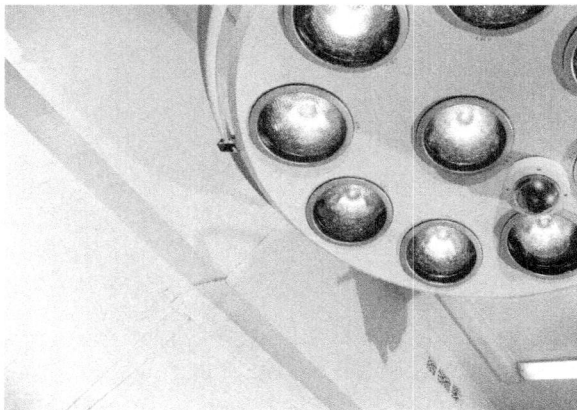

Are there other things I can do following a lumpectomy?

- **Watch for infection**
  Ask your care providers about symptoms.

- **Rest**
  You may feel tired after surgery, so try to get enough rest. Most patients get back into their normal routine after several days.

- **Arm exercises**
  Your surgeon, physical therapist, or other care team member may show you an exercise routine to reduce the probability of arm and shoulder stiffness after the surgery. Typically, you may begin light arm exercises the day after surgery, but some exercises should not be done while drains are in place. Please ask your surgeon about a routine that is appropriate for you. If you have had reconstruction surgery, please check with your surgeon for restrictions.

Breast-conserving surgery: Intermediate-term symptoms

Many patients report sensitivity to touch, some itchiness, or fleeting sharp, shooting pains. These symptoms typically resolve over time. If the discomfort persists, check with your care providers to see if you might be a candidate to take medicines such as acetaminophen or ibuprofen. Uncommonly, stronger pain medicines are needed.

Invasive

Management: Nodes

The axillary (underarm) lymph nodes receive approximately 85 percent of the lymph drainage from the breast. The remainder drains to the internal mammary nodes alongside the breast and paraclavicular (around the collarbone) nodes. A larger tumor size is associated with a higher probability of node involvement. Here are the odds for spread based on tumor substage:

T1a	5%
T1b	16%
T1c	28%
T2	47%
T3	68%
T4	86%

Grade

Axillary node involvement is also a function of the grade of invasive cancer: The higher the grade, the more likely there is to spread to regional lymph nodes.

For example, the US Surveillance and End Results (SEER) database showed that the probability of axillary spread for patients with low-grade cancer was only three percent. Compare this to 21 percent for those with high-grade cancer.

Location

Cancers closer to the axillary nodes have a higher probability of involvement of these nodes. For example, cancer in the upper outer quadrant of the breast is more likely to spread to axillary nodes than a cancer in the lower inner quadrant.

Management: Node assessment

Physical exam

A physical exam is a suboptimal way to assess the status of the axillary nodes, as involved nodes are often unable to be felt, and so-called reactive lymph nodes are easily mistaken as involved with cancer. Still, if we palpate something unusual in the axilla, there is a roughly 60 to 85 percent chance that cancer will be confirmed in the nodes. We depend primarily on the surgical removal of node(s) to determine the actual status of your nodes.

Axillary ultrasound

Axillary ultrasound with fine needle aspiration may help determine if you should proceed to a dissection of the underarm area rather than the less invasive axillary sentinel node removal procedure: If the nodes appear uninvolved by exam and imaging, we prefer the removal of a small number (often one or two) of nodes for invasive breast cancer; if we know the nodes to be involved, an axillary node dissection is performed.

Sentinel lymph node biopsy (SLNB)

A sentinel axillary lymph node biopsy is used clinically for patients with no known node involvement (using palpation and imaging). It allows for an assessment of the node(s) in a way that has lower complications compared to a more traditional axillary lymph node dissection. SLNB is usually done when the surgeon removes the primary tumor. However, the procedure can also be done before or after the primary tumor removal.

Your surgeon injects a radioactive substance, blue dye, or both near the tumor to find the sentinel node (everything must go through the sentinel: If it's clean, we can leave the other nodes alone). The surgeon then uses a device that detects radioactivity to find the sentinel node or looks for nodes stained with the blue dye. Once the surgeon identifies the sentinel lymph node, she makes a small incision (about 1/2 inch) in the overlying skin and removes the node.

The sentinel lymph node is then checked for the presence of cancer cells by a pathologist. If the surgeon finds cancer, she may remove additional lymph nodes during the same biopsy or a follow-up surgical procedure. Many patients do not need the removal of any more nodes, even if one or two sentinel nodes are involved with cancer.

Invasive

Management: Nodes - A fascinating history

Halsted: Breast cancer needs radical surgery

Managing regional lymph nodes has been an area of study for centuries. The oldest description of cancer was discovered in Egypt and dated back to 3000 BC. The Edwin Smith Papyrus describes eight cases of tumors or ulcers of the breast that were removed by a so-called fire drill. The authors note, however, that "there is no treatment."

In the late 1800s, the renowned surgeon William Halsted made the case that the axillary nodes serve as the gateway to distant spread. In this context, he proposed the removal of the breast, underlying chest muscle, and axillary nodes as optimal management for breast cancer. We call this a radical mastectomy.

But no survival advantage

We now have large randomized clinical trials that challenge Halsted's idea that such radical surgery was necessary. For example, the National Surgical Adjuvant Breast and Bowel Project (NSABP) B-04 trial randomized patients (with no cancer in the nodes) to have a radical mastectomy with removal of the breast, chest muscle, and nodes versus removal of the breast only.

The comparison group only had lymph nodes removed if they subsequently had cancer recurrence in that area. This trial showed that delayed treatment of the underarm (axillary) lymph nodes did not adversely affect survival. In essence, the trial pointed to the underarm nodes as *not* being a source of the future spread of cancer.

Sentinel node mapping

Kett and colleagues published the first results of lymph node mapping of the breast (after the injection of the areola region with blue dye). They found an isolated blue node, typically next to a vein (axillary vein). In 1993, Krag reported the identification of an isolated node using a tiny amount of radioactive material and a probe to find radioactivity (gamma probe).

266

Invasive

Management: Nodes

Axillary lymph node dissection (ALND)

An axillary lymph node dissection is used when the nodes are known to have cancer. For those with clinically uninvolved nodes (or for those with a palpable node but with a biopsy of that node not showing cancer), a sentinel lymph node biopsy can accurately predict the lymph node status.

Who needs an axillary lymph node dissection?

ALND is indicated for those with clinically involved ("positive") axillary nodes, either by fine needle aspiration or sentinel node biopsy.* The dissection extent is affected by the amount of cancer involvement. Note that the more extensive the dissection, the greater the potential side effects. These can include permanent lymphedema (significant swelling of your arm or breast), nerve injury, shoulder dysfunction, and loss of sensation. On the other hand, the risk of a recurrence in the axilla is inversely related to the number of nodes removed in a formal axillary lymph node dissection. The axillary failure rate when fewer than five nodes are removed is five to 21 percent, compared to only 3 to 5 percent when a surgeon removes more than five.

Does axillary node dissection affect survival?

Whether taking more nodes out influences survival remains uncertain. Some of the best data obtained in the modern era come in the form of a meta-analysis (a review of a collection of studies) that compared axillary dissection versus no dissection (and included a study of axillary radiation therapy versus no axillary radiation). No differences in overall survival, metastases, or local recurrence were associated with axillary treatment.

---

*Many patients with early (T1 or T2) tumors that are clinically node-negative with less than three involved sentinel nodes and who will be treated with whole breast radiation therapy do not need an axillary dissection.

Invasive

Management: Sentinel node(s)

You have about 20 to 40 axillary nodes. An axillary node dissection can remove ten or more, raising the specter of potential toxicities such as permanent arm swelling (lymphedema). Is there evidence that the less invasive sentinel lymph node biopsy yields survival as good as a dissection for those with no suggestion of node involvement? And what about axillary recurrence rates? The National Surgical Adjuvant Breast and Bowel Project (NSABP) B-32 and the subsequent American College of Surgeons Oncology Group study provides some answers.

Evidence

The NSABP B-32 trial randomly assigned women with clinically node-negative breast cancer to an axillary sentinel node biopsy (SNB) or SNB followed by an axillary lymph node dissection (ALND). Most (87.5 percent) had a lumpectomy; the rest had a mastectomy. Nearly 88 percent also received adjuvant systemic therapy (chemotherapy, endocrine therapy, or both), and 82 percent had radiation therapy to the affected breast. At ten years, the researchers found no differences in overall or disease-free survival between the two groups. Locoregional control rates were 96 percent for both groups.

The American College of Surgeons Oncology Group (ACOSOG) Z0011 trial tested whether women with an involved sentinel node (but no clinical evidence of axillary node involvement) could be safely treated with no further node surgery than an axillary sentinel lymph node biopsy. All of the women were treated with lumpectomy. More than 95 percent received systemic therapy (chemotherapy, anti-estrogen therapy, or both), and about 90 percent had external-beam radiation therapy to the affected breast.

At a median 6.3 year follow-up, the two groups of women had similar five-year overall survival (92.5 percent in the SLNB-only group versus 91.8 percent in the SLNB plus ALND group) and five-year disease-free survival (83.9 percent in the SLNB only set and 82.2 percent in the SLNB plus ALND group). There is **no benefit to an axillary lymph node dissection in patients with early-stage breast cancer who have only one or two involved sentinel nodes,** provided whole breast radiation therapy is given.

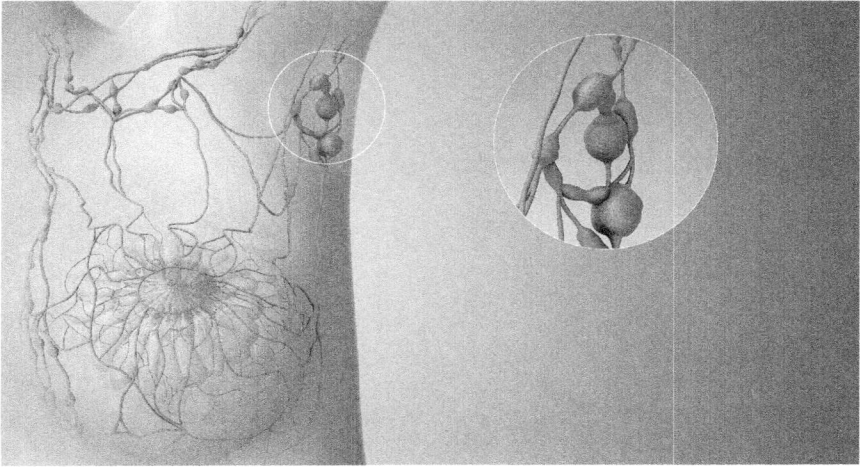

The European AMOROS clinical trial randomized 4823 patients with T1 or T2 breast cancer with positive sentinel nodes to an axillary node dissection of axillary radiation therapy. There were no differences in 5-year survival or disease-free survival. The axillary recurrence rates were 1.8 and 0.93 percent with RT versus node dissection. Lymphedema was less common in the radiotherapy group (11 versus 23 percent).

Sentinel lymph node biopsy: Logistics

Your surgeon injects a radioactive substance, a blue dye, or both near the tumor to find the sentinel lymph node. The surgeon then uses a device that detects radioactivity to find the sentinel node or looks for lymph nodes stained with the blue dye. Once the surgeon identifies the sentinel node, the surgeon makes a small incision (about 1/2 inch) in the overlying skin and removes the node.

The sentinel node is then checked for the presence of cancer cells by a pathologist. If the sentinel node has cancer, you may (or may not) need the removal of additional nodes during the same biopsy or a follow-up surgical procedure. The sentinel lymph node biopsy procedure may be done on an outpatient basis or may require a short stay in the hospital. It is typically done at the same time the primary tumor is removed (by lumpectomy or mastectomy). However, the procedure can also be done before or after the tumor's removal.

Invasive

Management: Sentinel node(s)

1 Assess

We begin by checking the axilla (underarm area) before surgery.

Palpable (we can feel it) nodes
If you or a care team member can feel (palpate) an enlarged node, you should proceed to a biopsy of the node; if you are known to have cancer in a known, you would typically proceed to a standard axillary lymph node dissection.

Abnormal nodes on imaging
Using ultrasound (non-invasive test that uses sound waves) can be an effective screening method for detecting abnormal nodes that we cannot feel. Those with abnormal nodes by imaging have a higher risk of having multiple nodes involved with cancer. Before surgery, the concerning nodes should have a biopsy.

2 Patient selection

Early breast cancer with uninvolved nodes before surgery
Here, sentinel node mapping is generally preferred, as it results in lower complication risk than a dissection of many nodes.

DCIS (non-invasive) with planned mastectomy or higher risk
High-risk includes larger DCIS (say, over 2 inches (5 centimeters) or palpable)

Who is *not* a candidate for the sentinel node procedure?
If you have node involvement (or have locally advanced or inflammatory breast cancer) before surgery, you should not have a sentinel lymph node biopsy. A standard removal of several nodes (axillary lymph node dissection) is needed. If knowing whether involvement of your nodes would not guide management, you may avoid a sentinel axillary node procedure. We do not routinely omit the procedure in those of advanced age but have a discussion in a Tumor Board with a team of clinicians before making a final decision.

Multicentric disease
If you have cancer in more than one quadrant of the breast multicentric breast cancer, you may still be a candidate for a sentinel lymph node mapping. In one study of 142 women with multicentric breast cancer, sentinel node mapping was successful in 91 percent of patients. Among only 4 percent, the procedure said there was no cancer in nodes when there was involvement.

Previous breast and axilla procedures for benign conditions
While a sentinel node mapping may be possible if you have had a lumpectomy in the past, we do not have high-level evidence to under stand its effectiveness for those who have undergone cosmetic breast surgery.

Recurrent breast cancer and previous axillary procedures
Suppose you have cancer return in the same breast (local recurrence). A sentinel node mapping with radioactive material may be possible. Still, there may be a higher probability of technical failure or a falsely negative result (the test says no cancer when cancer is present in the nodes).

Pregnancy
Pregnant women should avoid a sentinel lymph node biopsy, given the potential side effects of the dye or radioactive material on the fetus.

Male breast cancer
While there is limited data, using the same criteria for sentinel node mapping is reasonable as we use for females.

Invasive

Management: Sentinel node(s)

Complications

We have abundant evidence showing the sentinel lymph node biopsy to be associated with fewer side effects than the more invasive axillary lymph node dissection. For appropriately selected patients, the sentinel lymph node mapping does not compromise your survival or increase your risk of a recurrence in the axilla. Here are the results of 5611 patients enrolled in the National Surgical Adjuvant Breast and Bowel Project (NSABP) B-32 study.

	Sentinel	**Axillary dissection**
Limb swelling	8%	14%
Numbness	8%	31%
Arm movement deficits	13%	19%
Seroma	Not available	

A meta-analysis (a study of a collection of seven published reports) comparing an axillary lymph node dissection versus a sentinel lymph node biopsy showed a reduction in risk of infection, seroma, arm swelling, and numbness among patients with the sentinel node procedure. These results suggest that sentinel lymph node mapping is the new standard for staging most patients with no node involvement before surgery. Today, an axillary node dissection is only done if we know your nodes are involved before surgery or if it would be challenging to find the sentinel node (for example, with inflammatory breast cancer).

Axillary radiation therapy versus dissection

Three randomized trials compared axillary node dissection with axillary radiation. All of these investigations demonstrate low rates of axillary recurrence and no differences in survival probability. Radiation therapy that includes the nodes may be adequate for highly selected patients.

Older patients

Older patients may not require an axillary node sampling, particularly if the information gained would not influence cancer management or outcomes. The available data suggest that women who meet several criteria may dodge an immediate axillary surgery. These criteria include 1) a small (2 cm or smaller) cancer; clinically uninvolved nodes; 3) estrogen receptor (ER)-positive; 4) receiving anti-estrogen (endocrine) therapy.

Internal mammary nodes

Cancers of all quadrants of the breast can spread to nodes that lie alongside your breast bone or sternum. Perhaps not surprisingly, primary cancers in the parts of your breast closer to the internal mammary nodes are more likely to spread there. Isolated (that is, without accompanying involvement of the axillary nodes) is relatively unusual, however. Here are the results of one series of 7,000 patients:

Axillary + internal mammary nodes   22%

Internal mammary nodes *alone*   5%

Isolated internal mammary node recurrence appears to be more common for primary cancers in the medial (closer to the breastbone) cancers, compared to lateral ones (8 percent versus 3 percent). Still, the management of internal mammary nodes remains controversial. Here are some reasons why:

• Four randomized trials showed no survival benefit with an extended mastectomy (that included internal mammary nodes) compared to a more standard mastectomy (that did not include internal mammary nodes); *but*

• Randomized trials (and a meta-analysis or compilation of studies) show radiation therapy after mastectomy increases locoregional control and is associated with improved long-term survival odds. Such improvements have occurred only in trials that used systemic therapy, such as chemotherapy.

• Women who receive whole breast radiation therapy (following breast-conserving surgery) have better survival chances compared to those who did not have radiation therapy. Locoregional control improves survival chances.

Invasive

Management: Chemotherapy *before* surgery

Neoadjuvant (before surgery) chemotherapy

Can you have a sentinel lymph node mapping if you had neoadjuvant (before surgery) chemotherapy? As most patients will have no disease in the nodes after neoadjuvant chemotherapy, we would like to avoid the side effects associated with a standard axillary lymph node dissection. But, a sentinel node procedure may not be accurate in this clinical setting, with individual institutions reporting false-negative (the test says there is no cancer in the nodes when there is) rates of 15 to 30 percent. One of the best studies is the American College of Surgeons Oncology Group (ACOSOG) Z1071 trial.

The researchers examined women with known lymph node involvement (confirmed by biopsy) who underwent chemotherapy before surgery. After chemotherapy, patients had a sentinel lymph node biopsy followed by an axillary lymph node dissection. Here's what they found: 1) Surgeons successfully found the sentinel lymph node in 92.5% of patients; 2) among those who had node involvement that was moveable before chemotherapy and who, in addition, had at least two lymph nodes removed and examined, there was a false-negative rate of 12.8% (the goal had been 10%).

Here's one approach for chemotherapy before surgery: Before preoperative systemic therapy, perform axillary imaging with ultrasound and biopsy of any concerning axillary nodes. If the node biopsy shows no cancer, a sentinel lymph node biopsy (SLNB) can be performed before or after preoperative systemic therapy. If the node biopsy is positive for cancer, the axilla may be restaged after systemic (for example, chemotherapy) therapy. Then:

- Axillary lymph node dissection (ALND) should be performed if the axillary nodes are already known to contain cancer;

- Sentinel node biopsy or axillary node dissection can be performed if the axilla is clinically (by palpation; imaging) negative.

Management: Radiation therapy after mastectomy?

Most patients who have breast removal for invasive breast cancer will not need radiation therapy (RT). However, radiation therapy after mastectomy is indicated for patients who have conditions that place them at high risk for local recurrence:

- Four or more nodes involved: Radiation therapy should be given
- One to three to three nodes involved: Strongly consider radiation therapy
- Uninvolved nodes and tumor over 5 cm: Consider radiation therapy
- Margins involved (re-excision preferred; if not, strongly consider RT)
- Uninvolved axillary nodes and tumor 5 cm or less and margins close (under one millimeter): Consider radiation therapy.
- Uninvolved nodes *and* tumor 5 cm or less *and* margins at least 1 millimeter (mm): No radiation therapy.

In the case of micrometastasis (more than 0.2 to 2 millimeters) and no axillary node dissection, evaluate other patient risk factors when considering radiation therapy.

Radiotherapy improves mortality by 8 percent for node-positive patients

Post (after)-mastectomy radiation therapy (RT) for patients with lymph node involvement reduces the 10-year probability of any recurrence (including locoregional and distant) by 10% and the 20-year risk of breast cancer-related mortality by 8%. The benefits of RT are independent of the number of involved axillary lymph nodes and the use of systemic treatment. Therefore, while PMRT has historically been recommended for high-risk patients (including those with involved margins, four or more involved axillary nodes, and T3–T4 tumors independent of the nodal status), we should now routinely consider post-mastectomy radiation therapy for those with one to three involved axillary nodes.

After mastectomy: Radiation therapy target

Older randomized trials used broad locoregional RT fields encompassing the chest wall and all regional lymph nodes. Recent data support this tactic, especially when the lymph nodes are involved.

Invasive

Management: Radiation after lumpectomy

Locoregional control and survival improvements

Radiation therapy (RT) aims to eradicate any cancer remaining in the breast (and lymph nodes) following surgery for patients with a lumpectomy. RT can reduce the locoregional recurrence risk and improve your breast cancer-specific and overall survival chances.

Approaches

For the vast majority of women treated with breast-conserving surgery, we offer whole breast radiation therapy (WBRT). Selected low-risk patients may consider accelerated partial breast irradiation (APBI). There are some *exceptions* to the offering of whole breast radiation therapy:

- Select older patients (70 or older) with uninvolved nodes, pathologic T1 tumors that are hormone receptor-positive (and with acceptable surgical margins) may consider *not* having radiation therapy if they receive endocrine therapy. While the in-breast recurrence is higher without RT, there is no survival disadvantage.

- Select women at least age 50 with small (two centimeters or less), node-negative breast cancer with acceptable margins may be candidates for accelerated partial breast irradiation. Surgical margins should be at least two millimeters and there should be no lymphovascular invasion. Finally, the cancer should not be related to the breast cancer gene mutation BRCA.

Radiation therapy: Treating the whole breast followed by a "boost"

For many women who receive external beam radiation therapy to the whole breast, we also deliver a so-called "boost" of radiation therapy to the tumor bed (where the primary site used to be is the highest risk for recurrence area in the breast). And for those with lymph node involvement (or thought to be at higher risk for nodal involvement), we may add radiation fields covering the regional nodes.

Evidence supporting radiation therapy (RT)

Whole breast RT alone improves outcomes:

- Radiation therapy drops the 10-year risk of any first recurrence (including locoregional and distant) by 15 percent.
- Radiation therapy drops the 15-year risk of breast cancer-related death by four percent.
- Adding a boost of radiation therapy to the whole breast portion further halves the risk of recurrence in the breast.

Concerning the **boost**, I think it is especially important for those with unfavorable risk factors for local control. Such prognostic factors include young patients (for example, those under 50), those for whom the invasive cancer is associated with an extensive intraductal component (EIC), lymphovascular invasion, or focally involved margins. For the last, we often recommend a breast re-excision.

Radiation dose

Six weeks (approximately): The doses used to treat the breast, chest wall, and regional nodes have historically been 45 to 50 Gy ("Gray") in 25 to 28 daily fractions, given Monday through Friday. This whole breast radiation therapy is often followed by a boost of 10 to 16 Gy in 2 Gy single doses. My most given regimen is 23 treatments to the whole breast, followed by seven to the tumor bed (six weeks total). If there is a focally involved margin, the radiation boost dose may be higher than usual. For those without node involvement, shorter courses are often appropriate.

Shorter courses (hypo-fractionation): Recently, shorter fractionation schemes of 15 to 16 daily fractions with 2.5 to 2.67 Gy per treatment have shown similar effectiveness and comparable side effects for appropriately selected patients. These data need better validation for patients who have had a mastectomy or need radiation therapy to the regional nodes. These patients were either not included or under-represented in the relevant trials.

Currently, I consider hypo-fractionation for patients who don't require radiation therapy to regional nodes), and have acceptable margins. Let's look at the data supporting the use of a shorter course. We have a prospective randomized trial comparing five weeks of RT with three weeks plus a day (25 versus 16 treatments; neither approach incorporated a boost to the tumor bed.

Invasive

The Early Breast Cancer Trialists' Collaborative Group analyzed the results of patients participating in 10 trials randomizing to breast-conserving surgery with or without radiation therapy (RT). Here are the 5-year outcomes:

	No RT	RT
Local recurrence	**26%**	**7%**
Nodes uninvolved	23%	7%
Nodes involved	41%	11%
Breast cancer survival	**64%**	**70%**

Results of individual trials that have long-term results for breast-conserving surgery (BCS) with radiation therapy versus without it.

Study*	Follow-up	In-breast recurrence	
		BCS	BCS/RT
NSABP (USA)	20 years	39%	14%
Finland	12 years	27%	12%
Uppsala-Oreboro	10 years	24%	8%
German	10 years	34%	10%
Milan 3	10 years	23.5%	6%

Are three weeks as good as five weeks of radiation therapy?

The answer for appropriately selected patients with early, node-negative breast cancer appears to be yes. Researchers at the Ontario Clinical Oncology Group coordinating center (Canada) led a multicenter study to determine whether a hypo-fractionated three-week schedule of whole-breast irradiation would be as effective as a five-week schedule. Women with invasive breast cancer who had undergone breast-conserving surgery and for whom resection margins were clear (and axillary nodes uninvolved) were randomly assigned to receive whole-breast irradiation either at a standard dose of 50 Gy in 25 fractions over five weeks (the control group) or at a dose of 42.5 Gy in 16 fractions for three weeks and a day (the hypo-fractionated-radiation group). Here are the results at ten years, with half of the patients followed for at least 12 years:

	25 treatments	16 treatments
Local recurrence	6.7%	6.2%
Local recurrence, high-grade	**4.7%**	**15.6%**
Good/excellent cosmetic outcome	71%	70%
Survival	84.4%	84.6%

Researchers' conclusion: Ten years after treatment, accelerated, hypo-fractionated whole-breast irradiation was not inferior to standard radiation treatment in women who had undergone breast-conserving surgery for invasive breast cancer with clear surgical margins and negative axillary nodes.

My take: There are some limitations to this landmark study. The trial only entered highly select patients (node-negative, invasive breast cancer with clear margins after lumpectomy) and did not include patients with pure ductal carcinoma in situ (DCIS). Researchers excluded women with large breasts, and few patients received chemotherapy. Finally, the investigators did not know the value of boost radiation therapy at the study start. The separate START trials had a greater use of chemotherapy, and boost radiation therapy was allowed. There did not appear to be a higher complication rate in that trial.

The shorter course is an excellent approach for appropriately selected patients with early breast cancer. We have limited data on adding a "boost" to the short course of radiotherapy, but it is not uncommon to have a four to five-treatment boost to a small volume (the primary tumor bed).

Management: Radiation after lumpectomy

Radiation type

Radiation therapy typically involves the delivery of beams made of either electrons or photons (X-rays). Electrons deposit most of their dose with a limited depth, determined largely by the electron energy selected. On the other hand, photons pass completely through tissues, so we angle the beams to cover the target breast or chest wall to avoid critical organs such as the heart.

Radiation benefit

Whole breast external beam radiation therapy reduces the risk of a local or regional recurrence and is associated with a survival benefit. Prospective, randomized trials have shown a lowering of local recurrence chances by incorporating an additional boost dose of radiation therapy to the tumor bed.

Radiation treatment planning

Based on your cancer stage and other pathologic factors, we radiation oncologists define a target volume:

- The breast (or chest wall) is the primary target

- The axilla (underarm area) may be targeted

- Other regional nodes, including the internal mammary ones(located next to the breastbone/sternum on the same side of your body as the primary breast cancer) or nodes around the collarbone (supraclavicular/infraclavicular)

Simulation is the planning session that you have prior to beginning radiation therapy. During simulation, your radiation oncologist will carefully define the radiation target, taking care to minimize risk to surrounding structures such as the heart and lung. There are two types of simulation: Virtual versus clinical simulation. For the former, we use low-dose CT scans (typically without contrast) to reconstruct high resolution digital films that can be used for -

The simulation requires that you are in the treatment position while the radiation oncologist begins radiation planning. Most of the planning is done after completing your part of the process. For the simulation (treatment planning), some centers use a mold to hold you in the treatment position as you lie on your back (supine). A care team member may place markers to help define the targets (for example, a wire around the breast and on the lumpectomy scar).

You are then imaged using a CT scanner, typically with 3 mm slice spacing through the desired treatment volume. Modern scanners may complete the entire procedure in under 30 minutes. Once the simulation is complete, a team that includes your doctor, dosimetrist, and others then design the fields, shaping them with metal leaves in the head of the treatment machine. A dosimetrist creates a plan that optimizes the radiation distribution. Once your radiation oncologist approves the fields, plan, and prescription, treatment can proceed.

Special situations

Patients with very large breasts can represent a challenge in treatment planning. The radiation therapy dose can be inhomogeneous, creating hot spots in areas such as the underarm region. On some occasions, we treat patients in the prone (lying on their abdomen, with the breast hanging through a hole in the positioning device) position, allowing the breast to fall away from critical structures such as the lung. Treating the internal mammary nodes (which lie next to the sternum or breast bone) can also be challenging. Here, virtual simulation can allow your radiation oncologist to locate these lymph nodes with relative accuracy.

Management: Radiation after mastectomy

The simulation techniques to target the chest wall after mastectomy are similar to those we use for an entire breast. However, as the skin is usually an important target when radiation therapy is needed after mastectomy, your radiation oncologist may request that material is placed on your skin during the treatment to ensure that the full dose is given to the skin. This tissue-equivalent material feels like rubber and is known as a bolus. The radiation therapist may place the bolus on the skin daily or every other day, and your radiation oncologist may remove it before you complete your treatment.

The target includes the chest wall, mastectomy scar (and drain sites when indicted) for 25 to 28 treatments.. Regional nodes may be treated at the same time as the chest wall. A supplemental boost may be given to grossly involved or enlarged lymph nodes that have not been surgically addressed.

Management: Radiation after surgery

The challenge: Excess heart disease

Left breast or chest wall radiotherapy can deliver doses to the heart and coronary vessels, raising the risk of future cardiac events, including death. In an analysis of heart disease in a Nordic group of breast cancer survivors, researchers found a significant excess risk associated with radiation therapy, consistent with the risks seen in other radiotherapy-treated groups.

One potential solution: Respiratory gating

If radiation therapy hits the heart, it can potentially cause a heart attack or even cardiovascular death. We now have innovative means to protect the heart. Respiratory gating software can be integrated into the radiation treatment plan. For example, your radiation oncologist can then define a physical window (like a baseball strike zone) and deliver radiation therapy only when the target is in this strike zone as you breathe in and out. This technique can lead to sparing a greater amount of normal tissue, such as the heart.

Additional approaches can help reduce radiation dose to the heart (and the left anterior descending artery in particular - this blood vessel is commonly known as the "widow maker"):

Intensity modulated radiation therapy

Intensity-modulated radiation therapy (IMRT) is an innovative form of RT. IMRT uses photons (or, less commonly, proton) beams of varying intensities to target the breast and nodes with precision. The intensity of each radiation beam is controlled, and the beam shape changes during the treatment. Most patients do not need IMRT, but challenging body geometry can sometimes make it the preferred approach; for example, if we need to treat the left breast and regional nodes comprehensively.

Proton therapy

Proton beam scanning proton therapy delivers a narrow radiation beam that is magnetically swept across the target. The beam can approach the breast or chest wall target from multiple directions, creating a "U" shape around critical structures such as the heart.

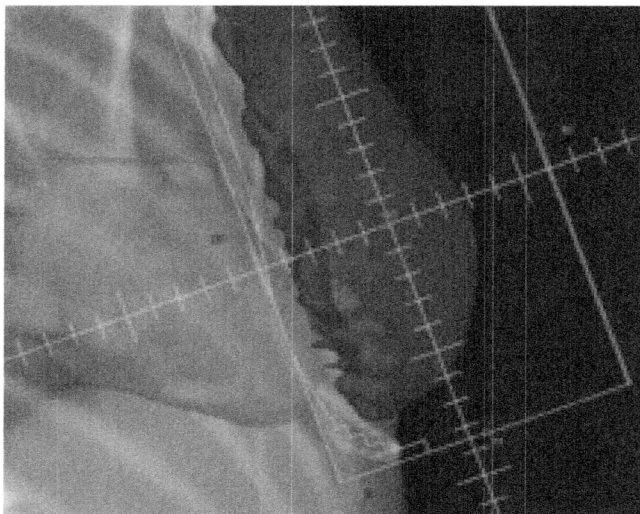

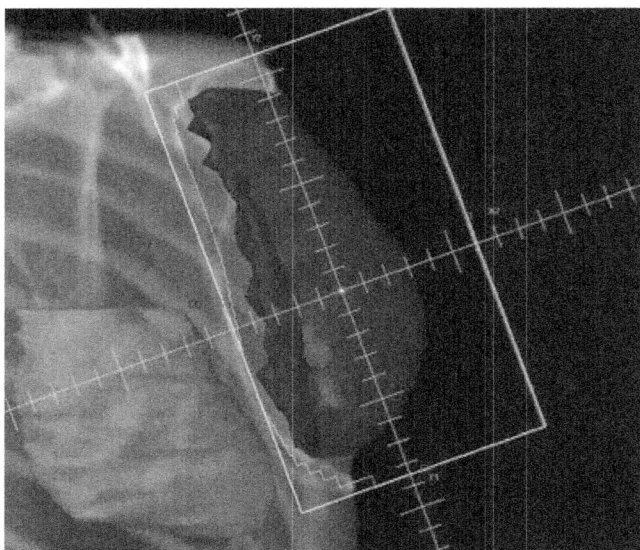

It is common for radiation therapy to follow chemotherapy when chemotherapy is indicated. Selected patients may receive oral chemotherapy (capecitabine) after RT, while those with a BRCA mutation may get olaparib.

Management: Radiation after preoperative systemic therapy and surgery

Breast-conserving surgery (with surgical axillary staging) possible

For those who had node involvement before treatment started, radiation therapy (after surgery) is recommended to the whole breast (with or without a boost to the tumor bed), with strong consideration of comprehensive radiation including the regional nodes.

If the nodes are involved at surgery, radiation should encompass the whole breast, with or without a boost to the tumor bed. There should also be comprehensive radiation therapy to include the regional nodes.

If the nodes were not involved before or after chemotherapy, radiation therapy targets the whole breast (with or without a boost to the tumor bed).

Breast-conserving surgery not possible

For those having a mastectomy and surgical axillary staging (with or without reconstruction), recommendations are as follow:

For those who had node involvement before chemotherapy and the nodes are uninvolved at surgery, we strongly consider radiation therapy to the chest wall and regional nodes.

For those with node involvement at surgery (after chemotherapy), radiation therapy should be offered to the chest wall and regional nodes.

If the nodes are uninvolved before and after chemotherapy (including an assessment with a sentinel lymph node biopsy or an axillary node dissection), no radiation therapy is needed.

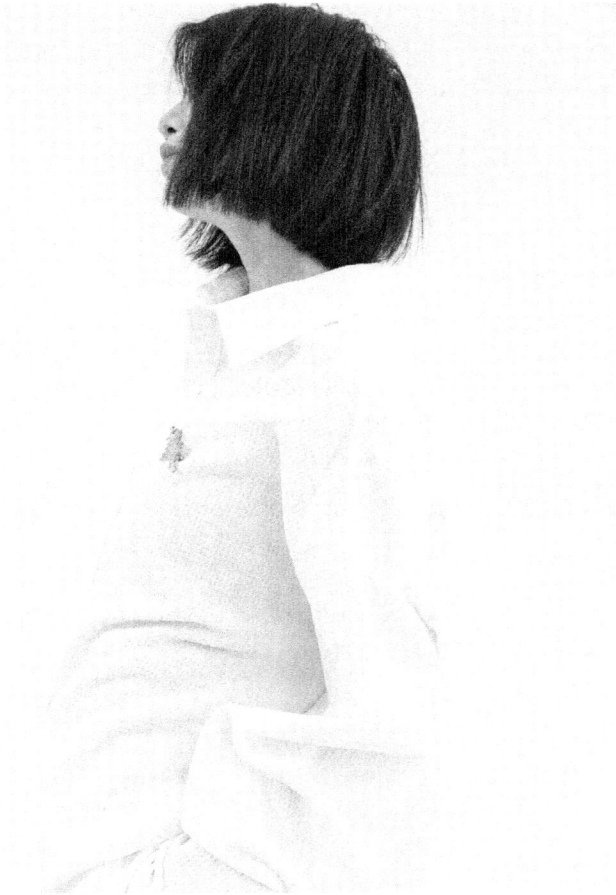

Invasive

Management: Radiation after lumpectomy

"Radiotherapy to the conserved breast halves the rate at which the disease recurs and reduces the breast cancer death rate by about a sixth."

> \- The Early Breast Cancer Trialists' Collaborative Group

RT: Whole breast + boost

For most women who receive external beam radiation therapy to the whole breast, we also deliver a so-called "boost" of radiation therapy to the tumor bed (where the primary site used to be is the highest risk for recurrence area in the breast). And for those with lymph node involvement (or thought to be at higher risk for nodal involvement), we add regional node RT.

Whole breast radiation therapy (with a traditional five-week course) alone improves outcomes:

- Radiation therapy drops the 10-year risk of any first recurrence (including locoregional and distant) by 15 percent.

- Radiation therapy drops the 15-year risk of breast cancer-related mortality by four percent.

- Adding a boost of radiation therapy to the whole breast portion further halves the risk of recurrence in the breast.

Radiation therapy "boost."

A boost dose of radiation therapy may be especially important for those with unfavorable risk factors. Such prognostic factors include young age (under 50), extensive intraductal component (EIC), lymphovascular invasion, or focally involved margins. For the last, we typically recommend a breast re-excision.

Radiation dose

Six weeks (approximately): The doses used to treat the breast, chest wall, and regional nodes have historically been 45 to 50 Gy ("Gray") in 25 to 28 daily fractions, given Monday through Friday. This treatment is often followed by a boost of 10 to 16 Gy in 2 Gy single doses. I often prescribe 23 treatments to the whole breast, followed by 7 to the tumor bed (over six weeks).

Shorter courses (hypo-fractionation): More recently, shorter fractionation schemes of 15 to 16 daily fractions with 2.5 to 2.67 Gy per fraction have shown similar effectiveness and comparable side effects for highly select patients. These data need to be well-validated in very young patients and among those who have had a mastectomy or need radiation therapy to regional nodes. These patients were either not included or under-represented in the clinical trials.

Radiation dose: Into the future

As hypo-fractionation in many places is being introduced for all patient subgroups and recognizing that we may never have randomized trials that will test this for particular subgroups of patients, I use hypofractionation for patients who have early breast cancer (that is, don't require radiation therapy to regional nodes), and acceptable margins. We have a prospective randomized trial comparing five weeks of RT with three weeks plus a day (25 versus 16 treatments; neither approach incorporated a boost to the tumor bed.

We are seeing great innovation in the radiation therapy fractionation realm. For example, the FAST clinical trial evaluated normal tissue effects and disease outcomes after five-fraction regiments. Researchers recruited 915 women from 18 United Kingdom centers from 2004 to 2007.

A once-weekly five fraction schedule of 28 Gy is estimated to be the equivalent of 50 Gy in 25 fractions in terms of late adverse effects at 10 years of follow-up. While the follow-up is short (three years) and the study was not powered for tumor control, in the future, we will hear more about innovative fractionation approaches to radiation therapy.

Invasive

Management: Radiation fields

How large should the radiation target be? Should we add comprehensive node radiation therapy (RT) to the usual breast RT? Comprehensive means treating the breast, reconstructed breast, or chest wall and aiming at the regional nodes. These typically include the axillary (underarm) and supraclavicular nodes (around the collarbone). Sometimes, the internal nodes next to the breast bone are added.

One study showed that adding regional nodal irradiation was associated with an improvement in the 5-year rate of disease-free survival compared with whole-breast irradiation alone (90% vs. 84%). The difference in the five-year rate of overall survival was not statistically significant (92% versus 91%) for these early-stage patients.

Here is the US National Comprehensive Cancer Network (NCCN) regarding radiation therapy after a mastectomy:

- Four or more nodes involved*: Radiation should include the breast (or chest wall), areas around the collarbone (supraclavicular and infraclavicular nodes), internal mammary nodes, and any part of the axilla at risk;

- One to three nodes involved*, we should treat the breast or chest wall and strongly consider targeting the regional nodes;

- If the nodes are not involved, we should target the breast or chest wall. Consider regional node radiation therapy for patients with central/medial tumors or tumors larger than two centimeters associated with high-risk features (young age or lymphovascular invasion.

Ongoing studies (including the NSABP B-51 clinical trial) should better define the optimal extent of radiotherapy fields following neoadjuvant chemotherapy, especially for those who get a complete pathologic response.

*Isolated tumor cells (ITCs) in nodes don't affect prognosis or treatment.

Short-term

Whole breast radiation therapy may be associated with side effects, including breast skin fibrosis/scarring (four percent) and decreased range of motion (1 percent). Mild generalized fatigue is common, often lasting for a month or two after the completion of radiation therapy.

Longer-term

• **Lymphedema:** Both surgery and radiation therapy can lead to early or delayed swelling of the breast, chest, or arm. Risks are highest among those who have a mastectomy with axillary node dissection followed by chest wall and axillary (underarm nodes) RT.

• **Nerve injury:** Uncommonly, RT can cause brachial plexopathy and damage to a nerve bundle at the top of your chest. Injury can cause weakness or a tingling/burning sensation in the arm or hand. RT to the nodes around the collarbone may cause nerve injury in less than 1 percent of patients.

• **Lungs:** RT to the breast region can result in lung inflammation (pneumonitis). Patients with it may present with a persistent dry cough or shortness of breath. With today's techniques, pneumonitis is rare.

• **Heart:** Incidental radiation to the heart (as a part of treatment to the breast or chest wall region for left-sided cancers) can result in myriad heart problems. These can include coronary artery disease, heart muscle injury, and valve problems. Technique matters greatly: Historic approaches often delivered relatively large doses to the heart or its vessels.

Once we recognized the radiation therapy side effects, we modified treatment techniques to reduce heart irradiation substantially. These changes are especially important for those who have received chemotherapy (or other drugs) that can damage the heart.

We have gotten better: In a study from the US Surveillance, Epidemiology, and End Results (SEER) database, the risk of death among those treated from 1973 to 1989 from ischemic heart disease was 13.1 versus 10.2 percent when comparing left breast cancers to right ones. From 1985 to 1989, the difference in 15-year death rates was not significantly different when comparing left and right breast radiation therapy.

Management: Radiation therapy (RT) side effects

The Early Breast Cancer Trialists Collaborative Group looked at nearly 20,000 women from 40 randomized trials of radiation versus no radiation therapy, with the trials initiated before 1990. Indeed, most clinical trials started before 1975 and used what we now consider suboptimal techniques. While radiation therapy decreased the risk of death from breast cancer by 13 percent, the death rate from other causes increased by 21 percent. The results of current radiation therapy have been much better.

• **Musculoskeletal:** Breast and axillary surgery can cause reduced arm mobility. RT can worsen surgery-related pain and motor restriction in the short- and long term. Rib fractures from radiation therapy are very uncommon, with a median time of about a year to its development.

• **Radiation therapy can cause cancer,** including a 1 in 1000 risk of an aggressive angiosarcoma. The risk increases with dose, length of time after RT, and younger age at the time of RT. We'll turn to other potential side effects of radiation therapy over the next couple of pages.

The most common cancer linked to radiation therapy is sarcoma (cancer of the connective tissue). For women who are long-term smokers, radiation therapy may also increase the risk of lung cancer. The risk of a second cancer is very small. The benefits of radiation therapy for appropriately selected patients almost always outweigh this risk.

Leukemia

While the risk of radiation therapy causing this blood cancer is very low, a large study gives us a sense of the risk magnitude. Researchers at Johns Hopkins Kimmel Cancer Center (USA) examined information from more than 20,000 women treated for early-stage breast cancer at eight USA cancer centers between 1998 and 2007. The recurrence rates and additional cancer diagnoses were recorded in a database by the National Comprehensive Cancer Center Network (NCCN).

Breast or chest wall region radiation therapy has been associated with a higher risk of leukemia and myelodysplastic syndrome. The risk, thankfully, is quite low.

Lung cancer

A study from 1992 to 2012 found that women who had breast cancer and got radiation therapy appeared to be more likely to develop lung cancer 20 years later than women who did not have breast cancer. The risk was small - three percent of those who had radiation therapy got lung cancer, compared to 2% of women who didn't have breast cancer. The increased risk appears approximately ten years after radiation therapy and can increase over time. The risk is higher for those who smoke cigarettes.

RT to the breast can result in pneumonitis, which usually manifests as a persistent dry cough or shortness of breath. Fortunately, with modern RT techniques, pneumonitis is rare [12]

Sarcoma

Radiation therapy to the breast/chest wall region can increase your risk of sarcoma of the blood vessels (angiosarcoma), bone (osteosarcoma), and other connective tissues in the radiation therapy volume. Fortunately, the risk is quite low.

Summary

Breast cancer treatment can sometimes cause cancer, although uncommonly. The risk of a new primary non-breast cancer after breast cancer treatment is nicely illustrated by a review of 58,068 Dutch patients diagnosed with invasive breast cancer between 1989 and 2003. With a median follow-up of 5.4 years, here is what they discovered:

Under 50 years old

Radiation therapy increased lung cancer risk by a factor of 2.31. Interestingly chemotherapy for this age group *decreased* second non-breast cancers (including colon and lung cancer) by about one-fifth (a relative 22 percent risk reduction).

Over 50 years old

Radiation therapy increased the second non-breast cancer risk by a factor of 3.43. Chemotherapy raised the risks of melanoma, uterus cancer, and a form of leukemia known as AML.

Invasive

Management: Accelerated partial breast irradiation

Accelerated partial breast irradiation (APBI) targets the tumor bed (the tumor location and not the whole breast) because most local recurrences occur in the vicinity of the primary tumor site.

Accelerated partial breast irradiation might be considered an acceptable treatment option in patients with a low risk for local recurrence, for example, those who are at least 50 years old with unicentric, unifocal, node-negative, nonlobular breast cancer, up to 3 cm without the presence of extensive intraductal components or vascular invasion, and with negative margins, especially if they will receive adjuvant hormonal treatment.

Patient selection and counseling should be performed in a multidisciplinary fashion, including collaboration between the treating surgeon and radiation oncologist.

The National Comprehensive Cancer Network (www.nccn.org) offers that local control rates in selected low-risk patients with early-stage breast cancer are comparable to those treated with standard whole breast radiation therapy. However, compared to standard whole breast radiation therapy, several studies show an inferior cosmetic outcome with external beam delivery methods of accelerated partial breast irradiation. Follow-up is limited, and studies are ongoing. The NCCN encourages clinical trial participation.

The NCCN panel indicates APBI is an option for any patient who is BRCA negative and meets these criteria:

- Age at least 50 years
- Invasive ductal carcinoma no more than two centimeters with margins of at least two millimeters, no lymphovascular invasion, and estrogen receptor-positive.
- Low or intermediate-grade, screening-detected DCIS measuring no more than 2.5 centimeters and with margins of at least three millimeters.

On the next page, you will see the guidelines of a different organization.

American Society of Breast Surgeons Guidelines 2022
Accelerated Partial Breast Irradiation (APBI)

Age	Minimum 45 years
Total tumor size (invasive and DCIS)	No more than three centimeters
Margins	• No tumor on ink for invasive cancers (including ones associated with DCIS)* • At least 2mm for DCIS*
Nodes	Uninvolved.**
Other	• Multifocal disease is allowed as long as the combined area of tumor is no more than 3 centimeters. • Tumor may be estrogen receptor positive or negative • Lymphovascular invasion is allowed as long as it is focal. • There is no evidence to support the use of accelerated partial breast irradiation in male patients. • Those with a history of ipsilateral (same side) should only be treated with accelerated partial breast irradiation as part of a specific clinical trial. • No contraindication to APBI in patients with a history of contralateral breast cancer.

* For those treated with intraoperative RT with unknown margin status: If margins are positive after intraoperative RT (IORT), you should consider a re-excision. If the re-excision margin is acceptable, your multidisciplinary, and you should consider whole breast radiation therapy. If whole breast irradiation is given after IORT, the IORT dose can substitute for the boost dose.

** Those treated with intraoperative RT (IORT) and subsequently found to have an involved sentinel lymph node should consider whole breast radiation therapy. If whole breast irradiation is administered after IORT, the IORT dose can be substituted for the boost dose

www.guidelinecentral.com/guideline/26105/#

Invasive

Management: Accelerated partial breast irradiation

Accelerated partial breast irradiation (APBI)

Accelerated partial breast irradiation uses focused radiation therapy on a limited portion of your breast. There are several options for the delivery of this localized form of radiation therapy:

- Conformal external beam radiation therapy (EBRT)
- Intensity-modulated radiation therapy (IMRT)
- Brachytherapy (interstitial versus intracavitary)
- Intraoperative radiation therapy (IORT)

Conformal external beam radiation therapy

This 3-D approach combines multiple radiation therapy fields to deliver a dose to the tumor bed region (the zone from which the surgeon removed primary cancer) while sparing most of your remaining breast tissue and solid organs. The approach preferred by the National Comprehensive Cancer Network is 30 Gy in 5 fractions, delivered every other day (for example, Monday, Wednesday, Friday, Monday, and Wednesday). Other approaches include radiation twice daily for five days versus 40 Gy in 15 fractions of three weeks.

For IMRT, we use a linear accelerator (treatment machine) to deliver highly focused small beams of radiation that allow the significant dose of radiation therapy to conform to the target tumor bed. The damage to surrounding tissue is less than for whole breast radiation. The use of IMRT for early breast cancer has been relatively limited and requires clinical expertise and physics support.

Local control

The ten-year local control rates in a randomized trial (APBI-IMRT-Florence) comparing whole and partial breast irradiation) appear similar at 97.5 and 96.3 percent, respectively. Acute and late treatment-related toxicity and cosmetic outcomes favor APBI.

Brachytherapy: Interstitial type

This specialized technique involves the placement of several small hollow catheters into the breast tissue surrounding the tumor bed. The radiation oncologist inserts high (or low) dose rate radioactive seeds into the catheters. The number of catheters used depends on the target size. The team removes the catheters at the end of the procedure.

Brachytherapy: Intracavitary type

A radiation oncologist inserts a delivery device into the tumor bed (where cancer used to be) cavity at the time of your lumpectomy ("open technique") or several days after under ultrasound guidance ("closed technique") in an office setting. Some patients may have a cavity evaluation device placed at the time of surgery, with the device exchanged for the treatment one later.

Intraoperative radiation therapy (IORT)

This form of RT reduces the entire dose into a single treatment administration, allowing surgery (lumpectomy) and radiation therapy to be completed in a single day. IORT permits the delivery of high doses of radiotherapy directly to the target tumor bed/surgical margins, while lowering dose to the skin and tissues just below the skin. IORT can lengthen the operative time, and we do not know the final surgical margins before the delivery of the radiation dose.

The TARGIT-IORT study randomized (in the United Kingdom, Europe, Australia, the USA, and Canada) to receive external beam radiation therapy for three to six weeks or intraoperative radiation therapy (IORT). With a median follow-up of 8.6 years, there appeared to be no significant difference in local recurrence, distant disease-free survival, or overall survival.

The local recurrence rate for TARGIT-IORT was 1.16 percent, compared with 0.95 percent for conventional external beam radiotherapy. If you are in a center that does IORT, discussing its use should occur when you and your caregivers are planning breast-conserving surgery.

Summary

A recent meta-analysis of randomized trials examined the effectiveness of partial breast irradiation compared with whole breast irradiation. Overall, whole breast irradiation was more effective than partial breast irradiation when given by external beam RT *without CT planning* or IORT. When properly planned, the absolute difference between groups for local recurrence appeared to be under one percent.

Management: Radiation after surgery

Accelerated Partial Breast Irradiation (APBI)

Here are radiation therapy schedules endorsed by the National Comprehensive Cancer Network:

Regimen	Method
30 Gy/5 fractions every other day (preferred)	External beam RT
40 Gy/15 fractions	
38.5 Gy/10 fractions BID	
34 Gy/10 fractions BID	Balloon/Interstitial

Newer approaches

Ultra-fractionated whole breast radiation therapy may be offered to highly select patients who are over 50 years following breast conserving surgery with pathologic Tis/T1/T2, node-negative breast cancer.

For example, 28.5 Gy may be delivered as a once-a-week approach for appropriately selected individuals. Here are the results from FAST, a randomized controlled trial of five-fraction whole breast radiation therapy for early breast cancer:

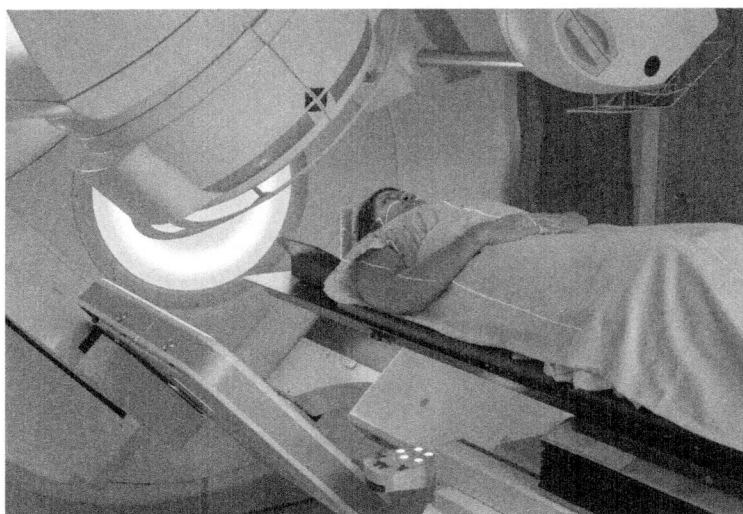

MANAGEMENT

Invasive breast cancer:
"Anti-estrogens"

Invasive

Management: Endocrine therapy

Action Point

High-level evidence (including meta-analyses of collections of research studies) shows endocrine ("anti-estrogen") therapy improves survival among those with non-metastatic, hormone receptor-positive (estrogen receptor or progesterone receptor positive) invasive breast cancer. There is consensus that women who fit this profile should receive endocrine therapy.

Background

Some breast cancer cells use estrogen or progesterone ("female" hormones produced in the body) to fuel their growth. When these hormones attach to proteins called hormone receptors, cancer cells that have these receptors grow. Your care team will check all breast cancers to see if they are estrogen receptor-positive (ER +) or ER -. The pathologist determines the hormone receptor status by testing the cancer removed during a biopsy or surgery. Most breast cancers are hormone receptor-positive. Clinicians only use hormone (endocrine) therapies if the breast cancer is hormone receptor-positive (estrogen receptor- and/or progesterone receptor-positive)

How do they work?

"Anti-estrogen" (endocrine) therapies stop or slow hormone receptor-positive cancer growth by preventing the cells from obtaining the hormones they need to grow. Some hormone therapies (for example, tamoxifen) attach to the receptor in the cancer cell, therefore blocking estrogen from attaching to the receptor. An alternative approach lowers estrogen levels in the body, depriving cancer cells of the estrogen they need to grow. The aromatase inhibitors are examples of this second approach.

300

0.7

THAT'S THE RELATIVE RISK OF BREAST CANCER DEATH
AMONG THOSE WHO TAKE TAMOXIFEN FOR 5
YEARS (COMPARED WITH NO ENDOCRINE
TREATMENT). THE RELATIVE RISK OF
BREAST CANCER RECURRENCE
IS 0.61.

Naming

I prefer the terms endocrine therapy or "anti-estrogen" treatment. Others use the somewhat confusing term "hormone therapy." The so-called hormone therapy used for breast cancer treatment is very different from that used as hormonal replacement therapy for women struggling with symptoms related to menopause.

Because the endocrine therapy approach can hinge on your menopausal status, we should first define menopause:

> **menopause** [men'-uh-pawz]. noun.
>
> The National Comprehensive Cancer Network (www.nccn.org) considers women 50 and older to be post-menopausal if they have not had periods for one year or more (in the absence of tamoxifen, chemotherapy, or ovarian suppression) and the estradiol blood level is in the post-menopausal range. Women are also post-menopausal if there have been no menstrual cycles while on tamoxifen and the estradiol blood levels are in the post-menopausal range.

There are several approaches to blocking hormones such as estrogen from driving the growth of estrogen receptor-positive breast cancer:

- Selective estrogen receptor modulator (tamoxifen)
- Aromatase inhibitors, which block the conversion of androgens ("male" hormone) to estrogens (for example, aromatase inhibitors such as anastrozole (Arimidex), letrozole (Femara), and exemestane.
- Reduction (or destruction) of ovary function

Aromatase inhibitors drugs are only for women in menopause, as they block the creation of estrogen in the body fat and adrenal glands but do not block estrogen production from the ovaries. Some women discontinue an aromatase inhibitor within the first five years. It is reasonable to then switch to tamoxifen after at least two years of the aromatase inhibitor drug have been completed.

Aromatase inhibitor (AI) benefits

Aromatase inhibitors versus tamoxifen	
AI (five years) versus tamoxifen (5 years)	From years 0 to one, the AI drops recurrence by 1/3 (relative risk 0.64); from years 2 to 4, the relative risk dropped by one-fifth. After five years, there was no further impact on recurrence.
Tamoxifen (five years) versus tamoxifen for 2-3 years, followed by AI (total of five years of endocrine therapy)	From years two to four, the AI-containing group had a recurrence drop by nearly 1/2 (relative risk 0.56); After five years, there was no further impact on recurrence. There appeared to be fewer deaths from breast cancer associated with the switch to an aromatase inhibitor.
AI (five years) versus tamoxifen (2-3 years) followed by an AI (total five years of endocrine therapy)	From years 0 to one, the AI lowered recurrence rates (relative risk 0.74) compared to tamoxifen. From years two to four, there were similar recurrence risks. Finally, using an AI alone led to a trend toward reduced breast cancer mortality, but it did not reach statistical significance (relative risk 0.89).

AIs and premenopausal women

Aromatase inhibitors (AIs) don't normally work in pre-menopausal women because their ovaries are still making estrogen, and the drugs don't block estrogen in the ovaries. However, some pre-menopausal women may take an aromatase inhibitor when combined with ovarian suppression (for example, drugs* that shut down the ovarian function), which shuts down the ovaries. Indeed, some findings suggest ovarian suppression plus an aromatase inhibitor may reduce breast cancer recurrence better than ovarian suppression plus tamoxifen (rates of freedom from breast cancer: 91 versus 87 percent at 68 months follow-up). This improvement is reflects reductions in local, regional, and contralateral breast events and in distant recurrence.

* examples include leuprolide (Lupron) and goserelin (Zoladex); alternatively, a surgeon can remove the ovaries.

Invasive

Management: Endocrine therapy

Action Point

An aromatase inhibitor pill is recommended for most women with post-menopausal breast cancer, as it improves recurrence and survival outcomes compared with tamoxifen. While five years of an AI is standard, emerging evidence suggests ten years might be better (albeit with increased complication risks).

Postmenopausal women

An aromatase inhibitor (AI) pill is appropriate for most women with post-menopausal breast cancer. The AIs are slightly better than tamoxifen at improving recurrence and survival odds. While the standard of care histori-cally has been a 5-year course of an aromatase inhibitor, we have some 2016 data to suggest that ten years might provide additional benefit (although with some increase in side effect risk).

Five years of aromatase inhibitor (AI) therapy, either as up-front treatment or after two to five years of tamoxifen, has become the standard of care for post-menopausal women with hormone receptor-positive early breast can-cer. The Canadian Cancer Trials Group MA.17R tested the benefit of extend-ing an aromatase inhibitor for an additional five years using letrozole.

Here are the results: 95 percent of the women in the 10-year letrozole group experienced disease-free survival, compared with 91 percent in the five-year group. However, women treated with the drug for ten years didn't live longer than those given a placebo (after the initial five years of endocrine therapy) in the study. Still, I think it is likely that a survival benefit will emerge in the data in the coming years.

Some women discontinue an aromatase inhibitor within the first five years. It is reasonable to switch to tamoxifen after at least two years of the AI have been completed.

Some women discontinue an aromatase inhibitor within the first five years. It is considered reasonable to then switch to tamoxifen after at least two years of the AI have been completed. Here are the result when an aromatase inhibitor (AI) was incorporated into endocrine therapy course:

	What did the AIs do, compared to tamoxifen?
AI (five years) versus tamoxifen (five years)	From years 0 to 1, the AI dropped recurrence risk by about one-third (relative risk 0.64); from years two to four, the relative risk dropped by one-fifth. After five years, there was no further impact on recurrence.
Tamoxifen (five years) versus tamoxifen for 2-3 years, followed by AI (total of five years of endocrine therapy)	From years two to four, the AI-containing group had a recurrence drop by nearly 1/2 (relative risk 0.56); After five years, there was no further impact on recurrence. There appeared to be fewer deaths from breast cancer associated with the switch to an aromatase inhibitor.
AI (five years) versus tamoxifen (two to three years) followed by of an AI (total five years of endocrine therapy)	From years 0 to 1, the AI lowered recurrence rates (relative risk 0.74) compared to tamoxifen. From years 2 to 4, there were similar recurrence risks. Finally, using AI alone led to a trend toward reduced breast cancer mortality, but it did not reach statistical significance (relative risk 0.89).

How long?

Approximately 70 percent of breast cancers are hormone receptor-positive. The recurrence risk among this population can persist for as long as 25 years or more after diagnosis. Five years of anti-estrogen (endocrine) therapy can reduce the risk of recurrence by about half and mortality by nearly a third. Recently, we got data from the ATLAS trial showing extending tamoxifen therapy to 10 years reduced the risk of breast cancer recurrence and breast cancer-related death.

However, the optimal length of treatment with aromatase inhibitors such as anastrozole (Arimidex) and letrozole (Femara) - often used instead of, or after, tamoxifen to stop estrogen production in post-menopausal women - is controversial. In support of extended treatment, the MA.17R trial showed ten years of letrozole reduced local recurrences and the development of cancer in the opposite breast compared to 5 years of the drug. On the other hand, the difference in distant recurrence (metastases) was quite small.

Invasive

Management: Endocrine therapy

Duration (continued)

Other studies have demonstrated less benefit from extended aromatase inhibitor therapy and more toxicity. Here are the disease-free survival chances among studies of extended aromatase therapy:

Study	Disease-free survival	Statistically significant?
MA.17R	95 vs. 91 percent	Yes
NSABP B-42	84 vs. 81 percent	Yes
DATA	83 vs. 79 percent	Borderline
IDEAL	88 vs. 88 percent	No

HemOnc Today April 10, 2017

Downsides

Aromatase inhibitor drugs are associated with an increased risk of adverse events, such as bone loss, fractures, bone and joint pain, hot flashes, and vaginal dryness. There are ways to reduce your chances of bone fracture and osteoporosis. Nevertheless, each individual and their clinicians will need to weigh the risks against the long-term projected benefits of extended anti-estrogen therapy beyond five years.

One clinician's take

Some patients will benefit from extended therapy, as we see recurrences 10 and 15 years after diagnosis. Still, it is something we should only recommend to some patients.

- V.K. Gadi, MD, Ph.D. (Fred Hutchinson Cancer Center, Seattle)

Invasive

Premenopausal women: Tamoxifen

For patients not at high risk for recurrence, tamoxifen represents the gold standard of care. While historically, the treatment lasted five years, extending tamoxifen to ten years should be considered for selected patients, for example, those at higher risk of recurrence.

An **aromatase inhibitor** (AI) pill is not appropriate as a single approach for women with intact ovarian function. This group includes women who lose their menstrual cycles due to chemotherapy, as they may resume menstruating during follow-up.

Ovarian suppression: Only for those at higher risk

For patients at higher risk for recurrence (under 35 or after those who received chemotherapy), consideration should be given to suppressing ovarian function (with injections) and adding an aromatase inhibitor (such as exemestane) instead of tamoxifen. Two clinical trials suggest that ovarian suppression with an aromatase inhibitor provides benefits behind those associated with tamoxifen, at least for higher-risk women. Here are the patients who benefited from the more aggressive approach, at least according to a combined analysis of two clinical trials (SOFT and TEXT)*:

Patients diagnosed under 35 years had a higher progression-free survival with ovarian suppression plus the aromatase inhibitor exemestane: Disease-free survival was 91% versus 87%, but there were no differences in overall survival odds. A subgroup analysis of the SOFT study suggested a benefit for the ovarian suppression-containing approach among patients treated with chemotherapy.

---

* Suppression of Ovarian Function Trial (SOFT) and Tamoxifen and Exemestane Trial (TEXT)

The decision to incorporate ovarian suppression for those at high-risk is challenging as there can be significant side effects associated with this approach. There does not appear to be a benefit for those *not* at higher risk of recurrence.

Side effects: Tamoxifen

A meta-analysis (of a collection of studies) from the 2011 Early Breast Cancer Trialists' Collaborative Group compared tamoxifen for five years versus no endocrine therapy. Here are some (but not all) of the major side effects found to be associated with tamoxifen:

- Deep venous thrombosis (blood clots, for example, in your calf)
- Uterus cancer (limited to women over 55 years of age)
- Hot flashes
- Vaginal discharge
- Sexual dysfunction
- Menstrual irregularities
- Stroke (not statistically significant)

Hot flashes

Hot flashes are among the most common and troublesome toxicities of tamoxifen. They may be due to a central nervous system anti-estrogen effect resulting in dysfunction of your body heat regulation system. Up to 80 percent of women on tamoxifen get hot flashes; 30 percent have severe hot flashes.

There is variability among individuals in hot flash risk associated with tamoxifen. For example, premenopausal women are more likely to get them than post-menopausal women. Genetics may play a role, too. In addition, some anti-depressant drugs known as SSRIs can decrease the conversion of tamoxifen to its most active by-product (endoxifen), influencing your chances of getting hot flashes. Examples include paroxetine and fluoxetine.

Blood clots

Tamoxifen can increase the risk of so-called thromboembolic disease, including pulmonary embolism (clots in the lung) and stroke. This elevated risk continues as long as you are on the drug. There may be an additional risk if one adds tamoxifen to chemotherapy, and the risk appears to rise if the tamoxifen use extends from five to 10 years.

Risk factors for developing clots in your veins also include prior surgery, fracture, and immobilization. Your doctor may counsel you to discontinue the tamoxifen for several days prior to prolonged immobilization from planned surgery or travel.

An analysis of trials of tamoxifen from the Early Breast Cancer Trialists Collaborative Group demonstrated a non-significant excess of stroke deaths (3 extra per 1000 women during the first 15 years), but this risk was exactly balanced by a reduction in heart-related deaths (3 fewer per 1000 women).

Endometrial (uterus) cancer

Tamoxifen can raise the risk of both the common type of uterus cancer and a less common one known as uterine sarcoma. In the Early Breast Cancer Trialists Collaborative Group overview analysis of 20 trials, researchers found tamoxifen to be associated with a 2.4 fold increased risk of uterus cancer, but there was no increase in death linked to this increase in risk. The rate in the Breast Cancer Prevention Trial was 2.3 per 1,000 women per year, compared to 0.9 for the placebo group.

With long-term follow-up, we now know that tamoxifen results in a very small increase in the incidence of an uncommon cancer of the uterus: Uterine sarcoma (carcinosarcoma or mixed Mullerian tumors) risk increases. The absolute risk of MMMT results in an additional 1.4 cases per 10,000 women per year.

Other tumors

While most individual clinical trials (including the largest one, the P-1 trial) looking at tamoxifen did *not* show an increases in non-uterine cancer, a meta-analysis of 16 randomized trials comparing tamoxifen with a placebo suggested a 1.3-fold increase in **gastrointestinal cancers.** We have some hints that tamoxifen may *lower* your risk of **ovarian cancer.** Still, we do not have high-level evidence to assert this with confidence.

Childbearing

Women of childbearing potential should use an effective means of contraception. Indeed, tamoxifen can induce ovulation. After stopping, check with your physician to see if you should be off the drug a minimum of a few months to ensure the drug has cleared your system.

Side effects: Tamoxifen (continued)

Coronary heart disease

Tamoxifen may not be associated with a beneficial or adverse cardiovascular effect among post-menopausal women. Still, the data are mixed. While tamoxifen can improve your lipid profile, it has not consistently been linked to a beneficial heart effect.

Eye problems

Tamoxifen has been found in some (but not all) studies to increase cataract risk. The drug may cause dry eye, irritation, and retinal deposits that may cause macular edema. However, these side effects are uncommon. Your first line of defense? A baseline eye exam.

Other

Tamoxifen can cause vaginal furlough, menstrual irregularities, sexual dysfunction, and other problems.

Childbearing age

Women of childbearing potential should use effective contraception while on tamoxifen, as the drug can induce ovulation and raise the risk of congenital abnormalities. After stopping tamoxifen, check with your physician to see if you should be off the drug for a minimum of a few months (before attempting to conceive a child) to ensure the drug has cleared out.

Side effects: Aromatase inhibitors (AIs)

- Musculoskeletal problems (bone pain, joint stiffness/achiness): Severe in about one-third of patients, although the difference between placebo (inactive "fake" pill) versus aromatase inhibitors in randomized trials appears to be about 5 to 8 percent. Still, 10 to 20% will quit the AI because of these symptoms.
- Sexual dysfunction, pain, or dissatisfaction
- Reduced vaginal lubrication; reduced sexual interest
- Cognitive problems (forgetfulness, for example)
- Fatigue

Musculoskeletal (muscle/bone) syndrome

Aromatase inhibitors can be associated with joint pain, stiffness, or muscle or bone pain. For about a third of patients, this symptom can be severe; on the other hand, if we look at the difference between aromatase inhibitor and placebo (inert), there is a 5 to 8 percent difference. The bottom line? Musculoskeletal symptoms lead 10 to 20 percent of patients to stop the medicine.

The good news? There appears to be a dose-response relationship between exercise and symptom severity, according to the Hormones and Physical Exercise (HOPE) trial. The exercise regimen consisted of twice-weekly supervised resistance and strength training plus moderate aerobic exercise for 150 minutes per week. Other patients use non-steroidal anti-inflammatory drugs but have their potential risks. Sometimes a switch to a different aromatase inhibitor can be beneficial. Some believe the anti-depressant and nerve pain medication duloxetine (Cymbalta) may relieve patients for whom a switch to a different AI doesn't help. Finally, vitamin D might help. One study used vitamin D2, 50,000 IU capsule per week, and found it helpful. Still, such high doses of vitamin D require close monitoring of blood levels.

Sexual dysfunction

Using an aromatase inhibitor can result in vaginal symptoms and sexual dysfunction. Some patients describe lower sexual interest, while others report diminished vaginal lubrication or pain with sex. Others mention orgasmic dysfunction and general dissatisfaction with their sex life.

Other side effects

Some women describe cognitive challenges associated with the use of an aromatase inhibitor. Predictors of discontinuation of the drug by one year included:

- Fatigue
- Forgetfulness
- Poor sleep

Compared to tamoxifen, aromatase inhibitor use can raise the risks of bone loss (osteoporosis), bone fractures, cardiovascular problems, and elevated cholesterol levels. On the positive side, aromatase inhibitor use can lead to a lower risk of venous thrombus (blood clots in your veins) and endometrial (uterus) cancer, at least as compared with tamoxifen.

Preferred aromatase inhibitor (AI)

The various aromatase inhibitors have equivalent effectiveness when used in the adjuvant setting (following surgery with curative intent).

Timing of aromatase inhibitor (AI)

No chemotherapy, no radiation therapy

If you have hormone receptor-positive breast cancer and are not scheduled to have chemotherapy or radiation therapy, most patients begin the AI about four to six weeks following surgery.

Chemotherapy

For patients getting chemotherapy, it is generally recommended to sequence the chemotherapy before the endocrine therapy, although a meta-analysis from the Early Breast Cancer Trialists' Collaborative Group that compared concurrently with sequential treatment found similar drops in the risk for recurrence.

Radiation therapy

For women receiving radiotherapy after surgery, some clinicians have you start the aromatase inhibitor during radiation, while others wait until radiation therapy is complete. This author is unaware of data showing a difference in survival based on the timing of AI initiation relative to radiation therapy.

HER-2 positive

In the original clinical trials showing tremendous value for adding trastuzumab (Herceptin) to chemotherapy for HER-2 overexpressing breast cancer, endocrine therapy was initiated (for hormone receptor-positive cancers) once the chemotherapy portion of treatment was complete.

Non-compliance

One study suggests that non-compliance with either tamoxifen or an aromatase inhibitor may increase your risk of death. However, there appeared to be no influence on breast cancer-specific mortality. We join the National Comprehensive Cancer Network (NCCN) in encouraging compliance.

Extending endocrine therapy - Role for genomic testing

For those with hormone receptor-positive (ER/PR +), HER2 negative breast cancer, the Breast Cancer Index can help determine whether extending endocrine therapy beyond five years has potential value.

Test	Risk*	Treatment implications
Breast Cancer Index (BCI)	BCI (H/I) **Low**	• For patients with T1 and T2 hormone receptor-positive, HER2-negative, and pN0 tumors, a BCI (H/I) in the low-risk range(0–5), regardless of T size, places the tumor into the same excellent prognostic category as T1a–T1b, N0, M0. • Patients with BCI (H/I) low demonstrated a lower risk of distant recurrence (compared to BCI [H/I] high) and no significant improvement in disease-free or overall survival compared to the control arm in terms of extending endocrine therapy duration.
	BCI (H/I) **High**	• For patients with T1 hormone receptor-positive, HER2-negative, and pN0 tumors, a BCI (H/I) high (5.1–10) demonstrated significant rates of late distant recurrence. • In secondary analyses of the MA.17, Trans-aTTom, and IDEAL trials, patients with HR-positive, T1–T3, pN0 or pN+ who had a BCI (H/I) high demonstrated significant improvements in disease-free survival when adjuvant endocrine therapy was extended, compared to the control arm. • In contrast, BCI (H/I) low patients derived no benefit from extended adjuvant therapy.

Extending tamoxifen to ten years improves disease-free survival

For those with hormone receptor-positive breast cancer, endocrine therapy (after surgery) is generally recommended for a minimum of five years. Given continuing risk after five years, researchers have looked at longer durations of endocrine therapy and discovered extending endocrine therapy can improve disease-free survival odds.

Extending tamoxifen from five to 10 years

The ATLAS trial randomized pre- and post-menopausal women to five versus ten years of tamoxifen. Extending the tamoxifen to ten years appeared to be associated with a lower recurrence risk and better breast cancer-specific survival odds:

	Tam 5 years	Tam 10 years
Recurrence in years 5 to 14	21.4%	25.1 %

The most significant side effects with 10 years of tamoxifen were a higher risk of uterus (endometrial) cancer and pulmonary embolism (lung blood clots).

Following tamoxifen with an AI improves outcomes

The MA-17 trial of 5187 patients who completed 4.5 to 6 years of tamoxifen showed that extended therapy with an aromatase inhibitor (letrozole) provides benefits for postmenopausal women with hormone receptor-positive, early breast cancer. The addition of the aromatase inhibitor greatly improved disease-free survival. No data are available regarding aromatase inhibitor use for more than five years.

The Austrian Breast and Colorectal Cancer Study Group Trial 6a randomized patients (who had completed five years of tamoxifen) to three years of the aromatase inhibitor anastrazole or no further therapy. At a median of 62.3 months, the use of anastrazole appeared to have a significant advantage in recurrence risk, dropping the relapse rate (38 percent relative risk reduction).

Tamoxifen, aromatase inhibitor, or both

The BIG 1-98 trial randomized patients to tamoxifen alone for five years, the aromatase inhibitor letrozole for for five years, tamoxifen for two years followed by letrozole for three years, or letrozole for two years followed by tamoxifen for   three years. Here are the key findings:

- **Five years of tamoxifen alone versus letrozole alone.** Letrozole had a slightly lower risk of contralateral breast cancer in the first 10 years, but this reversed beyond 10 years. Disease-free survival rates were similar when comparing tamoxifen against letrozole.

The incidence of significant cardiac adverse events was much higher with letrozole, while the incidence of blood clots was significantly higher in the tamoxifen arm. In addition, the letrozole group had a higher bone fracture rate (9.5 versus 6.5 percent). Finally, after a median 71 months of follow-up, there appeared to be no differences in disease-free survival with tamoxifen followed by letrozole or the reverse sequence, compared with letrozole alone.

- **Five years of tamoxifen followed by an AI (for three years).** An extension study of the Austrian Breast Cancer Study Group (ABCSG) trial 6 randomized hormone receptor-positive postmenopausal patients who completed five years of tamoxifen to three years of an aromatase inhibitor (anastrozole) or no further treatment. At a median of 62.3 months, the addition of the AI was associated with a significantly lower risk of recurrence (38 percent relative risk reduction).

Which aromatase inhibitor?

The National Comprehensive Cancer Network (www.nccn.org) finds no meaningful differences in effectiveness or toxicity when comparing the available aromatase inhibitors. Finally, there are no data suggesting that an aromatase for five years is better than 10 years of tamoxifen.

Invasive

Management: CDK4/6 inhibitors

> **Action Point**
>
> CDK4/6 inhibitors treat certain breast cancers that have spread to distant body parts (metastasized to organs such as the bones, lungs, or liver). These drugs block the process through which breast cancer cells divide and multiply.

CDK4/6 proteins are in healthy cells and cancer cells. Currently, there are three CDK4/6 inhibitors used to treat breast cancer:

- Ibrance (chemical name: Palbociclib)

- Kisqali (chemical name: Ribociclib)

- Verzenio (chemical name: Abemaciclib)

The CDK4/6 proteins in healthy and cancer cells control how quickly cells grow and divide. In metastatic breast cancer, these proteins in the cell nucleus can become overactive and cause the cancer cells to grow uncontrollably. CDK4/6 inhibitors interrupt these proteins to slow (or stop) the cancer cells from growing.

CDK4/6 inhibitors treat metastatic breast cancers that are hormone-receptor-positive and HER2-negative. The CDK4/6 inhibitors described above are pills taken by mouth.

Verzenio is a daily medicine taken either alone or with other treatments. It appears to affect the CDK4 protein more than the CDK6 protein. Ibrance and Kisqali affect both CDK4 and CDK6 and must be taken along with endocrine therapy. They are given in four-week cycles that include a week-long break — you take the medication for three weeks and then take a week off.

Outcomes with CDK4/6 inhibitors

As an example of improved outcomes, The MONALEESA-3 clinical trial looked at endocrine therapy (fulvestrant) with or without the CDK4/6 inhibitor ribociclib for metastatic disease. The overall survival rates at 3.5 years were 58 percent and 46 percent, in favor of the CDK4/6 inhibitor group.

CDK4/6 inhibitors for early breast cancer

CDK4/6 inhibitors improve outcomes for those with metastases. What about earlier diseases? In the PENELOPE-B clinical trial, adding palbociclib to adjuvant endocrine therapy did *not* improve invasive–disease–free survival in patients with estrogen receptor-positive, HER2-negative breast cancer and residual disease after neoadjuvant chemotherapy.

Only the MONARCH-E trial (which used abemaciclib) has shown a benefit in invasive disease-free survival. Here are the MONARCH-E trial details:

> • Patients with four or more positive nodes, or one to three nodes and either tumor size 5 cm or greater, grade 3, or Ki-67 level of at least 20 percent, were randomly assigned to standard-of-care adjuvant endocrine therapy with or without abemaciclib (150 milligrams twice daily for two years).

> • Abemaciclib plus endocrine therapy demonstrated superior invasive disease-free survival versus endocrine therapy alone, with two-year invasive disease-free survival rates of 92.2 versus 88.7 percent, respectively.

CDK4/6 inhibitor side effects

Like most cancer medicines, CDK4/6 inhibitors cause side effects, but they tend to be less intense than those caused by chemotherapy. The most common side effects of all three medicines are nausea, diarrhea, fatigue, and low blood counts (low white blood cell counts or neutropenia; anemia (low red blood cell counts); low platelet counts or thrombocytopenia.

Invasive

Management: Favorable cancers

Endocrine therapy

Here are some favorable subtypes of breast cancer:

- Pure tubular
- Pure mucinous
- Pure cribriform
- Encapsulated or solid papillary carcinoma

Here are the recommendations for those with pT1, pT2, or pT3 who also have either no node involvement or 2 millimeters or less cancer involvement (pN1mi):

For primary cancers less than one centimeter (cm), consider endocrine therapy for risk reduction. For tumors one to 2.9 cm, consider endocrine therapy. Those with tumors 3 cm or larger should receive endocrine therapy.

For those with nodal involvement more than 2 millimeters, adjuvant therapy should be given, with or without chemotherapy.

Other favorable breast cancer subtypes:

- Adenoid cystic and other salivary carcinomas
- Secretory carcinoma
- Rare low-grade forms of metaplastic carcinoma

There is limited data supporting local therapy (for example, a lumpectomy followed by radiation therapy) only. Those with node involvement may consider systemic or targeted therapy.

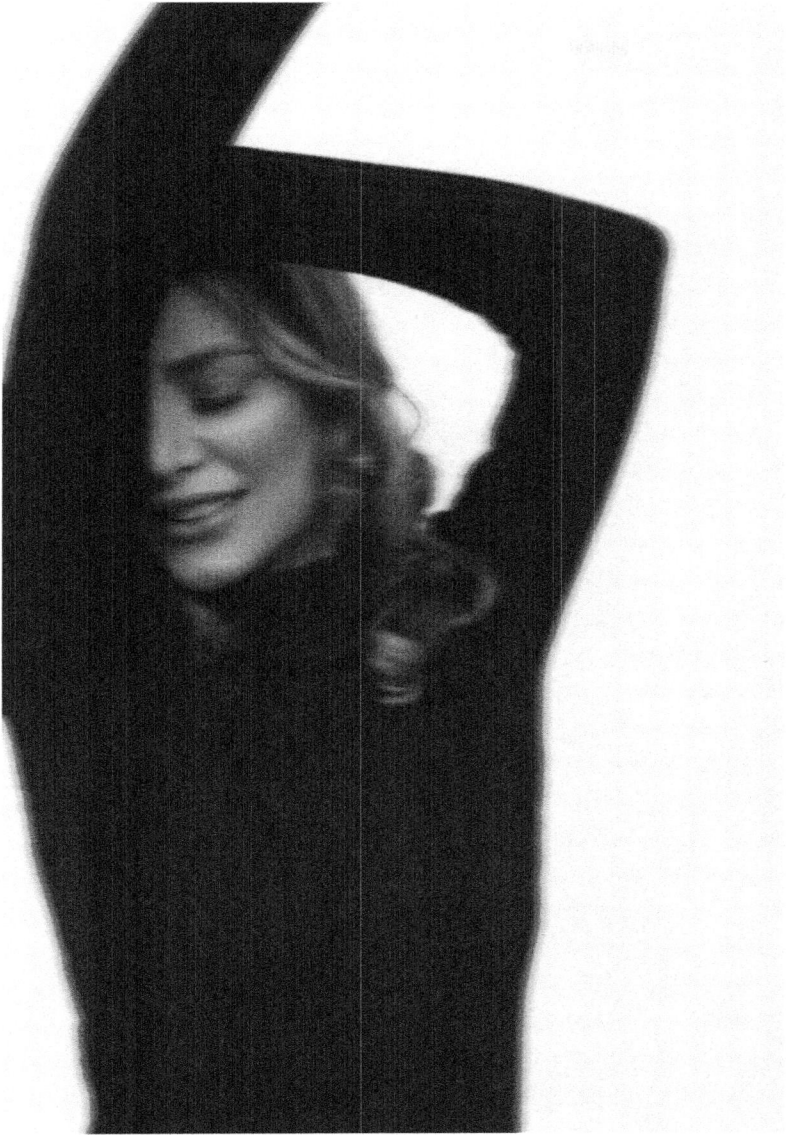

MANAGEMENT

Invasive breast cancer: Chemotherapy

Invasive

Management: Chemotherapy (chemo)

Treatment with cancer-killing drugs that may be injected into a vein or taken by mouth. The drugs travel through the bloodstream to destroy cancer cells in distant body parts such as the bones, lungs, and liver.

Most individuals with breast cancer will not need chemotherapy. The decision to offer adjuvant (after surgery) chemotherapy for breast cancer that has no distant spread is complex and incorporates several variables, including:

- Primary tumor size
- Number of nodes involved
- Measures of proliferation (grade; HER2 overexpression)
- Expression of estrogen receptors or progesterone receptors
- Patient age and medical fitness
- Higher risk features such as lymphovascular invasion
- Patient preference

Additional tools to aid in determining the value of chemotherapy include genomic analysis and benefit-risk calculators, especially among those with hormone receptor-positive (ER/PR +) breast cancer. Algorithms have been published estimating rates of recurrence. Predict (www.predict.uk/index.html) is an online tool where patients and clinicians can see how different early invasive breast cancer treatments might improve survival rates after surgery. The current version does not include all of the treatments that are currently available, and an appropriate clinician should advise you on all of your treatment options.

Over the next pages, we will look at different scenarios, including 1) HER2 overexpression; 2) triple-negative cancer; 3) lymph node involvement; 4) no lymph node involvement.

STEPS TO CHEMO

Chemotherapy is the use of drugs designed to kill cancer cells.

DEFINE

Risk

What is your chance of metastasis (distant spread)?

CHOOSE

Drugs

Should chemotherapy be used? If yes, what type? Should drugs such as Herceptin be added?

Invasive

Management: Chemotherapy - Benefits

Overall, chemotherapy added to surgery decreases the risk of recurrence and improves survival. Still, the absolute benefits for patients with a low risk of recurrence may be quite small (or even non-existent).

Oxford Overview: Chemotherapy benefits

The Early Breast Cancer Trialists' Collaborative Group (EBCTG) nicely addresses chemotherapy benefits. It performs a meta-analysis, an analysis of a collection of research studies, every five years. In the 2012 meta-analysis, the use of chemotherapy containing a type of drug known as an anthracycline (for example, doxorubicin or Adriamycin) compared to no chemotherapy resulted in the following:

	Chemo	No chemo
Risk of recurrence	47%	39%
Breast cancer mortality	36%	29%
Overall mortality	40%`	35%

Compared with no treatment, the use of a common regimen known as CMF (cyclophosphamide, methotrexate, fluorouracil) was also associated with improvement in these outcomes at the ten-year mark.

Which chemotherapy type?

Anthracycline-containing chemotherapy versus CMF? A separate Oxford overview suggests that an anthracycline-containing regimen is at least equivalent to the historical standard CMF and that the addition of taxane to an anthracycline-based regimen further improves outcomes.

Alternatives to anthracycline-based treatment

Many patients at higher risk for recurrence will have the aforementioned AC-T regimen. Selected patients who choose chemotherapy may have potential alternative options to regimens containing "harsh" drugs such as doxorubicin (Adriamycin) or epirubicin. The non-anthracycline regimen of docetaxel (Taxotere) and cyclophosphamide (Cytoxan), given over 12 weeks - also known as **TC** - may be an appropriate alternative for patients who have indications for chemotherapy but have a lower-risk disease. TC does not have the higher risks of congestive heart failure and secondary leukemias (blood cancer) associated with anthracyclines. There have been no direct head-to-head comparisons of AC, T versus TC.

In the US Oncology Trial 9735, researchers randomly assigned over 1000 women (with stages I to III, HER-2 negative breast cancer) to either AC or TC. After a median follow-up of 7 years, TC resulted in a slightly higher disease-free survival (81 versus 75 percent) and overall survival (87 versus 82 percent) compared with AC. Remember, this trial did not use the regimen that has yet to be beaten: Adriamycin and cyclophosphamide, incorporating paclitaxel (also known as AC-T or AC-Taxol).

Chemotherapy schedule: Dose-dense

"Dose-dense" chemotherapy means the drugs are given more frequently than historically. A meta-analysis of dose-dense versus standard dosing showed the dose-dense approach:

- Reduced the recurrence rate (relative risk 0.83).
- Improved survival (relative risk 0.86).
- Did not raise the chances of non-breast cancer mortality compared with standard dosing.

One commonly used dose-dense approach gives AC every two weeks four times, and then a so-called taxane.

Stem cell transplant (super high-dose chemotherapy)

A meta-analysis of 15 trials looking at bone marrow transplant (very high-dose chemotherapy) after surgery showed that those enrolled in the high-dose chemotherapy (stem cell transplant) arm did *not* have higher survival than those with more standard chemotherapy.

Invasive

Chemotherapy - Who?

Oncotype DX is a tumor profiling test that helps determine the benefit (if any) of chemotherapy in addition to endocrine therapy to manage some hormone receptor-positive breast cancers.

What

If you've been recently diagnosed with early, estrogen receptor-positive (ER+), HER2-negative breast cancer, the Oncotype DX Breast Recurrence Score (or other genomic test) can help you and your care team understand what management options are right for you — including whether you're likely to benefit from chemotherapy.

The Breast Recurrence Score test looks at several cancer-related genes in your tumor tissue. Because every woman's tumor is unique, understanding the biology of your specific tumor will help you and your doctor make more confident decisions about your care.

How the test works

The Breast Recurrence Score (RS) test looks at several cancer-related genes in your tumor tissue. Because every woman's tumor is unique, understanding the biology of your specific tumor will help you and your doctor make more informed decisions about your care.

Medicare and most private insurance carriers cover the Oncotype DX Breast Recurrence Score for eligible patients with early-stage invasive breast cancer. Since insurance coverage can vary across the country, it's a good idea to check with your insurer to ensure the test is covered.

Recurrence Score (RS)

Most results from the Oncotype DX Breast Recurrence Score test are available approximately two weeks after the laboratory receives the cancer sample. The results are sent to your doctor so they can discuss them with you and answer your questions.

You'll get a score between 0-100. A low score means cancer has a lower probability of returning, and you have a lower (albeit not zero) chance of benefiting from chemotherapy. A high score means cancer has a higher chance of recurring, and there is a higher chance that you will benefit from chemotherapy. she can discuss the results with you and answer your questions.

Let's look at the meaning of your Recurrence Score (RS):

> • **If you are over 50 years old,** there is no benefit to receiving chemotherapy if your score is 0 to 25. On the other hand, there is a more than 15 percent benefit if your RS is 26 to 100.

> • **If you are 50 or under,** there is no benefit to chemotherapy if your Recurrence Score is 0 to 15. On the other hand, if your RS is 16 to 20, the chemotherapy benefit is 1.6 percent, and if the RS is 21 to 25, it is 6.5 percent. Finally, for a Recurrence Score of 26 to 100, there is more than a 15 percent benefit associated with chemotherapy.

> • **When the recurrence score is low (0 to 10),** it is prognostic for a very low distant recurrence rate (two percent) at ten years.

Later in this chapter, we will look at the use of OncotypeDX for those with spread to regional lymph nodes (node-positive). Let's look at hother genomic tests.

EndoPredict

Other genomic tests can also guide the provision of chemotherapy. For those with estrogen receptor-positive, HER2-negative invasive breast cancer, EndoPredict calculates the chance that your cancer will return in the ten years after treatment, offering important information about how aggressive your cancer is.

EndoPredict can predict who might benefit from chemotherapy. If you fall into the low EPclin score group (less than 3.3), there appears to be no benefit to adding chemotherapy to endocrine therapy; on the other hand, patients with a higher EndoPredict score have a potential benefit from chemotherapy.

MammoPrint (Amsterdam 70-gene profile)

For those with early breast cancer, this test assesses the risk that cancer will spread to distant sites of the body. It gives a binary result, high-risk or low-risk, and can help your oncologist decide whether or not you would likely benefit from chemotherapy. Recent results from the MINDACT clinical trial provide the highest level of medical evidence, confirming the test's ability to identify Low-Risk patients based on the genomic fingerprint of cancer who are not likely to show a significant benefit from chemotherapy.

In the landmark MINDACT study, 46 percent of patients were identified as at high risk for recurrence according to traditional clinical and pathologic factors (and who would therefore have been candidates for chemotherapy) were classified as Low Risk by MammaPrint, and were not likely to have a significant benefit from chemotherapy.

The American Association of Clinical Oncology has suggested that Mamma-Print is one of several tests that may be used to determine the prognosis for those with high clinical risk, hormone receptor-positive, HER2 negative breast cancer and no or limited (one to three) involved noes in informing decisions regarding withholding chemotherapy.

Breast Cancer Index (BCI)

The BCI is an accurate predictor of responsiveness to endocrine therapy (such as letrozole), with lower-level evidence indicating that it may identify those who would benefit from extended endocrine therapy.

PAM50 risk of recurrence score

The Predictor Analysis of Microarray 50 (PAM50) test has prognostic utility: In the ABCSG-8 trial, the estimated 10-year distant relapse-free survival rates were about 98, 91, and 80 percent in the low-, intermediate-, and high-risk groups based on the ROR (risk of recurrence) score.

Other assays

While there are several other genomic assays, they are not ready for routine use outside a clinical trial.

Genomic assay: Profiling your cancer

Gene expression tests allow for personalized medicine. Testing can allow you to learn more about your cancer and to individualize your breast cancer management. Here are the National Comprehensive Cancer Network Guidelines' take: "Predictive" addresses the ability to estimate response to chemotherapy. "Prognosis" points to survival estimates.

Test	Predictive	Prognostic	Preference
Oncotype DX (no nodes +)	Yes	Yes	Preferred
Oncotype DX (0 or 1-3 nodes +)			
MammaPrint (0 or 1-3 nodes +)	Not determined	Yes	Premenopausal: Other
Prosigna (0 or 1-3 nodes +)	Not determined	Yes	Other
EndoPredict (0 or 1-3 nodes +)	Not determined	Yes	Other
Breast Cancer Index	Yes, of extended endocrine therapy after surgery	Yes	Other

These gene expression assays complement T, N, M, and biomarker information. Gene expression testing is not required for staging. The National Comprehensive Cancer Network (www.nccn.org) prefers the Oncotype DX test for prognosis and predicting chemotherapy benefits. Other prognostic gene expression assays can give prognosis information, but the ability to predict chemotherapy benefits is not as clear.

Chemotherapy - Who Needs It? Oncotype DX

Hormone receptor-positive (ER/PR +), HER2 negative breast cancer:

Test	RS*	Treatment implications
Oncotype DX Postmenopausal with 0 to 3 nodes involved	Under 26	Patients with T1b/c, pN0 cancer with RS 0-10 have a metastasis risk of less than 4%, and those with RS 11 to 25 have no benefit from adding chemo to endocrine therapy.
	26 or higher	Patients with pT1-3, pN0-1a cancer have a significant potential benefit from adding chemo to endocrine therapy.
Oncotype DX Premenopausal with no nodes involved	15 or lower	Premenopausal patients with T1b/c, pN0, with RS under 16 have no benefit from adding chemotherapy to endocrine therapy.
	16 to 25	There may be a small chemotherapy benefit; it is unclear if the benefit is due to ovarian suppression caused by chemo. Options include chemo followed by endocrine therapy versus ovarian function suppression combined with tamoxifen or an aromatase inhibitor.
	26 or higher	Chemotherapy, followed by endocrine therapy, is recommended.
Oncotype DX Premenopausal with 1 to 3 nodes involved	Under 26	There may be a small chemotherapy benefit; it is unclear if the benefit is due to ovarian suppression caused by chemo. Options include chemo followed by endocrine therapy versus ovarian function suppression combined with tamoxifen or an aromatase inhibitor.
	26 or higher	Chemotherapy, followed by endocrine therapy, is recommended.

* Recurrence Score (RS)

Test	Risk	Treatment implications
MammaPrint 0 to 3 nodes involved	Low	Low-risk patients have a 1.3 percent recurrence chance. High-risk patients have an 11.7 percent recurrence chance and have significantly better outcomes with chemotherapy. Nearly half of clinically high-risk patients were reclassified as MammaPrint Low Risk and could forgo chemo without compromising their outcomes.
	High	
Prosigna 0 to 3 nodes involved	Node negative: Low (0-40); Intermediate (41-60); High (61-100)	The average 10 year chance of metastases is: • Low-risk group 4 percent • Intermediate-risk group 11 percent • High-risk group 22 percent
	Node positive: Low (0-40)	The average 10 year chance of metastases is: • Low-risk group 6 percent • Intermediate-risk group 10 percent • High-risk group 28 percent
	Node positive: High (41-100)	
EndoPredict Premenopausal with 1 to 3 nodes involved	Low (3.3 or less)	Low-risk score: Regardless of the T size, the 10-year risk for those without node involvement was four percent (ANCSG 6/8) in clinical trials. Those with 1 to 3 nodes involved and a low score had a 5.6 percent distant recurrence rate in the TransATAC study. The test is prognostic in endocrine and chemo-endocrine-treated patients.
	High (over 3.3)	

Residual cancer following preoperative therapy

Patients with "triple-negative" breast cancer who have residual invasive cancer after receiving neoadjuvant (before surgery) chemotherapy for HER2-negative breast cancer have suboptimal prognoses: Among patients who did not have a pathological complete response, more than 20 percent have a relapse within five years. Now we have data from the CREATE-X clinical trial to inform patients whether additional chemotherapy might improve outcomes.

Create-X trial: Oral chemotherapy (Xeloda®) benefits some

Researchers randomly assigned 910 patients with HER2-negative residual invasive breast cancer after neoadjuvant chemotherapy (containing an anthracycline such as doxorubicin/Adriamycin or a taxane) to receive standard care after surgery, either with oral chemotherapy known as **capecitabine** (Xeloda) or without it. Here are the conclusions of the authors:

The Capecitabine for Residual Cancer as Adjuvant Therapy (CREATE-X) randomly assigned 900 patients with HER2-negative breast cancer and residual disease after chemotherapy had chemotherapy before surgery. The patients had anthracycline or taxane chemotherapy. They were then assigned to receive the oral chemotherapy capecitabine (Xeloda) or not.

The capecitabine group had better disease-free survival (74 versus 79 percent) and overall survival odds (89 versus 84 percent). A subgroup analysis suggested that improving disease-free survival with capecitabine resulted in better outcomes for those with triple-negative disease (70 versus 56 percent). For those with HER2-positive cancers who have residual disease after chemotherapy and Herceptin before surgery (neoadjuvant treatment), adding ado-trastuzumab emtansine or Kadcyla improves outcomes.

Capecitabine (Xeloda) downsides

The hand-foot syndrome was the most frequent side effect in 73 percent of patients, including 11.1 percent, for which it was rather severe. Over 40 percent of patients had drops in their blood counts. The most common non-blood side effects, fatigue, nausea, diarrhea, inflammation of the mouth, and increases in some blood markers, occurred in over 20 percent. All of the serious adverse events resolved and were non-fatal.

The National Comprehensive Cancer Network endorses post-operative capecitabine (Xeloda) for those with "triple-negative" breast cancer who do not have a complete response to preoperative systemic therapy. The standard approach for those with a BRCA mutation is olaparib for one year.

Not all studies have demonstrated improved outcomes with adding the oral chemotherapy agent capecitabine. For example, the GEICAM/2003-11 clinical trial found no improvements in disease-free survival when adding capecitabine (Xeloda) to standard chemotherapy for patients with early triple-negative breast cancer.

The GEICAM/2003-11 study authors note several research limitations. The trial was open-label; patients knew whether they were getting the drug. Second, the population enrolled demonstrated a much lower recurrence rate than expected. This latter finding can compromise the ability to show a difference between treatment approaches.

Olaparib (Lynparza™)

For post-operative treatment of those with high-risk early breast cancer who have a deleterious BRCA mutation (and have been treated with chemotherapy before or after surgery), olaparib (a pill) is recommended. Those with BRCA mutations and metastases may also use the drug.

The most common side effects include nausea, fatigue, anemia, vomiting, diarrhea, diminished appetite, headache, taste changes, cough, neutropenia, shortness of breath, dizziness, and white blood cell and platelet decreases.

> The National Comprehensive Cancer Network Guidelines, version 4.2022, offer that for those with triple-negative breast cancer (who have systemic therapy before surgery) if there is any residual cancer in the breast or nodes, options include:
>
> - Capecitabine (Xeloda) for six to eight cycles
> - Olaparib for one year, if there is a germline BRCA mutation
> - Immunotherapy (pembrolizumab/Keytruda) for those who had pembrolizumab preoperatively.

For those with triple-negative breast cancer with a complete pathological response to preoperative systemic therapy, the care team may offer additional immunotherapy to those at high risk (Stages II/III) who received it before surgery.

Invasive

Management: Chemotherapy - Special populations

Older patients (over 65)

If the risk of recurrence is sufficiently high (and the patient has a good performance status), chemotherapy may be valuable. Older patients should have a geriatric assessment before committing to chemotherapy, however. We have less information for those over 70, but performance status and other health conditions can be invaluable in decision-making.

The HOPE clinical trial evaluated women with high-risk early breast cancer aged 65 years and older who were initiating chemotherapy before or after surgery. With a median follow-up of four years, here are the findings:

  • Twenty-one percent of patients received less than 85 percent of the relative dose intensity. This lower chemotherapy intensity was associated with older age, lower performance status, and the chemotherapy regimen (anthracycline versus CMF).

  • Dose reduction, treatment delays, or early discontinuation of therapy was associated with inferior survival outcomes.

Male breast cancer

The same factors used for women with breast cancer inform chemotherapy decisions for males.

Breast cancer in pregnancy (gestational pregnancy)

We define **gestational breast cancer** (pregnancy-associated breast cancer) as breast cancer discovered during pregnancy, in the first year after delivery of the baby, or any time during lactation. Modern studies suggest no negative impact on survival compared to non-pregnancy breast cancer. It appears safe to administer many breast cancer drugs after the first trimester.

We have the most data for anthracycline-based chemotherapy, such as with Adriamycin. An emerging body of literature suggests that taxanes are safe during the second and third trimesters of pregnancy.

Timing of chemotherapy administration is critical; the medical oncologist will take care of your blood counts to reduce your risk of infection or bleeding. In general, chemotherapy is not given three to four weeks before the baby is due to be born. Herceptin (trastuzumab) is avoided during pregnancy, and we don't know if the other anti-HER2 drugs are safe.

Many chemotherapy drugs are excreted in breast milk, and some studies have even found infants to have drops in the white blood cell count, a condition known as neutropenia. Out of caution, your doctor will likely recommend that breastfeeding be avoided in women receiving drugs such as chemotherapy, trastuzumab (Herceptin), endocrine therapy (tamoxifen, for example), and others.

Women should avoid drugs such as tamoxifen during pregnancy. Aromatase inhibitors (AIs) are not used for pre-menopausal women, but some may go on them if they have ovarian suppression. Pregnant women should not take an AI. Nursing mothers usually avoid tamoxifen as it can suppress lactation and potentially harm the child.

Obese women

Obesity is associated with lower survival among those with hormone

receptor-positive and HER2-negative breast cancer. Obesity alone (without other concerning factors raising the risk for recurrence) is not an indication of the receipt of chemotherapy.

Women of childbearing age

You may wish to consider a discussion with your doctor regarding the preservation of fertility.

Invasive

Management: Chemotherapy details

How

- Chemotherapy is most commonly injected into a vein. Less commonly, it may be given in pill form or injected into the muscle or fat tissue below the skin.

When

- After surgery (adjuvant chemotherapy) or, less commonly, before surgery (neoadjuvant chemotherapy). Neoadjuvant chemotherapy (NACT) for breast cancer can make breast-conserving surgery more feasible for those with larger cancers. The timing of chemotherapy does not affect your survival chances, but large cancers downsized by neoadjuvant treatment might have a higher local recurrence chance after breast-conserving therapy than tumors of the same size in women who have not received neoadjuvant treatment.

- Chemotherapy typically starts within 4 to 8 weeks after surgery.

- Drugs are often given on a 14, 21, or 28-day cycle.

- Total treatment length varies but often lasts from 3 to 6 months.

What

- Chemotherapy often works best with combinations of drugs. There are many chemotherapy regimens, and you and your medical oncologist will select one based on factors such as your age and health, cancer characteristics (including grade, HER2 status, and estrogen receptors), and stage.

- Some drug combinations are illustrated on the next page.

Chemotherapy drugs

Chemo	Names
CMF	cyclophosphamide (Cytoxan), methotrexate (Rheumatrex), 5-fluorouracil (Adrucil)
CAF (FAC)	cyclophosphamide (Cytoxan), doxorubicin (Adriamycin), 5-fluorouracil (Adrucil)
AC	doxorubicin (Adriamycin), cyclophosphamide (Cytoxan)
TAC	docetaxel (Taxotere), doxorubicin (Adriamycin), and cyclophosphamide (Cytoxan)
AC, T	doxorubicin (Adriamycin) and cyclophosphamide (Cytoxan), followed by paclitaxel (Taxol) or docetaxel (Taxotere)
TC	docetaxel (Taxotere), cyclophosphamide (Cytoxan)

Invasive

Management: HER-2 positive

Breast cancer is a group of diseases with several biologic subtypes. One subtype is known as HER2-overexpressing. HER2/neu (human epidermal growth factor receptor 2) is a growth-promoting protein that sticks out of the cell surface like an antenna. About 20 percent of breast cancers will have overexpression of the oncogene and are called HER2-positive. At diagnosis, your doctor will check your cancer to see if it has higher levels than normal (overexpression) of HER2. We have powerful treatment tools for this aggressive subtype of breast cancer, including chemotherapy combined with drugs (such as trastuzumab (Herceptin)) that target the HER2 pathway.

What qualifies as HER2 positive?

Your cancer (biopsy or surgical material) is tested for HER2 overexpression, typically by one of these tests:

- Immunohistochemistry (IHC) test: Score of 3+ (the scale is 0 to 3)*

- Fluorescent *in situ* hybridization (FISH)

Herceptin-based treatment: Who needs it?

The clinical trials that established the benefit of adding Herceptin-containing systemic therapy included women with lymph node involvement by cancer or those without such involvement but thought to be at high risk for recurrence. This latter group included women with primary cancers over one centimeter in size. Still, there is lower level evidence to suggest that there may be significant benefit from Herceptin with chemotherapy for patients with smaller primary cancers.

---

* If the result is 0 or 1+, the cancer is HER2-negative (and generally does not respond to drugs targeting HER2); if the result is 2+, the HER2 status is not clear ("equivocal"), and we need to do a FISH test to get an answer. For metastatic disease, cancers that have Her2 scores 1+, 2+, or 3+ may respond.

Background

In 1996, the US Food and Drug Administration approved Herceptin as part of a treatment containing doxorubicin (Adriamycin), cyclophosphamide, and paclitaxel chemotherapy as adjuvant treatment of patients with HER2-positive, node-positive breast cancer. The history of this revolutionary drug, and the critical role played by leaders such as Dr. Dennis Slamon, are detailed in Robert Bazell's book Her-2: The Making of Herceptin, a Revolutionary Treatment for Breast Cancer. The book is a medical thriller, and I think it is well worth the read. Check out Living Proof with Harry Connick Jr for those who prefer film.

The evidence

Several large clinical trials have demonstrated the effectiveness of chemotherapy plus Herceptin (trastuzumab). We can divide the approaches into ones that contain a type of chemotherapy known as anthracyclines (Adriamycin/doxorubicin is an example) and non-anthracycline ones. Here are two landmark trials that established Herceptin as a breakthrough drug for those whose tumors overexpress HER-2.

	Who	What
NSABP B-31	HER-2 overexpressing and nodes involved with cancer	Chemotherapy (AC) 4 times, followed by paclitaxel chemotherapy, with or without Herceptin beginning with the first treatment of paclitaxel
NCCTG N-9831	HER-2 overexpressing and nodes involved *or* High risk*, but nodes uninvolved	Chemotherapy (AC) 4 times, followed by weekly paclitaxel (T) chemotherapy for 12 weeks (no Herceptin) *or* AC then T chemotherapy followed by Herceptin *or* AC then TH, followed by Herceptin

* Estrogen receptor-negative and primary size over one centimeters versus node-negative or estrogen receptor- positive and primary over two centimeters.

339

Researchers combined the two large studies examining whether Herceptin (trastuzumab) improved outcomes. There were 4,045 patients included in the joint analysis, with a median follow-up of 3.9 years. The inclusion of Herceptin led to a near-halving of the risk of recurrence (hazard ratio 0.61) and a more than a third (39 percent) reduction in the risk of death. Researchers found similar benefits to Herceptin when they looked at the studies separately.

Downsides

There are some downsides. Patients treated with trastuzumab had a higher chance of suffering from cardiac toxicity. The rates of congestive heart failure (CHF) or cardiac-related death range from 0% (Fin-HER trial) to 4.1 percent (NSABP trial). In comparison, the NCCTG trial found the three-year congestive heart failure or cardiac death incidence to be 0.3 percent with no Herceptin, 2.8 percent with Herceptin following chemotherapy, and 3.3 percent in the Herceptin initially combined with paclitaxel chemotherapy groups. These findings point to the need for careful (and ongoing) monitoring of cardiac problems.

Tremendous benefits

A 2012 analysis of eight trials confirmed the benefits of adding trastuzumab (Herceptin) to chemotherapy for patients with HER2- positive breast cancer:

- *Improvement in disease-free survival*

  Patients with HER2 overexpression were **nearly half as likely to recur if they had Herceptin added to chemotherapy** (hazard ratio for relapse 0.6). This benefit appears whether the Herceptin is given during and after chemotherapy or after chemotherapy alone. However, only the first approach yielded a survival improvement; sequential chemotherapy followed by Herceptin did not provide the same benefit.

- *Improvement in overall survival*

  Patients with Herceptin added to chemotherapy were one-third less likely to die than those not receiving Herceptin. While Herceptin for six months seemed to provide some benefit, the improvement was smaller than for one year.

For patients with estrogen receptor-positive breast cancer, endocrine therapy begins after the chemotherapy portion of treatment is complete; the "anti-estrogen" drugs begin during (and after) the continuing Herceptin.

1/2

That's the approximate reduction in the risk
or recurrence with Herceptin combined with
chemotherapy, compared to chemotherapy alone.

Herceptin benefits long-lasting

The benefits of Herceptin are long-lasting. The combined North Central Cancer Treatment Group and National Surgical Adjuvant Breast and Bowel Project studies published data at a median follow-up of 8.4 years. The addition of Herceptin led to a 37 percent improvement in overall survival and a 40 percent improvement in disease-free survival.

How is Herceptin given?

Your medical oncology nurse will typically administer Herceptin through a vein. In the period after chemotherapy, Herceptin is given once every three weeks and is generally well-tolerated. The infusion itself is typically much quicker than with chemotherapy.

How long will I be on Herceptin?

The 2012 meta-analysis (review of a collection of studies) supports using one year of Herceptin rather than shorter periods. Here are some results from studies looking at various durations of Herceptin:

- Herceptin: One versus two years

    The Herceptin Adjuvant (HERA) trial included 5,090 women with HER2-positive breast cancer who had completed chemotherapy. They randomly assigned the patients to observation or Herceptin for one or two years. There were no differences in disease-free or overall survival odds at the eight-year follow-up.

- Herceptin: Six versus 12 months

    The Protocol for Herceptin as Adjuvant therapy with Reduced Exposure (PHARE) trial randomly assigned 3,380 women to 6 versus 12 months of Herceptin. At a median follow-up of 42.5 months, treatment for six months resulted in a lower two-year disease-free survival (91 percent, compared to 94 percent for one year of Herceptin). The shorter-duration patients also were nearly 1.5 times more likely to die of the disease.

I had chemotherapy and Herceptin before surgery.

Herceptin typically continues for a cumulative one year. However, suppose you have residual cancer in the breast or regional nodes. Recent data suggests a significant benefit from adding trastuzumab emtansine (also known as ado-trastuzumab emtansine or Kadcyla) after surgery.

Kadcyla for those with residual disease after preoperative systemic therapy

After receiving neoadjuvant chemotherapy and Herceptin, patients with **residual breast cancer** have a worse prognosis than those without residual cancer. Kadcyla (T-DM1 or ado-trastuzumab emtansine) benefits patients with metastatic breast cancer previously treated with chemotherapy plus HER2-targeted therapy. In this context, researchers conducted a randomized trial for patients with HER2-positive early breast cancer who had residual invasive disease in the breast or axillary nodes at surgery.

Patients were randomly assigned to receive Kadcyla (T-DM1) or Herceptin. The estimated percentage of patients free of invasive disease at three years was 88.3% in the T-DM1 group and 77 percent in the Herceptin group. Distant recurrence as the first invasive-disease event occurred in 10.5 percent of patients in the T-DM1 group and 15.9 percent in the trastuzumab group.

In conclusion, for those with residual disease at surgery following neoadjuvant chemotherapy and Herceptin, switching from Herceptin to Kadcyla after surgery improves outcomes.

Newer Treatments (HER2-positive)

Enhertu

The US Food and Drug Administration approved Enhertu (fam-trastuzumab deruteçan-nxki) In 2019 for treating HER2-positive breast cancer. Enhertu is for patients who have had at least two other treatments for their HER2-positive breast cancer that has metastasized or cannot be surgically removed.

Enhertu is composed of three components:

- Fam-trastazumab, an anti-HER2 medication

- DXd, a so-called topoisomerase inhibitor that prevents cancer cells from dividing

- A compound that links the other components

In a clinical study of 184 women, most people treated with Enhertu saw their tumors shrink. Some (about 4 percent) had a complete response - imaging could no longer demonstrate cancer. Most (56 percent) got a partial response, meaning their tumor shrank by at least 30 percent.

Overall, 97 percent saw their tumor shrink, stop growing, or slow growth rate. Half of the people who responded to Enhertu maintained their response for nearly 15 months.

Nerlynx (neratinib)

The US Food and Drug Administration approved neratinib in 2017 for early-stage breast cancer (and in 2020 for metastatic cancer) in combination with the pill chemotherapy drug capecitabine (Xeloda). Your medical oncologist may offer neratinib if you have had at least two other treatments for HER2-positive breast cancer.

The NALA clinical trial randomized those with metastatic HER2-positive disease to neratinib plus capecitabine (oral drugs) or lapatinib plus capecitabine. The one-year progression-free rate was 29 percent versus 15 percent, favoring neratinib.

Special situations

I'm a male with Her2-positive breast cancer.
The Herceptin-based recommendations are the same as for women.

Pregnancy
Herceptin may not be used during pregnancy, as we don't have sufficient evidence to know if it is safe. It is also recommended not to breastfeed while on the drug. Selected patients may have *chemotherapy* after the first trimester.

Pre-existing heart issues
It is especially important to have close monitoring of cardiac function. Some potential factors that may increase your risk include age over 50, pre-existing cardiac problems, being overweight, and high blood pressure.

Breast cancer is small, and nodes are uninvolved
The clinical trials that established Herceptin benefits limited eligibility to women with either node-positive or high-risk, node-negative tumors. What should you do if your primary cancer is one centimeter or less, and your nodes are uninvolved? That answer is not entirely clear, but the available research suggests that such patients are at a higher risk of recurrence than similar patients with node-negative breast cancer.

The benefits of Herceptin for patients with small (31 percent had primary cancer 6-10 mm; 17 percent had cancers 5 mm or smaller), HER2-positive cancer were evaluated in a non-randomized trial (all patients were treated with paclitaxel chemotherapy and Herceptin). The three-year invasive cancer-free survival was 98.7 percent, and recurrence-free survival was 99.2 percent.

While this was not a randomized trial (and therefore only provides low-level evidence), these outcomes suggest a potential role for chemotherapy and Herceptin for small cancers, even if they are not associated with spread to regional nodes.

CAR-T cells
Researchers at City of Hope (USA) have opened a first-in-human clinical trial to assess the use of chimeric antigen receptor T-cell (CAR-T) therapy for patients with HER2-positive breast cancer that has spread to the brain. Here, immune system cells are removed from the body, genetically re-engineered to be more effective, and injected back in.

Invasive

Management: "Triple-negative"

Cell receptors are antennae-like structures that receive messages from substances (such as estrogen) in your bloodstream. The receptors then guide the cell's behavior. For example, hormone receptors inside (and on the surface of) the cell may receive messages from the hormones estrogen and progesterone. About two-thirds of breast cancer will be positive for estrogen- and progesterone receptors. A smaller percentage of patients with breast cancer will have too many HER2 receptors. Fortunately, we have therapies that target these receptors, at least for those whose cancers have them.

Aggressive

Approximately 15 to 20 percent of patients will have breast cancer that does not have receptors for estrogen, progesterone, or HER2. Such cancers are known as "triple negative." As these cells lack these receptors, we cannot target them with anti-estrogen or anti-HER2 drugs. In addition, triple-negative breast cancers tend to be more aggressive than other types of breast cancer. The cells tend to be higher grade than other breast cancer types. Generally, this breast cancer subtype has the greatest risk of distant metastases. The distant recurrence chances peaks at three years and decline rapidly after that.

Systemic therapy

For individuals with triple-negative breast cancer, treatment may include some combination of surgery, radiation therapy, and systemic therapy such as chemotherapy. For most of those with triple-negative breast cancer, chemotherapy is recommended. The primary goal is to reduce the probability of metastasis (cancer spreads to distant body parts such as the bones, liver, lungs, or brain).

Details

Chemotherapy may be given before (neoadjuvant) or after (adjuvant) surgery. The neoadjuvant approach may be used if your primary cancer is large, the in-inflammatory type, or if there is a significant disease burden in regional nodes. This approach can lead to tumor shrinkage and help your doctors better understand how sensitive it is to chemotherapy.

346

Your chemotherapy may (or may not) be the same type given to individuals with hormone receptor-positive or HER2-positive breast cancer. Studies show chemotherapy often works better against triple-negative breast cancer than hormone receptor-positive disease.

Your medical oncologist may not recommend that you receive chemotherapy; for example, if you have a very low-grade tumor, if the tumor is very small, or if the risks of chemotherapy outweigh the benefits. Because chemotherapy is a common treatment for triple-negative breast cancer, your medical oncologist will likely recommend it.

National Comprehensive Cancer Network Guidelines, 4.2022

If the estrogen and progesterone receptor statuses were determined from a biopsy (non-surgical), the tests might be repeated on the surgical specimen. This approach reduces the chance of a sampling error for a heterogeneous tumor.

Triple-negative with nodes involved: Chemotherapy recommended

For those with node involvement, chemotherapy is a Category 1 recommendation, meaning there is consensus based on high-level evidence. There should also be consideration of adjuvant (after surgery) "bone hardening drugs" - bisphosphonates - for risk reduction of distant metastases for three to five years in postmenopausal patients. Adding of one year of olaparib (after chemotherapy) is an option for select patients with BRCA mutations. Those with residual disease after neoadjuvant chemotherapy may consider oral chemotherapy (capecitabine for six to eight cycles) or continue immunotherapy (if given before surgery. Finally, those with a germline BRCA mutation have olaparib for one year.

You should consider adjuvant (after surgery) chemotherapy if the tumor is five millimeters or smaller (but there is a microscopic spread to a node (pN1mi).

Triple-negative with no nodes involved

- For those with tumors 5 millimeters and no node involvement, no drugs are recommended.

- For those with tumors six to 10 millimeters, you should consider chemotherapy.

- For those with more than one-centimeter tumors, the chemotherapy recommendation is based on high-level evidence.

Invasive cancer

Immunotherapy

Immunotherapy medicines unleash the power of your body's immune system to attack cancer cells. Immunotherapy drugs for breast cancer haven't demonstrated results as strong as for other cancers.

Immunotherapy medicines include:

> • **Keytruda** (chemical name: pembrolizumab) is a checkpoint inhibitor immunotherapy drug used to treat some metastatic breast cancers. Pembrolizumab is given by vein (through an IV).

Pembrolizumab (Keytruda) targets PD-1 (a protein on immune system T cells that normally helps keep them from attacking other cells in the body). By blocking PD-1, these drugs boost the immune response against breast cancer cells. Immunotherapy may be used with chemotherapy to treat "triple-negative" breast cancer:

- Before surgery (neoadjuvant) for stage II or III breast cancer

- After surgery (adjuvant) for stage II or III breast cancer

- For cancer that has come back (recurred) locally but a surgeon cannot remove it.

- For metastatic (spread to distant sites) breast cancer

Pembrolizumab is given by vein, typically every three or six weeks. Sometimes, your doctor will test your cancer cells to see the levels of the PD-L1 protein, an indicator or likelihood to respond to immunotherapy.

Immunotherapy: Potential side effects

Potential side effects of these drugs can include cough, nausea, fatigue, skin rash, constipation, diarrhea, and poor appetite. More serious possible complications include the following:

Infusion reactions (uncommon)

While receiving the drug, individuals may have an allergic-lie reaction to immunotherapy. Symptoms may include rash, itchy skin, fever, chills, flushing face, dizziness, wheezing, and difficulty breathing.

Autoimmune reactions

Immunotherapy removes one of the immune system's protections (a checkpoint). Immunotherapy can allow the immune system to attack other body parts, including the intestines, liver, lungs, hormone-producing glands (such as the thyroid), or other organs.

You may hear terms such as colitis (colon inflammation), pneumonitis (lung inflammation), or thyroiditis (thyroid inflammation).

Please immediately inform your healthcare team if you experience any of these symptoms. Treatment must sometimes stop; some patients need high doses of corticosteroids to suppress the immune system.

Invasive

Chemotherapy: Lymph node involvement

Patients with node involvement are often offered chemotherapy. In addition, if the cancer is estrogen- or progesterone receptor-positive, endocrine therapy is taken (after completion of chemotherapy). For those who have HER2 overexpression, therapy targeting HER-2 is added to chemotherapy. Select patients who are HER2 negative and have only 1 to 3 nodes involved may consider a breast cancer assay (such as Oncotype DX) to help guide decision-making regarding the addition of chemotherapy to endocrine therapy.

Not all individuals with hormone receptor-positive with one to three nodes involved will need chemotherapy

Some patients with axillary node involvement derive no benefit from chemotherapy. These include postmenopausal women with one to three nodes involved who have a low recurrence score.

The RxPONDER study found that **postmenopausal** women with hormone receptor-positive, HER2-negative breast cancer with one to three positive nodes and a 21-gene (Oncotype DX) Recurrence Score of 25 or less derived no further benefit from chemotherapy added to endocrine therapy.

On the other hand, **premenopausal** women with the same characteristics had a nearly halving (45 percent reduction) in the risk of invasive disease events with the addition of chemotherapy. Premenopausal patients with one to three positive nodes and an RS of 25 or less should consider chemotherapy. The invasive disease-free survival rate improved by 5 percent with chemotherapy in this group.

The 2022 updated analysis shows that postmenopausal women with a recurrence score of 0 to 25 continue to *not* benefit from the addition of chemotherapy to endocrine therapy. But premenopausal women with a recurrence score of 0 to 25 benefit from adjuvant chemotherapy, which is associated with a near halving (44 to 46 percent) decrease in invasive disease–free survival, distant recurrence–free survival, and disease recurrence–free interval events."

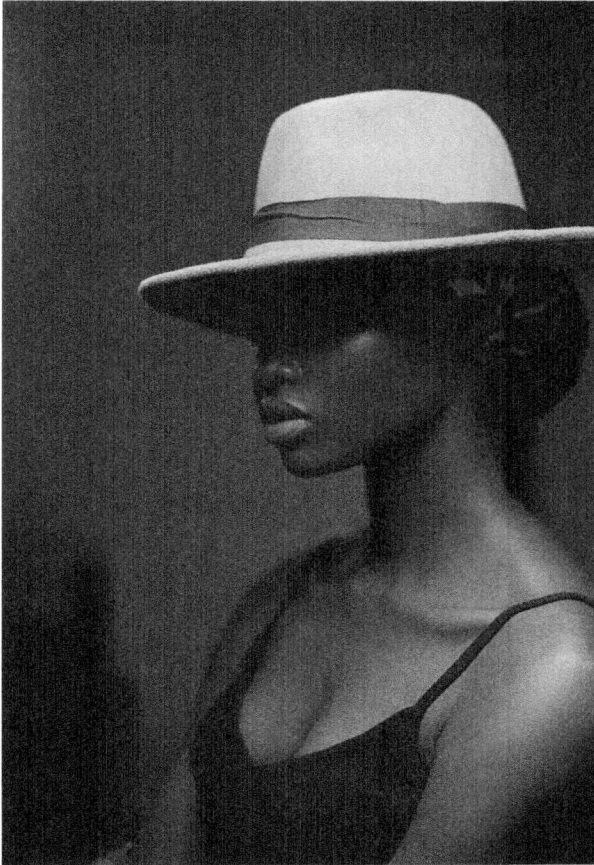

RxPONDER showed a benefit from adding chemotherapy to the surgery, radiation, and standard endocrine therapy given to premenopausal women with 1 to 3 involved axillary nodes and Oncotype recurrence scores (RS) less than 26.

The 2022 update showed an invasive disease-free survival absolute benefit of 4.9 percent and a distant recurrence-free survival absolute benefit of 2.5 percent.

Mouth and throat sores

Chemotherapy preferentially affects rapidly growing cells. Given the cells in our mouth and throat turn over regularly, it is perhaps not surprising that some chemotherapy drugs can cause problems such as sores or dryness in your lips or mouth (including your tongue, gums, roof or floor of mouth). Such drugs include (but are not limited to) capecitabine (Xeloda), fluorouracil, methotrexate, and doxorubicin.

Begin with a dental evaluation before you begin chemotherapy. During your course of chemotherapy, brushing your teeth (with a soft toothbrush) after each meal and before bedtime can be helpful, as can toothpaste with baking soda and peroxide. Try to floss daily. If you smoke, stop. Finally, ask your medical oncologist if you can eat a diet rich in fruits and vegetables. Avoid alcohol-containing mouthwashes.

Many patients who receive fluorouracil (5-FU) as a part of their chemotherapy find it helpful to swish ice chips or cold water in their mouths during the first 30 minutes of treatment: The cold appears to reduce the amount of drug that reaches your mouth. If you develop mouth sores, ask a care team member whether medications that coat the lining of your mouth might be appropriate for you. Some patients benefit from painkillers applied directly to the sore spot, which can cause numbness (so be especially careful when eating or brushing your teeth).

Other helpful strategies may include avoidance of acidic, spicy, and hot (temperature) foods. Sharp and crunchy foods such as crackers, pretzels, and chips can be challenging for many. You should avoid alcohol as well. On the positive side, try eating small meals more frequently (cutting food into small pieces and eating slowly). Consider using a straw to keep liquids away from mouth sores. Finally, try rinsing your mouth several times daily with a weak salt water solution or a combination of baking soda and warm water.

Hair loss (alopecia)

During chemotherapy, your hair may thin or fall out, depending on which drug(s) you receive. By hair, I also mean your eyebrows, eyelashes, and body. While the hair typically regrows soon after completion of chemotherapy, the color or texture can change. Many patients will choose to cut their hair short beforehand, providing some degree of control. Others turn to mild shampoos and hair brushes and use low heat when drying their hair.

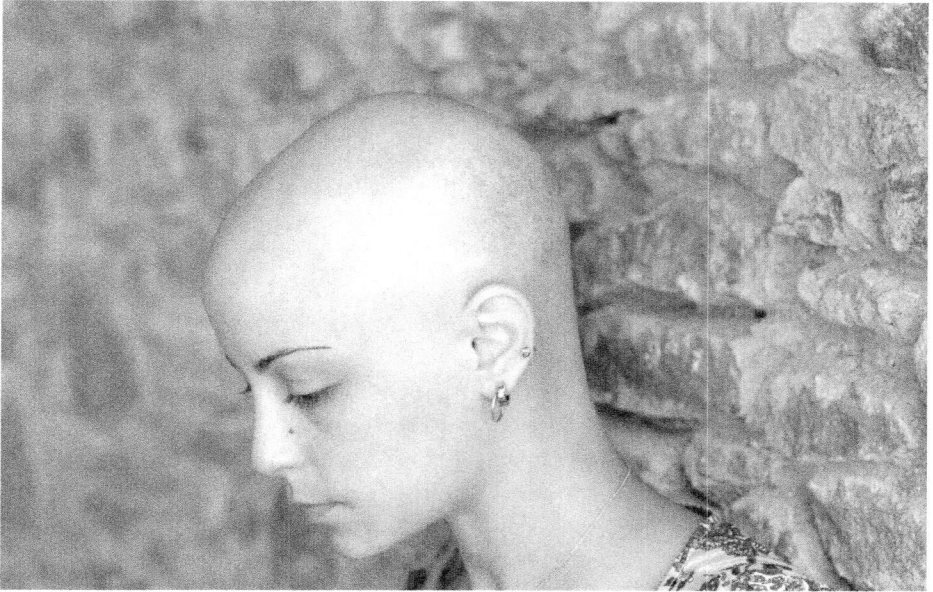

Hair loss

Within weeks after chemotherapy begins, many notice hair loss upon awakening, seeing it on their pillow. With brushing, they may see hair come out in clumps. This hair loss can be quite emotionally challenging. For many, wearing a wig, scarf, or cap can help them to feel more attractive. You can begin planning before chemotherapy if you are told that your hair will likely fall out.

- Wigs: If you want to wear a wig, you may want to shop before treatment to match your hair color.

- American Cancer Society can direct women to places to help them with wigs, and some ACS offices offer wigs. Some insurance plans will help cover the cost of a wig.

- Hats, turbans, and scarves can also help hide hair loss, although some prefer to leave their heads uncovered. But, if you go bareheaded, don't forget the sunscreen for your scalp if you go outside.

- Cutting your hair short may ease the inconvenience of shedding lots of hair and may make watching your hair fall out a bit less traumatic.

Scalp cooling for hair loss

Hair loss can be a devastating side effect of chemotherapy. Still, the recent US Food and Drug Administration (FDA) approval of the DigniCap Cooling System may improve the quality of life for many chemotherapy patients. Historically, scalp cooling has not been available in the United States, partly because of concerns that it wasn't effective at preventing hair loss and about potential scalp metastases and thermal injury.

Scalp cooling devices lower the scalp temperature to prevent hair loss during chemotherapy. There are several methods to do this, but typically a hypothermia cap is connected to a computer-controlled cooling unit. A coolant circulates through channels in the cap, and sensors help keep the temperature in the appropriate range. The scalp cooling results in your blood vessels in the scalp constricting, reducing blood flow to the hair follicles while the chemotherapy is at its maximum. As a result, your hair follicles are less exposed to chemotherapy.

There are downsides. In the short term, many patients complain about a cold sensation ("brain freeze") and headaches from the scalp cooling. Inflammation of the scalp and skin injuries are rare with device types that don't involve frozen caps. Fortunately, the data suggests no increased risk of scalp metastases, at least at an average follow-up of 2.5 years in a USA study. In that study, the DigniCap system prevented hair loss in 66.3% of patients with breast cancer (compared to those who did not have the cap). Of note, the patients in the research had Stage I/II breast cancer and were receiving taxane-based chemotherapy. Those getting an anthracycline such as doxorubicin (Adriamycin) were excluded. While scalp cooling doesn't prevent you from losing some hair, it may reduce volume loss. Still, cost remains a significant issue in the United States, as you likely would have to pay out of pocket.

Other side effects
- Fever or infection
- Neutropenia or thrombocytopenia (drops in white blood cells or platelets)
- Thrombocytopenia (drops in platelets)
- Dehydration or disturbances in blood chemistries
- Malnutrition
- Deep venous thrombosis or pulmonary embolism (clots that can spread to the lungs, sometimes becoming life-threatening)

⚠ Don't perm or color your hair during chemotherapy. Chemical treatments can enhance hair loss. Once your hair has begun to grow back (after completion of chemotherapy), you may perm or dye your hair.

Eyebrows and eyelashes

Some patients also feel upset about losing their eyebrows and eyelashes. The American Cancer Society offers a program called "Look Good, Feel Better," which teaches women makeup techniques to improve their appearance during cancer treatment, including tips for eyebrows and eyelashes.

Nail weakness

Some chemotherapy drugs can cause damage to your fingernails and toenails. Your nails may become brittle and sore and may even fall off. Fortunately, these problems are typically temporary. Still, if you develop nail inflammation or a rash that becomes open or is associated with a discharge, check in with your medical oncology team. The nail could be infected and, if needed, treated with antibiotics. Those who develop an infection in separated nails may be recommended to soak their fingers or toes in a solution of white vinegar and water for 15 minutes every night. It can help kill bacteria while drying the area out.

Infections

Chemotherapy may reduce the number of your infection-fighting white blood cells (WBCs), raising your infection risk. In this context, it is wise to wash your hands often and to stay away from others who are ill. Your physician should check your blood cell count before each treatment to ensure that you have enough white blood cells (platelets and red blood cells) to give you chemotherapy. If you get a small cut or nick of the skin, please clean it immediately.

⚠ Please notify your doctor immediately if you have any signs of infection (such as a fever or shaking chills).

Skin

Chemotherapy often causes dry and irritated skin. You may wish to be proactive: One week before chemotherapy, begin measures to optimize your skin condition. Itching is common and can stem from multiple causes: the chemotherapy drug, a patient's naturally dry skin (particularly in people over 50), or as a symptom of cancer itself. While many use over-the-counter hydrocortisone creams, they're often too weak to be effective, says Lacouture. Instead, doctors can treat itching with steroids or anesthetic medications applied to the skin. If itching interferes with sleep, oral medications might work.

Skin color changes can occur during chemotherapy, particularly with breast cancer treatment. The hands or face may be affected, making some feel self-conscious. If this happens, bleaching creams and exfoliants with salicylic acid are available. Here is advice from Dr. Lacouture (Memorial Sloan-Kettering Cancer Center), who focuses on treating side effects related to the skin, hair, and nails:

- Avoid long, hot showers or baths.

- Use gentle, fragrance-free soaps and laundry detergent.

- Use moisturizers, preferably creams or ointments rather than lotions (The thicker consistency is better at preventing skin dehydration). Apply the cream or ointment within 15 minutes of showering. Reapply at night, and moisturize your hands each time you wash them.

- If your skin is very dry and flaky, ammonium lactate cream can increase moisture. These are available by prescription and over the counter.

- Some chemotherapy drugs make skin more susceptible to sunburn. Use a sunscreen with at least an SPF 30, and make sure that it protects against both UVA and UVB rays. Protection against UVA requires ingredients such as zinc oxide, titanium dioxide, or avobenzone. Chemotherapy patients need to be smart about sun exposure. Use a broad-brimmed hat, sun-protective clothing, and an SPF of 30 reapplied every two hours if you're out side, more if you are swimming or sweating.

Side effects (toxicity): Collateral damage

Nausea and vomiting: Additional tips

Here are some tips for managing nausea, courtesy of the wonderful website www.breastcancer.org:

- Eat small amounts of food daily, so you don't feel full too quickly.

- Eat dry foods less likely to upset your stomach, like crackers, toast,

and cereal.

- Stay away from greasy foods that might disagree with your stomach.

- Try ginger-based foods to help ease nausea. These include ginger ale, ginger tea, or crystallized ginger eaten as a snack.

- Sit up after eating -- lying down after meals may disrupt digestion.
- Rinse your mouth before and after meals to eliminate bad tastes that may make you nauseous.

- Ask someone to cook for you or order take-out so you can avoid

strong smells that may be unpleasant for you.
- Ask your doctor about anti-nausea medications you can take before or after breast cancer treatment. You can also take anti-nausea medications with pain medications that nauseate you.

- Consider complementary and holistic techniques such as acupuncture, relaxation, and visualization to reduce nausea.

- Read tips on how to manage vomiting.

Check with your doctor, but swimming is fine for patients receiving chemotherapy as long as there are no open sores on your skin. However, hot tubs aren't a good idea. They can cause more blood flow to the skin, leading to greater blood flow to areas of inflammation. "There's no study that a hot tub will make it worse, but we tend to err on the cautious side," Dr. Lacouture offers.

Weight gain

Weight gain is commonly associated with chemotherapy for breast cancer. While the reasons are not entirely clear, chemotherapy can bring on menopause, which in turn can result in your gaining more body fat and losing lean muscle. Chemotherapy can also slow your metabolism, making it more challenging to keep weight off. Some women receive corticosteroids to help with chemotherapy-induced nausea and swelling. These drugs can stimulate appetite, increase body fat, and result in loss of muscle mass in your upper arms and legs.

Try to eat well and get some physical activity: Aim for a minimum of the equivalent of a brisk walk for 30 minutes daily. If that is not achievable, try to do what you can.

Fluid retention

If steroids are a part of your chemotherapy program, you may develop water retention. Fluid retention can also promote weight gain. Fluid retention is usually only temporary. Here are some suggestions for management:

- Elevate your feet as often as possible
- Don't stand for long periods
- Try not to sit with your legs crossed
- Avoid tight clothing
- Reduce your salt intake
- Weigh yourself daily

Dehydration

Staying hydrated can help alleviate some of the symptoms associated with receiving chemotherapy.

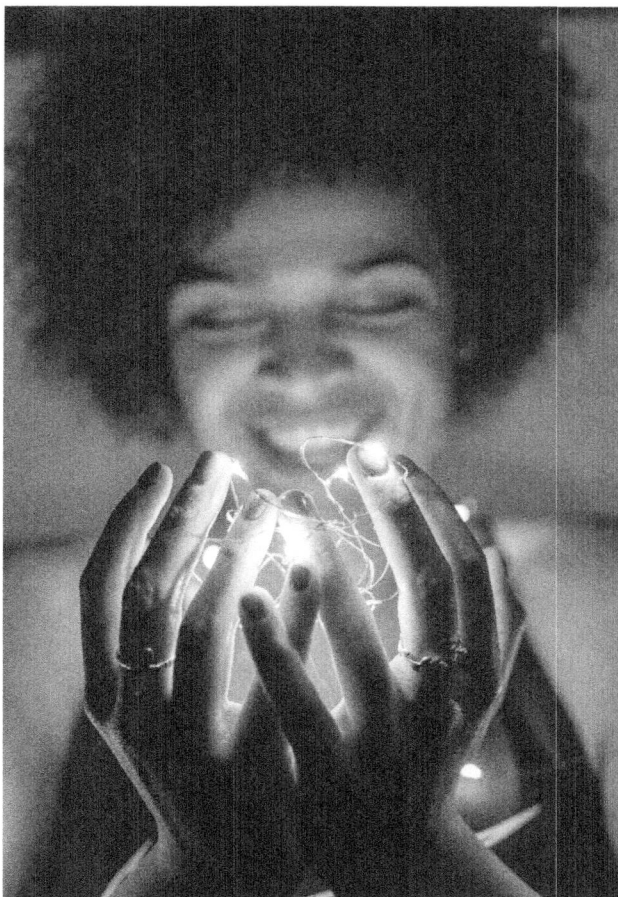

Invasive

Management: "Bone hardening" drugs

Bisphosphonates and RANK-ligand inhibitors

Bone-modifying agents (including bisphosphonates and the so-called RANK-ligand inhibitor denosumab) have a clear role in the management of patients with breast cancer spread to the bones and are even used to reduce the risk for bone fractures among high-risk populations without cancer. What is not entirely clear is the role of these drugs as a component of treatment for early-stage breast cancer.

A recent analysis of randomized trials suggests a role for these agents in women with breast cancer who have gone through menopause. Let's look at the takeaway lessons from this meta-analysis that included data from 18,766 women in 26 clinical trials:

- **Bisphosphonates**
  In consultation between the patient and oncologist, bisphosphonates should be considered for women after menopause with breast cancer who are considered candidates for systemic therapy. Disease characteristics and risk factors for the breakdown of the jaw bone (osteonecrosis) and kidney function impairment influence recommendations.

- **Zoledronic acid**
  Every 6 months for 3 to 5 years versus clodronate (daily) are the recommended bisphophonates.

- **Dental**
  An assessment is recommended before starting bisphophosphonate therapies.

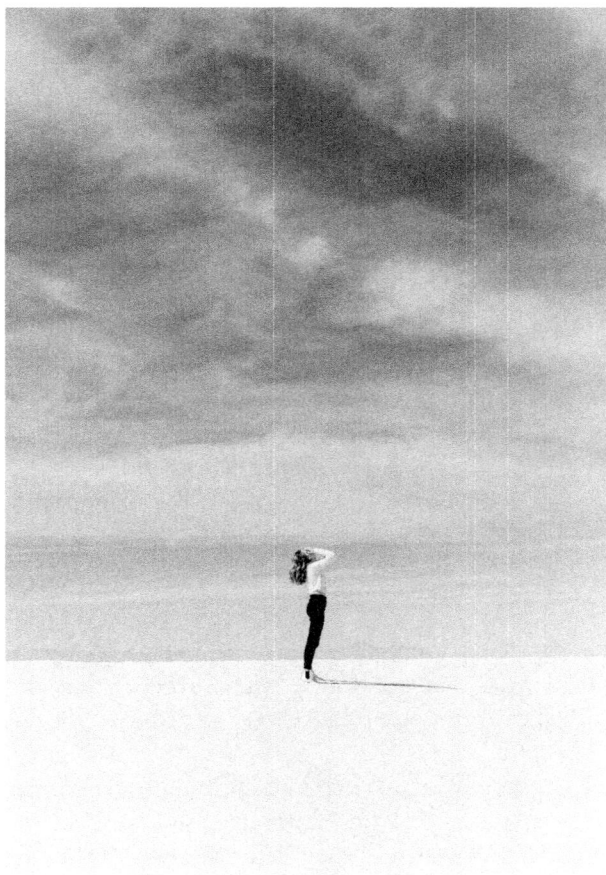

Invasive

Management: Olaparib

The so-called PARP inhibitor **olaparib** targets defects in cancers with BRCA mutations. The drug is for patients with BRCA mutations with metastatic breast cancer. More recently, we got study results showing that the drug also helps selected patients with earlier breast cancer.

The OlympiA study shows that adding olaparib after surgery can significantly extend invasive and distant disease-free survival among high-risk, HER2-negative early breast cancer patients. The study randomly assigned patients to receive either one year of olaparib (300 milligrams taken by mouth twice daily) for one year. Here are the exciting results after 2.5 years of follow-up:

For those on olaparib, 86 percent remained free of invasive cancer, compared with 77 percent in the control group. Distant disease-free survival also favored the olaparib group at 87.5 percent versus 80.4 percent.

Details

The study looked at 1836 patients with stage II or stage III breast cancer who had surgery and chemotherapy (before or after surgery), with or without radiation therapy. Just over one-quarter received platinum-type chemotherapy.

For the 82 percent who had "triple negative" breast cancer, all had high-risk disease, defined as pathologic T2 or greater disease or nodal involvement before chemotherapy. Not getting a complete response to chemotherapy also puts them into the high-risk category. The remaining patients with hormone receptor-positive breast cancer had four or more positive nodes involved before chemotherapy or failed to get a complete pathologic response and met special criteria for residual disease.

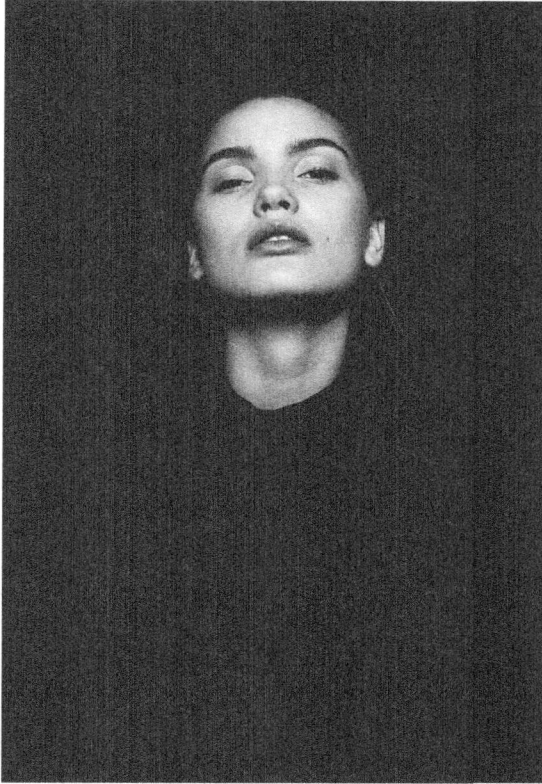

The **OlympiA study** showed a comparable incidence (eight percent) of serious side effects when comparing olaparib and placebo-treated patients.

Invasive

Special considerations

Fertility

If having children is important, you should talk to your care providers about your fertility options. Unfortunately, many physicians do not provide sufficient information about the risk of infertility associated with various treatments for breast cancer, and many patients concerned about fertility are not referred to fertility specialists for counseling before cancer treatment.

The optimal time to begin fertility planning is at the same time as you initiate breast cancer treatment planning. Here is the problem: The very treatments designed to save or extend your life have varying probabilities of taking away your ability to conceive a child. Here are some examples:

Chemotherapy and fertility

The medical oncologist may recommend chemotherapy for selected women at higher risk for breast cancer recurrence. Chemotherapy drugs can result in the permanent loss of your menstrual cycles (periods). The risk, however, depends on the specific drugs administered. Risk increases with age: Women under 40 are more likely than older women to have a resumption of their periods after chemotherapy.

Tamoxifen ("anti-estrogen pills") and fertility

With tamoxifen, periods may return after treatment ends, although cycles may be irregular. Unfortunately, even if menstrual cycles return, treatment can shorten the time to have children. In addition, women on tamoxifen should not become pregnant, as the medicine has a risk of inducing congenital disabilities. Typically, tamoxifen is for five or more years; during this period, the probability of natural fertility may decrease.

Storing embryos

What are some steps you may take before starting treatment to preserve fertility? One potential option is storing embryos. Here, eggs are collected over several menstrual cycles, fertilized, and then frozen. After your treatment, the embryos can be thawed and implanted into your uterus. Unfortunately, the collection of eggs can delay the initiation of treatment, so check with your physician to see how long is acceptable. In addition, a sperm donor is needed to fertilize the eggs before they are stored. Alternatively, unfertilized eggs (no sperm donor required) may be frozen and stored. In the contemporary era, freezing unfertilized eggs may yield pregnancy rates similar to those achieved with fertilized eggs.

Protecting the ovaries

Chemotherapy acts on fast-growing cells. Still, there can be collateral damage to normal cells in your body, including the egg-containing ovaries. We have some drugs that can attempt to shut down the ovaries during chemotherapy while reducing the probability of early menopause. These include goserelin (Zoladex), leuprolide (Lupron), and triptorelin.

A meta-analysis found the drugs to be associated with a higher recovery rate of regular menses after six months (2.4 times as likely, compared to those not on such drugs) and at least 12 months (1.85 times as likely) following the last chemotherapy cycle. In addition, these drugs were associated with a higher number of pregnancies (1.85-fold increase). However, this outcome was not uniformly reported, and the pregnancy rate was not the primary outcome in any trials.

RELAPSE

Local or regional recurrence

Locoregional recurrence

Work-up:
National Comprehensive Cancer Network Guidelines

Initial evaluation

- History and physical exam

- Discuss goals of therapy, adopt shared decision-making, and document course of care

- Blood tests (complete blood count; comprehensive metabolic panel), including liver function tests and alkaline phosphatase

- Chest diagnostic CT scan with contrast

- Abdominal ± pelvic diagnostic CT with contrast or MRI with contrast

- Brain MRI with contrast if concerning symptoms

- Spine MRI with contrast if back pain or symptoms of cord compression

- Bones can or sodium fluoride PET/CT (lower level recommendation)

- Standard PET/CT scan (optional)

- X-rays of symptomatic bones and long and weight-bearing bones abnormal on bone scan

- The first recurrence of disease should be biopsied; determination of tumor estrogen- and progesterone receptor status and HER2 status on recurrent site

- For patients with HER2-negative tumors eligible for single-agent drugs, strongly consider germline breast cancer gene (BRCA 1/2) testing

- Genetic counseling if you are at high risk for hereditary breast cancer

Treatment: Local

Local recurrence*

If you initially had a lumpectomy and radiation therapy and then had the cancer return in the breast, management consists of a breast removal)total mastectomy) with some axillary lymph nodes removed (if not previously done). On the other hand, if you have a recurrence after a breast removal and axillary node dissection (of lower underarm nodes, including at levels I and II), then you should have surgical resection of the recurrence if possible. Radiation therapy should then be added. Even if you had radiation therapy previously, you may (or may not) be a candidate for re-irradiation.

Regional (node) recurrence*

What should you do if cancer comes back in the axillary lymph nodes? Surgery should be done, if possible, and then followed by radiation therapy (also if possible). On the other hand, recurrences in the lymph nodes around the collarbone (supraclavicular region) in the internal mammary nodes right next to the breastbone (sternum) are typically managed with radiation therapy if possible.

In-breast recurrence: Can a sentinel node sampling be done?

Breast removal represents the standard of care for those who have a local in-breast relapse. But what about the axillary nodes? Can you repeat a sentinel lymph node mapping? We do not have high-level evidence to guide us, but here are some results from expert surgeons:

	Mapping success	Axillary recurrence
Memorial Sloan-Kettering	55%	0 (2.2 years)
Milan	93%*	4%

Experienced surgeons can sometimes pull off a repeat sentinel node mapping. Most studies suggest that using radioactive dye (as opposed to blue dye) may optimize the technique.

* For local or regional recurrences (without distant metastases), systemic therapy - such as chemotherapy may be offered before or after surgery. For those with a local or regional recurrence who also have distant metastases, radiation therapy should be considered, in addition to systemic therapy.

** Eight percent mapped to nodes outside of the axilla

Locoregional recurrence

Management: Drugs

Prior endocrine therapy within one year

Premenopausal. Ovarian removal or suppression, plus endocrine therapy (with or without a drug designed to help overcome cell resistance that has developed to endocrine therapy; examples are CDK4/6 or mTOR inhibitors) for post-menopausal women.

Postmenopausal. Consider a different endocrine therapy (with or without a drug designed to help overcome cell resistance to endocrine therapy; examples are so-called CDK4/6 or mTOR inhibitors) for postmenopausal women.

No prior endocrine therapy within one year

Premenopausal. Ovarian removal or suppression, plus endocrine therapy (with or without a drug designed to help overcome cell resistance that has developed to endocrine therapy; examples are so-called CDK4/6 or mTOR inhibitors) as for postmenopausal women.

Postmenopausal. Options include aromatase inhibitor (or other) drugs or other endocrine approaches, such as a CDK 4/6 inhibitor with an aromatase inhibitor or fulvestrant.

Chemotherapy

The CALOR trial examined chemotherapy's potential role in managing isolated (that is, with no associated distant metastases) local recurrences. Here are the results:

• *Estrogen receptor positive recurrence:* No benefit to chemotherapy.

• *Estrogen receptor negative recurrence:* Chemotherapy improved 10-year disease-free survival from 34 to 70 percent.

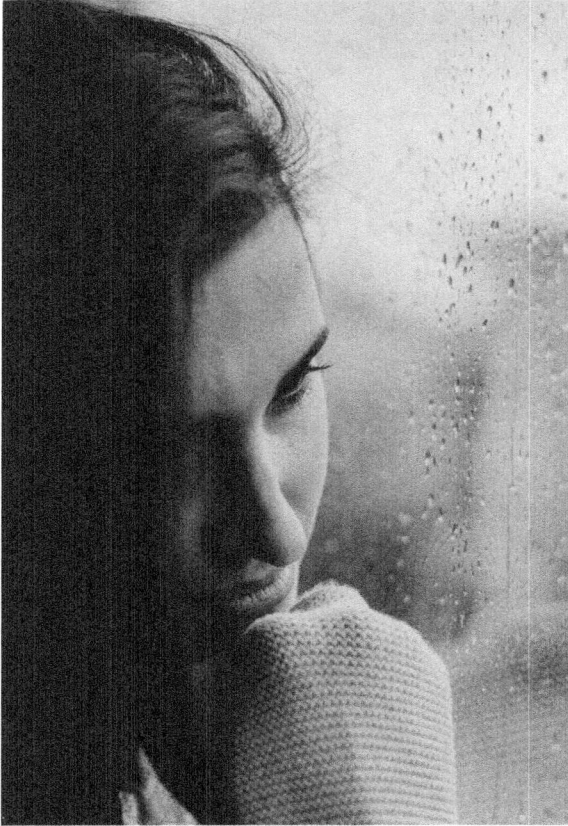

MANAGEMENT

Metastases

Metastases

Distant spread of cancer

Metastasis [muh-TAS-tuh-sis]: the development of secondary cancer growths at a distance from a primary site of cancer.

We sometimes refer to the distant spread of cancer as advanced, metastatic, or stage IV (4) breast cancer. All refer to cancer spreading from the breast's original site to more distant body parts. The most common sites of spread include the bones, liver, and lungs. Cancer can also spread to the brain or other body parts, however. In addition, metastatic cancer can affect one or more locations simultaneously. Spread to regional regions such as the axillary (underarm) nodes, paraclavicular (above or below the collarbone) nodes, or internal mammary nodes (next to the breastbone or sternum) may occur. Still, these are regional (and not distant) sites of spread.

How does distant spread occur?

Metastatic breast cancer develops when cells from the original cancer in the breast travel to distant parts of the body through the blood or lymphatic system. This new cancer is still known as breast cancer, even though it is in a different body part. Sometimes the cancer is present in distant sites at diagnoses, either macroscopically (we know about the metastases) or microscopically (our tests cannot show the distant spread, but it is present in small amounts). Alternatively, some cancer cells may survive treatment for what is initially non-metastatic cancer.

We have long believed that cancer metastasizes (spreads) when a single cancer cell escapes from the original tumor, travels through the bloodstream, and sets up shop in distant organs. However, a growing body of evidence suggests that these bad actors don't travel alone; instead, cancer cells migrate through the body in cellular clusters, like gangs. Roaming tumor clumps are led by a gang member fueled by a type of cellular kryptonite: a highly expressed protein called keratin 14. Understanding the molecular basis of collective dissemination may enable novel prognostics and therapies to improve patient outcomes.

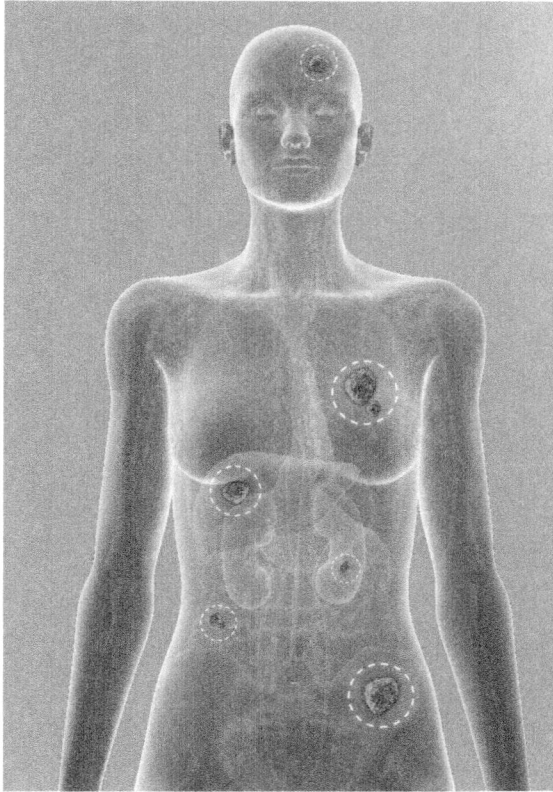

Metastases

Distant spread of cancer

Initial shock

You may be understandably devastated by the news that you have a distant spread of cancer or metastases. Some individuals experience anger, shock, or fear. It is understandable to have fears about your future and those of loved ones. Some women find a small amount of comfort in the knowledge that some women with metastases have lived for many years, experiencing long stretches of relative wellness.

No cure

While we do not yet have a cure for metastatic breast cancer, recent management advances mean that it may be controlled, often for years. For individuals with a good response to treatment, the disease can sometimes be managed akin to a chronic illness: Cancer can sometimes be associated with periodic flares but with extended times of wellness between these times of progression.

"How long do I have?"

Upon hearing that they have metastatic disease, many individuals initially ask, "How long do I have to live?" This question is always difficult to answer, as every patient's experience is unique and individual, and treatment factors can greatly affect survival. Whatever your situation, please know that treatments are continually improving, and many women live for years.

Coping

- *Be informed*

  Being informed can help you to understand your options for management.

- *Talk to a loved one*

  Let someone who cares about you know how you are feeling. This might help take off some of the burdens of trying to keep a lid on everything.

- *Challenge unhelpful thought patterns*

  Check-in with your care team about support resources such as social workers, mental health professionals, and other women in a similar situation) available to you. Many benefit from allowing themselves to be the center of their world, choosing with whom to interact and when to do so.

- *One step at a time*

  Working out how you now want to live your life may take a while. Some women prefer to carry on with their usual daily routine, while others will want to alter their life completely. It can help to talk to those around you or a health professional before making big changes. Try to take one step at a time and remember there is no need to rush into big decisions.

- *Share*

  Talking to others who have experienced secondary breast cancer may help –they may understand what you're going through. Every woman's needs are different. You can choose how much or how little information you need. Let your doctor know how you're feeling so s/he can help you manage any side effects early.

Metastases

Distant spread of cancer

Management overview

The type of treatment recommended to you will depend on the features of your metastatic breast cancer. Relevant factors include where cancer has spread and the special features (pathology) of your cancer. Important factors include whether your breast cancer is hormone positive, if it is HER2 positive, or if you have triple-negative breast cancer.

Tools

While the management of metastatic breast cancer is highly individualized, commonly used treatment tools include::

- Chemotherapy
- Radiation therapy
- Targeted therapy (trastuzumab (Herceptin) is an example)
- Endocrine ("anti-estrogen") therapy
- Surgery is less commonly used, although there are times when it may be recommended for you; for example, to treat or prevent a bone fracture or to remove a single tumor in the brain.

Treatment options are tailored to you as an individual, but offer hope: While survival rates vary greatly from person to person, one study found that about 37 percent of women lived at least 3 years after diagnosis with metastatic breast cancer [2]. Some women may live 10 or more years beyond diagnosis [3]. It is important to note that survival data are based on women diagnosed before some of the newer treatments for metastatic breast cancer were available. Modern treatments have improved survival for women diagnosed today.

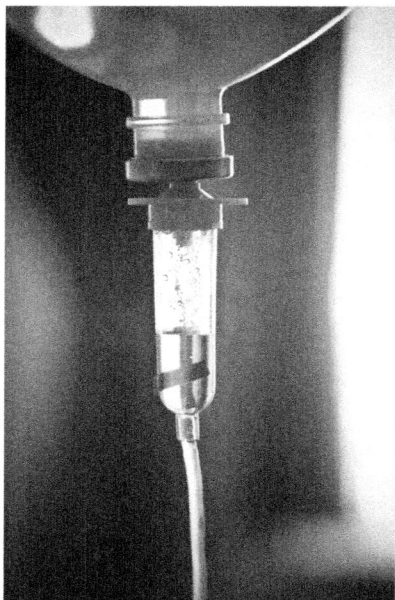

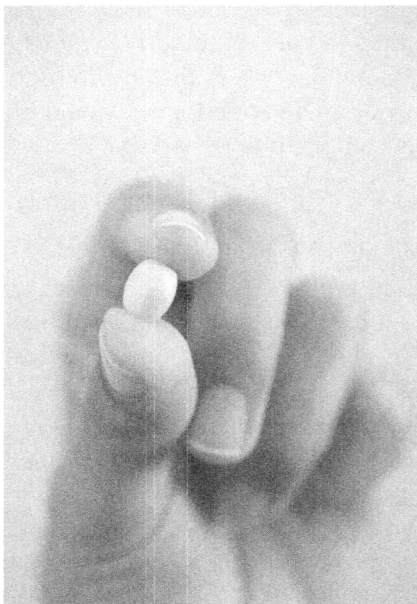

Metastases

Distant spread of cancer

Goals

Here are some of the primary goals of systemic treatment for the treatment of metastatic breast cancer:

- Survival prolongation
- Symptom relief (palliation)
- Quality of life maintenance

While the median survival is 18 to 24 months, many variables can affect the length (including cancer subtype, specific metastatic disease sites, and cancer volume). Some patients will even achieve long-term survival. Unfortunately, we do not have randomized clinical trials to prove that systemic therapy (such as chemotherapy, endocrine therapy, or anti-HER2 strategies) prolongs survival compared to the best supportive care.

A role for repeat biopsy

Sometimes, the biology of metastases is different from primary breast cancer. This finding suggests a potential role for a repeat biopsy to reassess molecular markers such as estrogen receptors (ER), progesterone receptors (PR), and HER2 overexpression. A biopsy may be especially important when the primary cancer is negative for these markers, as a change to positive would likely modify treatment recommendations significantly.

How often do molecular markers such as ER, PR, and HER2 change? A pooled analysis of two prospective trials showed discordance in ER, PR, and HER between the primary and recurrent cancer to be 13, 31, and 5.5 percent, respectively. A separate study found similar results, with 13, 28, and 3 percent discordance rates for ER, PR, and HER2.

Circulating tumor cells (CTCs) and tumor markers

Your doctor may (or may not) order blood tests to look for either tumor markers or cancer itself in the body. We can measure in-blood proteins that your cancer may produce; alternatively, circulating tumor cells that have broken away from initial cancer and have moved into the bloodstream may be measured. Both protein markers and circulating tumor cells are measured using a blood test. Here are some commonly used tumor markers:

- CA 15.3

- TRU-QUANT or CA 27.29

- CA125

- CEA (carcinoembryonic antigen)

- Circulating tumor cells (CellSearch test is approved by the US Food and Drug Administration)

While these tests may have some value, they are imperfect: If the tumor marker is great, it doesn't mean there is no cancer hiding; on the other hand, if the result is not good, it doesn't necessarily mean the cancer is progressing. The tests can be expensive, cause anxiety, and have not been associated with survival improvements for metastatic breast cancer patients. Still, some find them helpful for looking at trends over time and assessing responses to treatment.

Metastases

Distant spread of cancer

Prognosis

Factors that can influence your prognosis if you have metastatic breast cancer:

Interval from initial therapy to relapse

A relapse-free interval of two or more years is associated with a bet-   ter prognosis, at least when compared to those with a shorter time   to relapse.

Sites of metastases

If your metastases predominantly involve the bones, you may have prolonged progression-free and overall survival compared to those with liver or lung disease. Those with a very high volume of disease in the liver, bone marrow replacement, or carcinomatous meningitis may have a poorer prognosis.

Cancer markers (ER, PR, HER2)

Hormone receptor (estrogen- and progesterone)-positive metastases are associated with longer survival than ER/PR-negative disease. Those with HER2 overexpression or triple (ER/PR/HER2) negative breast cancer had shorter median survival, especially historically (when we did not have effective targeted therapies such as Herceptin).

Other adverse prognostic factors

- Poor performance status (your day-to-day activity level).
- Significant weight loss.
- An elevation in your blood levels of serum lactic dehydrogenase (LDH).

Work-up

The National Comprehensive Cancer Network (NCCN) offers the following a work-up for those with distant spread of cancer:

- History and physical exam

- CBC

- Liver function tests and alkaline phosphatase

- Chest diagnostic CT scan

- Abdominal ± pelvic diagnostic CT or MRI

- Brain MRI if neurologic symptoms

- Bone scan or sodium fluoride PET/CT (if FDG PET/CT is performed and indicates bone metastasis on both the PET and CT components, bone scan or sodium fluoride PET/CT may not be needed).

- FDG PET/CT scan (optional, with PET/CT most helpful in situations where standard staging studies are unclear or suspicious)

- X-rays of symptomatic bones and long and weight-bearing bones abnormal on bone scan

- The first recurrence of the disease should be biopsied

- Determination of tumor ER/PR and HER2 status on metastatic site*

- Genetic counseling if you are at high risk for hereditary breast cancer

---

* In clinical situations where a biopsy cannot safely be obtained, but the clinical evidence strongly supports recurrence, treatment may commence based on the primary tumor's ER/PR/HER2 status.

Metastases

Distant spread of cancer

Bone involvement

Drugs

Your oncologist will likely recommend using drugs to reduce your risk of developing fractures, bone pain, and potential compression of your spinal cord. Examples include bisphosphonates, medicines used to prevent or treat osteoporosis. They work by limiting the activity of bone cells called osteoclasts. This action can help strengthen the bone and reduce the breakdown that leads to osteoporosis. But bisphosphonates have another important role: They may help prevent breast cancer from spreading to your bones by making it more challenging for cancer to grow there.

Reduction in bone problems, but no survival advantage

Drugs that target the breakdown of bone cells by metastatic cancer can lower the risk of bones breaking (fractures), reduce the chances that you will need radiation therapy to treat bone pain, and drop the chances you will develop levels of blood calcium that are too high. In addition, using these drugs can also reduce the chances you would develop cancer spread that jeopardizes your spinal cord (spinal cord compression). We have no evidence that these drugs lengthen your overall survival time.

Should I take one of these drugs?

They should be considered if you have bone metastasis, especially the lytic (hole punching) type, or are in a weight-bearing bone if you have an expected survival of 3 months or longer, and if your kidney function is adequate.

Selected drugs for bone metastases

- **Denosumab (Prolia; Xgeva)**
  Denosumab is given under the skin (subcutaneous) injection every four weeks. The optimal duration remains to be determined.

- **Zoledronic acid (Reclast; Zometa)**
  Monthly by vein for a year, then every three months for a total of up to two years. Longer may be better, but we need more high-level evidence. These drugs should be accompanied by calcium (1200 to 1500 milligrams daily) and vitamin D (400 to 800 IU daily).

- **Pamidronate** (given by vein)
  Monthly for a year, then every three months for a total of up to two years. Longer may be better, but we need more high-level evidence. Pamidronate is slowly injected into a vein over two to 24 hours or as directed by your doctor. Pamidronate is generally accompanied by calcium (1200 to 1500 mg daily) and vitamin D (400 to 800 IU daily).

- **Ibandonate (Boniva):** Pill or by vein

- **Clodronate (Bonefos):** Pill

Zoledronic acid and pamidronate should be accompanied by calcium (1200 to 1500 mg daily) and vitamin D (400 to 800 IU daily). Bisphosphonates are typically given in addition to chemotherapy or endocrine therapy. Zoledronic acid may be superior to pamidronate for those with lytic bone metastasis. Finally, a 2012 meta-analysis found that the **newer drug denosumab was better than placebo, zoledronic acid, and pamidronate in reducing the risk of fractures.**

Improved recurrence risk (for postmenopausal women)

Early research results were mixed on whether bisphosphonates help reduce recurrence risk. More recent data suggest that these drugs reduce relapse risk, but only among postmenopausal women (or women who have been made postmenopausal through ovarian suppression).

Metastases

Distant spread of cancer

Bone involvement

Is one bisphosphonate better than the others?

A randomized trial looked at Bonefos, Boniva, and zoledronic acid. After 5.4 years of follow-up, 88% of the women lived and had no recurrence. This rate was the same no matter which bisphosphonate the women got. There appeared to be similar benefits among the bisphosphonate drugs by cancer subtype. Finally, the 5-year overall survival rate was 93%, with no survival differences seen when comparing the drugs.

Despite differences in the types of side effects, the overall severity of toxicity differed little when comparing the treatments. Patients generally prefer oral drugs.

Side effects (toxicity): Collateral damage

While I will not discuss the potential side effects of these drugs, there are some that I want to discuss. Some individuals on bisphosphonate drugs or denosumab will develop bone, muscle, or joint pain. Please immediately inform your healthcare provider if you develop any of these. Some individuals who take bisphosphonates require an increase in vitamin D and calcium intake. If you develop muscle twitching or an increase in your level of anxiety, ask your care provider if you need to take vitamin D and calcium supplements.

⚠ A rare but serious complication is jaw bone breakdown (osteonecrosis). It is important to have a full dental exam before starting treatment and to talk with your oncologist before getting any dental procedure while on bisphosphonates or denosumab.

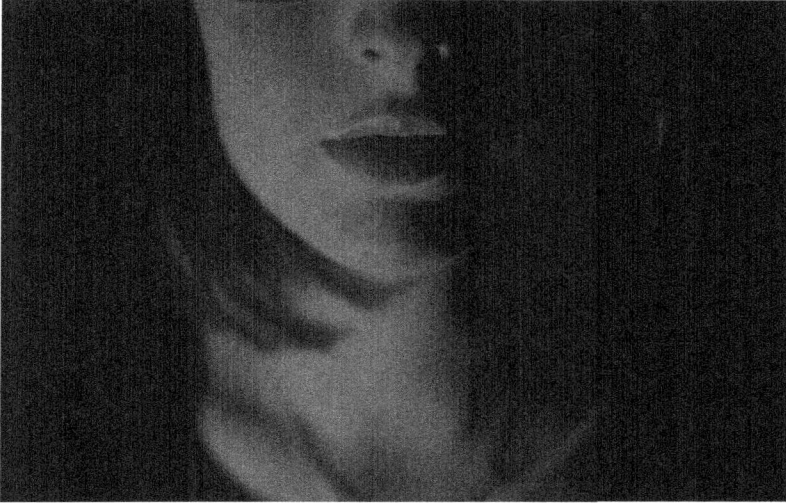

Bisphosphonates taken by mouth may irritate your esophagus. When taking these pills, follow the directions carefully. They should be taken on an empty stomach with plenty of plain water while sitting or standing. After taking a bisphosphonate, please remain upright for at least 30 minutes and avoid eating, drinking, or taking other medicines. Be careful with the use of antacids.

Downsides of bisphosphonates and denosumab include jaw breakdown (osteonecrosis). In this context, patients should have a dental examination with preventive dentistry before staring one of these drugs. Individuals taking these agents should also avoid (if possible) dental procedures that are invasive of gum or bone during treatment.

Preexisting low levels of calcium and vitamin D should be corrected before treatment. Ongoing assessment is indicated during therapy given the risk of a condition known as secondary hyperparathyroidism.

Metastases

Distant spread of cancer

Bone involvement

Is there a potential role for surgery for bone metastases?

If bone metastases weaken a leg or arm bone, you may need an orthopedic surgeon to place a metal rod in the bone. This intervention can drop the chances of the bone breaking; if your bone has already fractured, you will likely need surgical stabilization. Several weeks later, a short course of radiation therapy is typically given to destroy cancer in that region. If the radiation removes cancer in that zone, the bone can rebuild.

And if the cancer is destroying in my spine?

While not commonly needed, some patients have surgery for cancer that spreads to the spine. Other interventions may include the injection of bone cement into cracks (vertebroplasty). Kyphoplasty involves the insertion of a balloon first to widen the space inside the crack before the bone cement is injected. Such interventions are then usually followed by a short course of radiation therapy.

My blood calcium level is much too high. What are my options?

Your doctor offers that you have hypercalcemia, a condition with too much calcium in your blood. Sometimes cancer can cause it; in other cases, cancer's effects on the bone can allow calcium to slip out into the bloodstream. Even some cancer treatments can result in an elevation of your calcium levels.

Unfortunately, having too much calcium can be a major problem. Potential interventions include: 1) giving you extra fluids; or 2) using drugs that reduce the calcium coming out of the bone into the bloodstream. Examples of such drugs include pamidronate/pamidronic acid (Aredia), zoledronic acid (Zometa; Reclast), and denosumab (Xgeva).

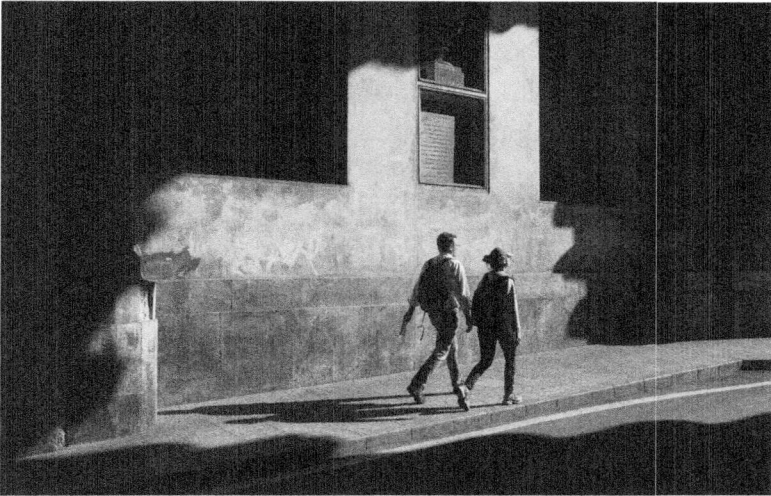

Systemic treatment of breast cancer recurrence or Stage IV disease generally prolongs survival and improves quality of life, but is not curative. Those with such disease are first stratified according to whether there are bone metastases. The next stratification is by tumor hormone receptor and HER2 status.

Metastases

Distant spread of cancer

Bone involvement

Is there a potential radiation therapy (RT) role for bone metastases?

Yes, radiation therapy is the most common local treatment for cancer spread to the bone, and **RT can be especially effective for pain relief.** Radiation therapy can also lower the risk of breaking a bone weakened from cancer. In essence, high-energy X-rays can destroy cancer cells in the local area, permitting the bones to have a chance to rebuild. As discussed in the previous page, surgery is sometimes offered before radiation therapy, particularly if a leg or arm is seriously weakened.

Radiation therapy uses high-energy X-rays (or particles, far less commonly) to try to destroy cancer cells. We typically aim a radiation beam at the target using a machine outside your body. RT is often given in either one large dose or over 5 to 10 days (Monday through Friday typically). The one-large treatment approach is convenient and offers an equal chance for pain relief. On the other hand, the longer course is associated with a slightly lower chance of your needing re-treatment to the same area, as described below.

Only slightly better long-term control with multiple radiation treatments

The American Society for Radiation Oncology (ASTRO) Guideline statement is clear: Multiple randomized trials have shown pain relief equivalency for dosing schema including 30 Gy ("gray") in 10 fractions (a fraction is a single treatment), 24 Gy in 6 fractions, 20 Gy in 5 fractions, and a single 8 Gy fraction for patients with previously not irradiated painful bone metastases. Fractionated treatment courses are associated with an 8% re-treatment to the same anatomic site due to recurrent pain versus 20% after a single fraction. In contrast, the single fraction treatment approach optimizes patient and caregiver convenience.

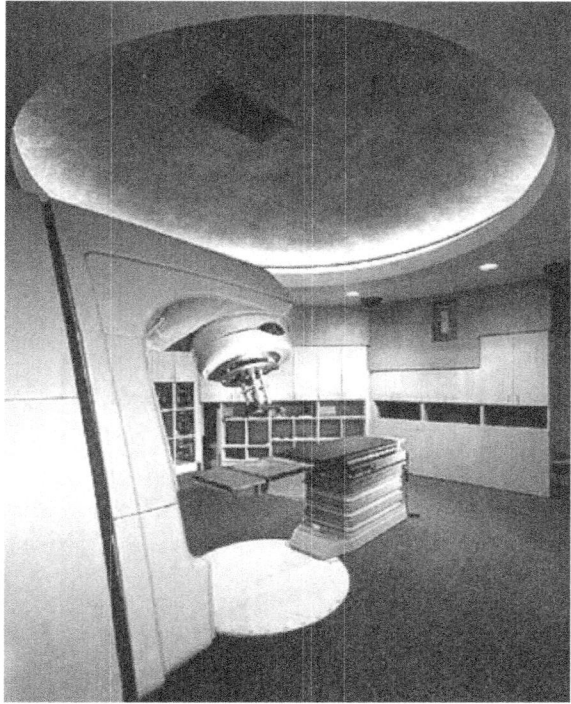

Stereotactic body radiation therapy (SBRT)

Stereotactic body radiation therapy (also known as stereotactic ablative radiation therapy or SABR) is a special form of external beam radiation therapy that gives large doses of radiation therapy for only one (or a few) days. A linear accelerator aims several X-ray beams at the cancer target from different angles. You do not feel anything during the delivery of the radiation therapy.

Side effects (toxicity): Collateral damage

Mild to moderate general fatigue is commonly associated with receiving radiation therapy, which may last for a month or two. Other potential side effects are limited to the volume being hit by the radiation therapy. For example, you may get a sore throat if we need to treat your cervical spine (neck). If we target bones such as the ribs, arms, or legs, many individuals experience no side effects other than general tiredness.

Metastases

Distant spread of cancer

Spinal cord compression: An emergency

Once diagnosed, spinal cord compression is a medical emergency. Spinal cord compression is a terrible complication of cancer spreading to the spine. Many patients experience motor weakness and loss of sensation and may even have bladder dysfunction. If not managed appropriately, the neurologic problems can progress rapidly to paralysis. If your care provider suspects you may have a compression, you will likely proceed immediately to an MRI imaging study of the spine.

Surgery: Suddenly Can't Walk?

You may be a candidate for surgery if you have a life expectancy of at least three months. The surgeon may approach the spine from the front, back, or a combination of the two (depending on the location of the problem). Surgery followed by a short course of radiation therapy can be quite effective in relieving spinal cord compression and its associated symptoms. Here are the results of the only randomized trial addressing whether surgery plus radiation therapy (RT) is better than radiation therapy alone, with the trial including several types of cancer:

	Surgery + RT	Radiation therapy
Regained walking	84%	57%
Kept walking	122 days	13 days

The study excluded patients with neurologic deficits for more than 24 hours, multiple spinal tumors, and prior radiation therapy. In addition, the in-hospital death rate was nearly 6 percent, and the complication rate was 22 percent.

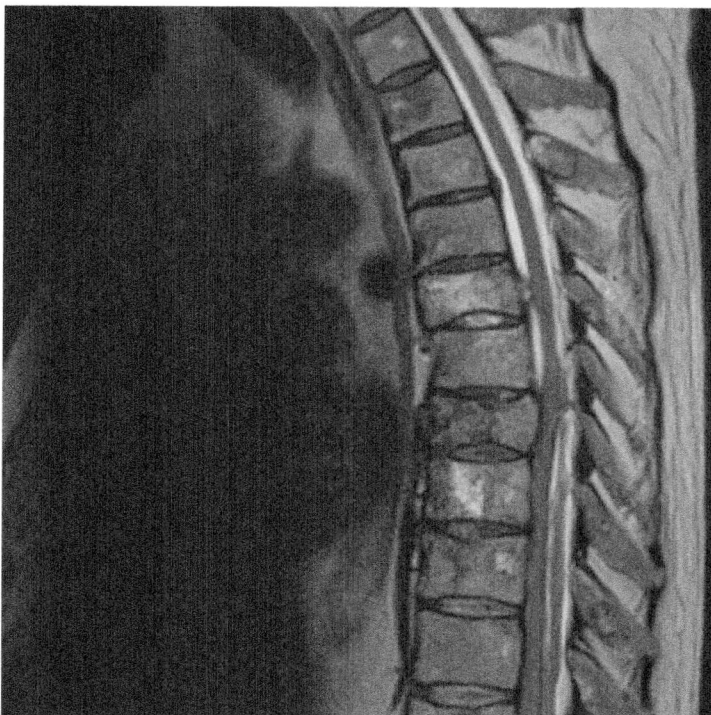

Spinal cord compression: Radiation therapy

Radiation therapy has long played a central role in managing spinal cord compression. In the modern era, surgery may be used (particularly if you cannot walk), with radiation therapy offered after that. To allow for healing, we generally wait one to three weeks after the surgery before irradiating patients.

Radiation therapy can be quite effective, especially for breast cancer. In one study using radiation therapy (without surgery), 70 percent of patients who could not walk regained the ability to ambulate, and the majority experienced pain relief. A typical course spans two weeks (10 treatments, with appointment times of 15 to 20 minutes).

Metastases

Distant spread of cancer

Systemic treatment

Management of metastatic breast cancer is individualized, taking into account your tumor biology, clinical factors, and your goals. In general, those with only one site of cancer spread may benefit from an intense approach to controlling that lesion added to systemic treatment (such as with chemotherapy or anti-estrogen drugs).

Goals

- Survival prolongation
- Symptom relief (palliation)
- Maintenance or improvement of quality of life

Selecting: Anti-estrogen drugs versus chemotherapy

Many doctors believe that chemotherapy is associated with a higher probability of cancer response for those with hormone receptor-positive breast cancer (especially for those with cancer in organs such as the liver and lung), compared with anti-estrogen (endocrine) therapy. We don't have recent high-level evidence to confirm that belief conclusively.

A historic meta-analysis (collection of studies) looked at several studies, all published before 1995. The researchers found higher response rates with chemotherapy by a factor of 1.25. Still, there were no differences in survival length when comparing the two management approaches. Over the next several pages, we will look at the various systemic therapy approaches for metastatic (secondary) breast cancer.

We have limited data regarding the effectiveness of endocrine therapy for those with estrogen receptor-low (1 to 10 percent) cancers. The ER-low-positive group is heterogeneous with biologic behavior often similar to ER-negative cancers.

Management: Drugs

Prior endocrine therapy within one year

Premenopausal Ovarian removal or suppression, plus endocrine therapy (with or without a drug designed to help overcome cell resistance that has developed to endocrine therapy; examples are so-called CDK4/6 or mTOR inhibitors) as for post-menopausal women.

Postmenopausal Consider a different endocrine therapy (with or without a drug designed to help overcome cell resistance to endocrine therapy; examples are so-called CDK4/6 or mTOR inhibitors) for postmenopausal women.

Visceral crisis Consider initial chemotherapy if the in organs such as the liver or lungs is particularly threatening.

No prior endocrine therapy within one year

Premenopausal Ovarian removal or suppression, plus endocrine therapy (with or without a drug designed to help overcome cell resistance to endocrine therapy; examples are so-called CDK4/6 or mTOR inhibitors) as for post-menopausal women.

Postmenopausal Options include aromatase inhibitor (or other) drugs or other endocrine approaches, such as a CDK 4/6 inhibitors with an aromatase inhibitor or fulvestrant.

Metastases

CDK4/6 inhibitor drugs for hormone receptor-positive

CDK4/6 inhibitor drugs target cell enzymes called CDK4 and CDK6, enzymes important for cell division. The increased activity of these proteins inside the nucleus causes a loss of cell cycle control, which leads to cells growing and dividing too fast. CDK4/6 inhibitor drugs include the following:

- Abemaciclib (Verzenio) pills
- Palbociclib (Ibrance) pills
- Ribociclib (Kisqali) pills

The CDK4/6 inhibitors are used in combination with endocrine therapy to treat hormone receptor-positive, HER2-negative metastatic breast cancers. Abemaciclib may be used alone.

Why combine a CDK4/6 inhibitor with endocrine therapy?

Endocrine therapy combined with a CDK4/6 inhibitor can improve progression-free survival, more than endocrine therapy alone. Here are some selected examples:

For example, the MONALEESA-3 clinical trial compared endocrine therapy (fulvestrant) with or without ribociclib. The overall response rates were better with the inclusion ribociclib at 32 versus 22 percent. The combination also appeared to be associated with higher 5-year survival rates (46 versus 31 percent).

The MONARCH 2 study also showed better response rates to be linked with combining endocrine therapy with a CDK4/6 inhibitor (abemaciclib): 48 percent versus 21 percent.

The MONARCH 3 study showed the power of combining abemaciclib with the endocrine therapy pill letrozole (Femara). The response rates were 48 percent with the combination, compared with 35 percent for letrozole alone.

CDK4/6 inhibitor	Possible side effects
Abemaciclib (Verzenio)	Diarrhea, low white blood cell counts, low red blood cell counts (anemia), blood clots, fatigue, nausea, vomiting, and abdominal pain. Abemaciclib can cause liver problems, so your medical oncologist will check your liver function before and during treatment. Rarely, abemaciclib can cause lung inflammation (pneumonitis). Please immediately tell your healthcare provider if you experience shortness of breath or other breathing problems while taking the drug.
Palbociclib (Ibrance)	Low white blood cell counts, low red blood cell counts (anemia), fatigue, nausea, vomiting, constipation, headache, back pain, and in rare cases, blood clots. Rarely, abemaciclib can cause lung inflammation (pneumonitis). Please immediately tell your healthcare provider if you experience shortness of breath or other breathing problems while taking the drug.
Ribociclib	Low white blood cell counts, nausea, vomiting, fatigue, diarrhea, hair loss, constipation, headache, and back pain. Rarely, ribociclib can cause EKG (electrocardiogram) changes. You will have an EKG before treatment. Rarely, abemaciclib can cause lung inflammation (pneumonitis). Please immediately tell your healthcare provider if you experience shortness of breath or other breathing problems while taking the drug.

Metastases (BRCA-mutation)

PARP inhibitors

Metastatic triple-negative breast cancer

Triple-negative breast cancers are:

- Estrogen receptor-negative
- Progesterone receptor-negative
- HER2- negative

PARP stands for poly adenosine diphosphate-ribose polymerase, a type of enzyme that helps repair DNA damage in cells. PARP inhibitors block the action of the PARP enzymes: PARP-1, PARP-2, and PARP-3. These all help repair damaged DNA in cells.

PARP inhibitors can keep cancer cells from repairing, and if they cannot repair, they die.

- Olaparib
- Talazoparib

The PARP inhibitors are for the treatment of advanced (metastatic) HER-2-negative breast cancer for those with a BRCA mutation. The efficacy of PARP inhibitors has been demonstrated in two clinical trials.

In the OlympiAD study, olaparib had a 58 percent response rate, compared with 22 percent for chemotherapy. The median progression-free survival also favored the PARP inhibitor (7 versus 4.2 months). Median survival lengths appeared similar at 19.3 and 17.1 months for olaparib and chemotherapy, respectively.

The EMBRACA study examined talazoparib versus chemotherapy. Again, the PARP inhibitor had an advantage over chemotherapy. The response rates were 63 percent for talazoparib versus 27 percent for chemotherapy. The median progression-free survivals were 8.6 and 5.6 months, respectively. Finally, the median survival appeared similar at around 19 months. The PARP inhibitors also appear associated with better quality of life.

PARP inhibitors	Possible side effects
Olaparib (Lynparza) pills twice daily **or** **Talazoparib (Talzenna) pills once daily**	Nausea, vomiting, diarrhea, fatigue, appetite loss, taste changes, stomach pain, and muscle and joint pain. PARP inhibitors can also reduce levels of red blood cells, white blood cells, and platelets. Blood counts are routinely checked before treatment and then monthly. Rarely, PARP inhibitors can cause cancer to develop in the blood (Acute Myeloid Leukemia or AML). Myelodysplastic syndrome is a serious bone marrow condition that can develop. Other uncommon side effects include blood clots in a deep vein (usually in the leg) or lungs (pulmonary embolism), which may be severe or lead to death. Please tell your healthcare provider right away if you have pain, swelling in an extremity, shortness of breath, chest pain, breathing that is faster than normal, or heart beats faster than normal. Your healthcare provider will do blood tests to check you blood cell counts before treatment, every month while on the drug, and weekly (if you have low blood counts that last a long time). These are not all the possible side effects. Please call your healthcare provider for medical advice about side effects.

Avoid grapefruit, grapefruit juice, Seville oranges, and Seville orange juice during treatment with olaparib since they may increase blood levels of the drug.

www.lynparza.com
www.talzenna.pfizerpro.com

Metastases (triple-negative)

Treatment overview

Triple-negative breast cancers are:

- Estrogen receptor-negative
- Progesterone receptor-negative
- HER2- negative

Chemotherapy

Chemotherapy options include numerous drugs described to the right. Chemo is often the first management approach for metastatic triple-negative breast cancer. Commonly used drugs include anthracyclines, taxanes, the oral chemotherapy agent capecitabine (Xeloda), gemcitabine, eribulin and others. Chemotherapy may be given as a single or multiple drugs.

Immunotherapy

For metastatic triple-negative breast cancer who have a germline (inherited) breast cancer gene mutation (BRCA1/2), if the cancer no longer responds to chemotherapy, other platinum drugs (such as carboplatin or cisplatin) may be an option. Alternatively,, targeted drugs known as PARP inhibitors (for example, olaparib/Lynparza or talazoparb/Talzenna may be options.

PARP inhibitors

For those with triple-negative breast cancer sho have a BRCA mutation (and whose cancer no longer responds to chemotherapy), targeted drugs known as PARP inhibitors may be considered. Examples include olaparib and talazoparib.

Antibody-drug conjugates

For metastatic triple-negative breast cancer for which at least two other drug treatments have been used, the antibody-drug conjugate sacituzumab govitecan (Trodelvy) might be a treatment option.

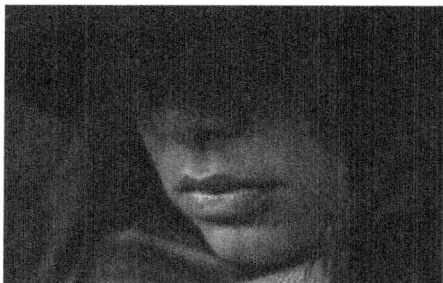

Chemotherapy

Drugs include anthracyclines (doxorubicin/Adriamycin; Abraxane), taxanes (paclitaxel), anti-metabolites (Xeloda; gemcitabine), microtubule inhibitors (vinorelbine; eribulin), and platinum drugs (cisplatin; carboplatin).

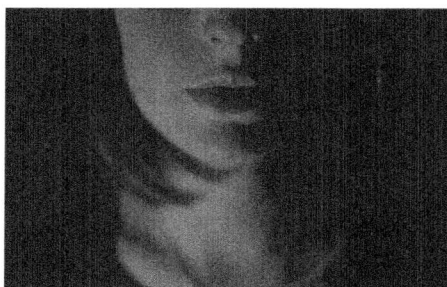

Immunotherapy

Currently used for triple-negative breast cancer, with studies ongoing for other breast cancer subtypes. Approved for those with a Combined Positive Score (CPS) of at least 10. Pembrolizumab (Keytruda) is an example.

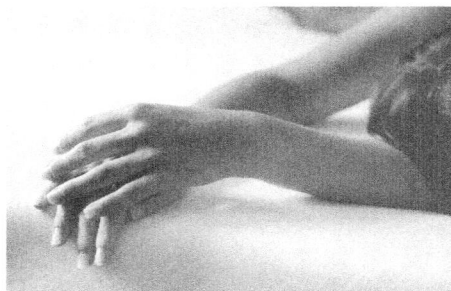

PARP inhibitors

PARP inhibition causes double-strand breaks in DNA. Can cause catastrophic DNA damage and cell death, especially in cells with BRCA 1/2 mutations.

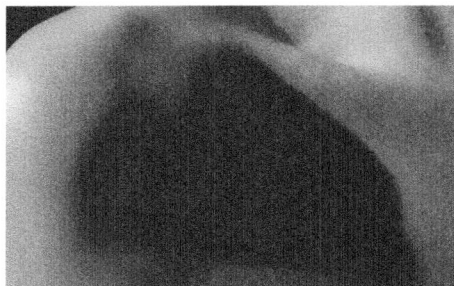

Antibody-drug conjugates

Exploit the cancer cell-specific targeting of a monoclonal antibody towards a cancer cell surface protein (TROP-2) to deliver a payload of chemotherapy that kills cancer cells. Sacituzumab govitecan is an example of this medicine class.

Metastases (triple negative)

Sacituzumab govitecan (Trodelvy)

Triple-negative breast cancer

Triple-negative breast cancer is aggressive and represents 15 to 20 percent of all breast cancers. Its prevalence is particularly high among premenopausal women with breast cancer and those of African American and Hispanic descents. TNBC lacks estrogen and progesterone receptors and has low expression of HER2. Metastatic TNBC management is challenging; we need more effective treatment options.

Antibody-drug conjugates: "Smart bombs"

Sacituzumab govitecan (Trodelvy) is used to treat metastatic triple-negative breast cancers that have already been treated with at least two drug therapies in the metastatic setting.

Antibody-drug conjugates deliver toxic drugs (a payload) directly to cancer cells. One potential target, a protein known as Trop-2, is present at high levels in triple-negative breast cancers. A variety of human cancer cells (including breast, lung, bladder, and others) overexpress Trop-2.

The antibody component binds to a specific protein on the cancer cell surface: Trop-2 in the case of sacituzumab govitecan. When the antibody and Trop-2 interact, the entire antibody-drug conjugate is taken into the interior of the cancer cell. Once inside, the payload (a chemotherapy drug known as SN-38) is released and kills the cancer cell.

For breast cancer, Trop-2 mRNA is a strong predictor of nodal involvement and distant metastasis. While Trop--2 expression is seen with all of the major breast cancer subtypes, overexpression appears more common in triple-negative breast cancer.

	Possible side effects
Sacituzumab govitecan (Trodelvy)	Possible side effects include **diarrhea**, nausea, vomiting, fatigue, anemia (low red blood cell counts), hair loss, constipation and rash. Sacituzumab govitecan increases the risk of having a low white blood cell count. Your blood cell counts will be monitored while taking sacituzumab govitecan. Premedication for the prevention of infusion reactions and chemotherapy-induced nausea or vomiting.

Sacituzumab may improve survival length

The TROPICS-02 study compared sacituzumab govitecan versus chemotherapy. Response rates appeared higher with sacituzumab (21 versus 14 percent), but survival appeared similar between the two approaches.

The ASCENT study used the same approach as the TROPICS-02 study. Response rates appeared higher with sacituzumab (31 versus 4 percent). Compared to people who got chemotherapy, those who got sacituzumab appeared half less likely to die. For those who did not have brain metastases, the one-year survival was 46 percent with sacituzumab and 19 percent with chemotherapy.

Overall, sacituzumab govitecan is well-tolerated - less than three percent in the a landmark clinical trial (published in the *New England Journal of Medicine* in 2019) discontinuing the drug because of toxicity. The responses appeared durable for patients with heavily pre-treated metastatic triple-negative breast cancer.

Triple-negative breast cancer: Into the future

Triple-negative breast cancer does not have estrogen or progesterone receptors nor the excessive HER2 receptors that drive other subtypes of breast cancer. There are currently no drugs specifically designed to target triple-negative breast cancer. Because triple-negative breast cancer does not have a primary driver we have historically targeted, we have largely depended on treatments we have had for decades, including chemotherapy, surgery, and radiation therapy. We finally have the first generation of therapies specifically targeting metastatic triple-negative breast cancer.

Turning your immune system against the cancer

Researchers combined the new drug atezolizumab with a chemotherapy called nab-paclitaxel for patients with metastatic triple negative breast cancer. Atezolizumab is immunotherapy; it is a so-called PD-L1 inhibitor that counteracts a cancer's ability to hide itself from your immune system. Basically, your immune system's T cells have PD1 receptors that, when activated, turn off a T cell's cell-killing activity. Many cancers express PD-L1.

Many cancers express PD-L1, a receptor that counters PD-1. Atezolizumab blocks the ability of PD1 receptors to bind PD-L1, thus leaving T cells able to target tumor tissue. In other words, when PD-L1 is blocked, cancer cells can no longer hide from T cells. This blockade can lead to a greater anti-cancer effect than chemotherapy alone. In a study of 24 patients, 42 percent responded to treatment, with most responders achieving stable disease.

No endocrine (anti-estrogen) therapy

As triple-negative breast cancers do not have estrogen or progesterone receptors, anti-estrogen therapy (such as tamoxifen or an aromatase inhibitor) is not recommended.

1 Cancer cell presses the STOP button of the immune T cell to stop the attack.

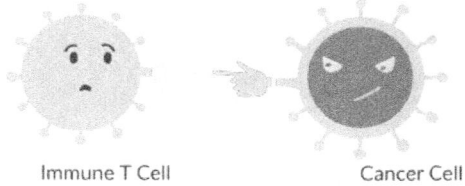

Immune T Cell   Cancer Cell

2 Checkpoint inhibitor blocks the STOP button, "taking the brakes off immune."

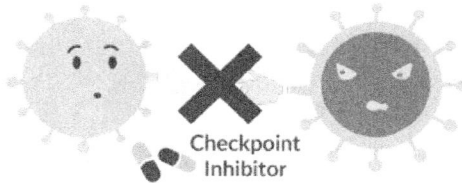

Checkpoint Inhibitor

3 Immune T cell is re-activated and can start attacking cancer cells.

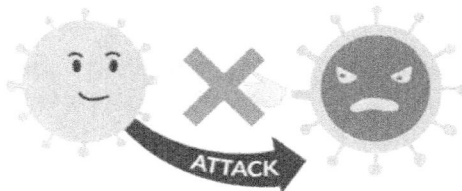

ATTACK

http://www.actgenomics.com/en/about

Metastases (triple-negative)

Immunotherapy

Metastatic triple-negative breast cancer

Triple-negative breast cancers are:

- Estrogen receptor-negative
- Progesterone receptor-negative
- HER2- negative

Pembrolizumab is a checkpoint inhibitor immunotherapy drug. The immunotherapy is combined with chemotherapy for treat metastatic triple-negative breast cancers that have a marker suggesting a possible response. This marker is known as programmed cell death ligand 1 (PD-L1). All metastatic triple-negative breast cancers should be tested to see if they are PD-L1-positive.

Compared with chemotherapy alone, combining immunotherapy with chemotherapy may prolong the time for cancer progression. The KEYNOTE-355 study is illustrative, showing the benefits of adding pembrolizumab immunotherapy to chemotherapy (Abraxane*, paclitaxel, or gemcitabine-carboplatin).

Response rates higher with immunotherapy plus chemotherapy

The objective response rate, or percent who responded to treatment, was 53 percent with chemotherapy plus immunotherapy, compared with 41 percent for chemotherapy alone. The clinical trial included women with triple negative breast cancers that were **PD-L1 positive, defined as a combined positive score (CPS) of 10 or more.** A high tumor mutational burden means that there are a high number of gene mutations in the metastatic breast cancer.

---

* nanoparticle albumin-bound paclitaxel

	Possible side effects
Immunotherapy: Pembrolizumab (Keytruda) - given by vein (through an IV)	Fatigue, decreased appetite, muscle pain, itchiness, nausea, diarrhea, rash, and constipation. Pembrolizumab can cause inflammation of the colon, a condition known as colitis. Other potential issues include liver problems and hormone gland problems. Rarely, abemaciclib can cause lung inflammation (pneumonitis) that can be life-threatening. . Please immediately tell your healthcare provider if you experience shortness of breath or other breathing problems while taking this drug. Some of these side effects can be permanent.

Immunotherapy added to chemotherapy improves survival

The KEYNOTE-355 clinical trial also demonstrated immunotherapy to be associated with a survival advantage (compared with chemotherapy). For those with a CPS score of at least 10, pembrolizumab appeared associated with a median survival of 23 months (versus 16.1 with chemotherapy). The median progression-free survival improved, too: 9.7 versus 5.6 months.

Metastases (HER2-low)

Trastuzumab deruxtecan

HER2-low triple-negative breast cancer

Triple-negative breast cancers are:

- Estrogen receptor-negative
- Progesterone receptor-negative
- HER2- negative

Trastuzumab deruxtecan (Enhertu) has been used for HER2-positive disease. New data shows its use for those with HER2-low triple-negative breast cancer improves outcomes. Approximately two of three patients with triple-negative breast cancer have a HER2-low status.

The DESTINY-Breast04 clinical trial demonstrated the effectiveness of targeting HER2 in HER2-low triple-negative breast cancer. Compared with chemotherapy, trastuzumab deruxtecan improved the median progression-free survival (9.9 versus 5.1 months) for the overall population.

For those with hormone receptor-negative breast cancer, the median progression survival was also better with trastazumab-deruxtecan (8.5 versus 2.9 months).

It is exciting to see new agents available for those selected patients with triple-negative breast cancer.

	Possible side effects
Trastuzumab deruxtecan (Enhertu) - given by vein (through an IV)	Potential serious side effects include: • Lung problems that may be severe or life-threatening. Please immediately tell your healthcare provider right away if you get a cough, fever, trouble breathing, or other worsening breathing symptoms (such as chest tightness or wheezing). • Low white blood cell counts (neutropenia), sometimes severe. Your healthcare provider will check you blood cell counts before staring the drug and before starting each dose. • Heart problems. Please let your healthcare provider know right away if you get any of these symptoms: New or worsening shortness of breath, coughing, feeling tired, ankle or leg swelling, irregular heartbeat, sudden weight gain, dizziness or feeling lightheaded, or loss of consciousness.

Enhertu improves survival (compared to chemotherapy)

The KEYNOTE-355 clinical trial also demonstrated immunotherapy to be associated with a survival advantage (compared with chemotherapy). For those with a CPS score of at least 10, pembrolizumab appeared associated with a median survival of 23 months (versus 16.1 with chemotherapy). The median progression-free survival improved, too: 9.7 versus 5.6 months.

Metastasis management: MTOR inhibitors

MTOR inhibitors are drugs that help reverse the resistance your cancer cells may develop to endocrine therapy. The development of such resistance among women taking endocrine therapy for hormone receptor-positive breast cancer is common.

Resistance

One mechanism of resistance to endocrine therapy is activation of the a growth-triggering pathway known as the mammalian target of rapamycin (mTOR) signal transduction pathway. Can we inhibit this mTOR pathway to regain the cancer-slowing properties of endocrine therapy? The answer is yes.

Research findings

Several randomized studies have investigated the use of aromatase inhibition in combination with inhibitors of the mTOR pathway. One such trial looked at postmenopausal women with metastatic (advanced), hormone receptor positive breast cancer who had not received prior endocrine therapy for their metastases. Researchers randomized patients to receive letrozole (Femara), with or without the mTOR inhibitor **temsirolimus**. The study was negative, with no differences in progression free survival seen.

On the other hand, the so-called BOLERO-2 trial had positive results. Once again, postmenopausal women with hormone receptor-positive advanced breast cancer (that had progressed or recurred during treatment with an aromatase inhibitor) were randomized to exemestane, with or without the mTOR inhibitor **everolimus**. Here are the results after half of patients had been followed for at least 18 months: The median progression free survival was significantly longer with everolimus plus exemestane at 11 versus 4.1 months.

Side effects more common in the everolimus group included infections, rash, lung inflammation, elevated blood sugar and stomatitis (inflammation of the mouth and lips). Elderly patients treated with an everolimus-containing regimen had similar incidences of these adverse events, but the younger patients had more on-treatment deaths.

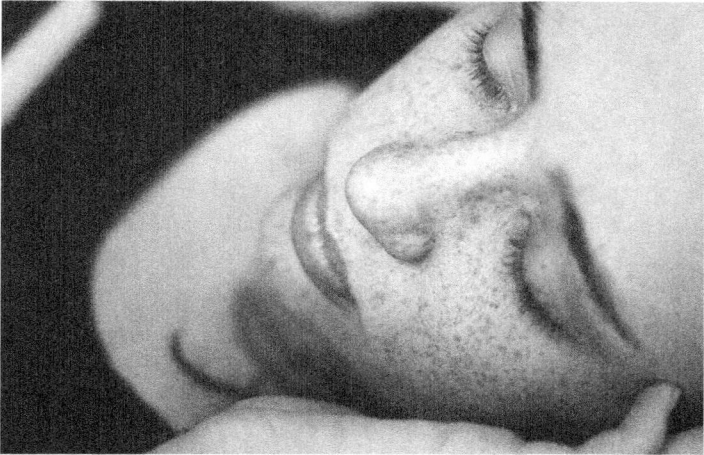

Management: Drugs

HER2-positive metastatic disease

Several HER2-directed agents may be used in the management of HER2-positive breast cancer, either in the first-line or later-line setting:

• **Trastuzumab emtansine (Herceptin)** - This monoclonal antibody binds the part of HER2 that is sticking outside of the cell.

• **Pertuzumab (Perjeta)** - This monoclonal antibody interferes with the ability of HER2 to bind itself to other HER2 receptors or other members of the EGFR family (HER1, 3, or 4). It is given with Herceptin.

• **Ado-trastuzumab emtansine (T-DM1; Kadcyla)** Ado-trastuzumab emtansine (is an antibody-drug combination composed of Herceptin, a linker, and DM1 (which targets the cell skeleton or microtubules). In essence the chemotherapy is built into it, so no additional chemotherapy is needed.

• **Fam-trastuzumab deruxtecan (trastuzumab deruxtecan, or DS-8201** - Fam-trastuzumab deruxtecan is an antibody-drug group composed of an anti-HER2 antibody, a linker, and a cell-killing topoisomerase I inhibitor. As with T-DM1, this combination drug incorporates a cytotoxic agent, and chemotherapy is not added.

• **Tucatinib** – Tucatinib is an oral tyrosine kinase inhibitor. It is used in combination with the oral chemotherapy capecitabine plus Herceptin.

• **Lapatinib** – Lapatinib is a tyrosine kinase inhibitor against EGFR1 and HER2 that results in inhibition of signaling pathways downstream of HER2, used in combinations with trastuzumab or capecitabine.

• **Neratinib** – Neratinib is an irreversible inhibitor of HER, used in combination with the oral chemotherapy capecitabine.

• **Margetuximab** – Margetuximab is an Fc-engineered anti-HER2-receptor monoclonal antibody used in combination with chemotherapy.

Trastuzumab Deruxtecan versus Trastuzumab Emtansine

Trastuzumab deruxtecan (ENHERTU) use yielded better progression-free survival (and a trend toward better overall survival) when compared to the historical gold standard, trastuzumab emtansine (T-DM1/Kadcyla). Researchers compared the two drugs (given every three weeks) for those with HER2-positive metastatic breast cancer previously treated with trastuzumab emtansine and a taxane.

The progression-free survival at 12 months was 76 percent with trastuzumab deruxtecan and 34 percent with trastuzumab emtansine

524 patients with unresectable or metastatic HER2-positive breast cancer who had previously received Herceptin and a taxane in the advanced/metastatic setting were randomized to receive trastuzumab deruxtecan or trastuzumab emtansine (Kadcyla) once every 3 weeks.

Drug-related interstitial lung disease or inflammation (pneumonitis) occurred in 10.5 percent of the patients in the trastuzumab deruxtecan group and in 1.9 percent of those in the trastuzumab emtansine group

HER-2 positive metastatic disease

A small Chinese study suggests that for advanced, HER2-positive breast cancer, Herceptin plus endocrine therapy is not inferior to Herceptin plus chemotherapy. Researchers presented the sysucc-002 randomized clinical trial results at the American Society of Clinical Oncology 2021 annual meeting.

Metastases

Distant spread of cancer

Visceral disease (for example, in the lungs or liver)

Chemotherapy is often perceived as being associated with a higher response rate than anti-estrogen (endocrine) approaches. Still, endocrine therapy is sometimes offered to select patients with disease in solid organs such as the liver or lungs, provided the patient is not in a crisis.

Endocrine therapy (if you cancer is hormone receptor positive*)

In crisis

If you are in a crisis (for example, you have replacement of your bone marrow with cancer, carcinomatous meningitis*, a significant volume of cancer in your liver, or lymphangitic lung metastases**), chemotherapy is generally recommended in order to try to achieve rapid symptom relief.

Not in crisis

The National Comprehensive Cancer Network (NCCN) observes that because systemic treatment of metastatic breast cancer can improve survival and enhance quality of life (but is not curative), use of anti-estrogen (endocrine) therapy is *preferred*, when reasonable. Still, if you have symptoms from spread to organs such as the lung or liver, chemotherapy should be strongly considered.

Estrogen receptor positive and/or progesterone receptor positive (ER+ and/or PR+)

Metastases: Distant spread of cancer

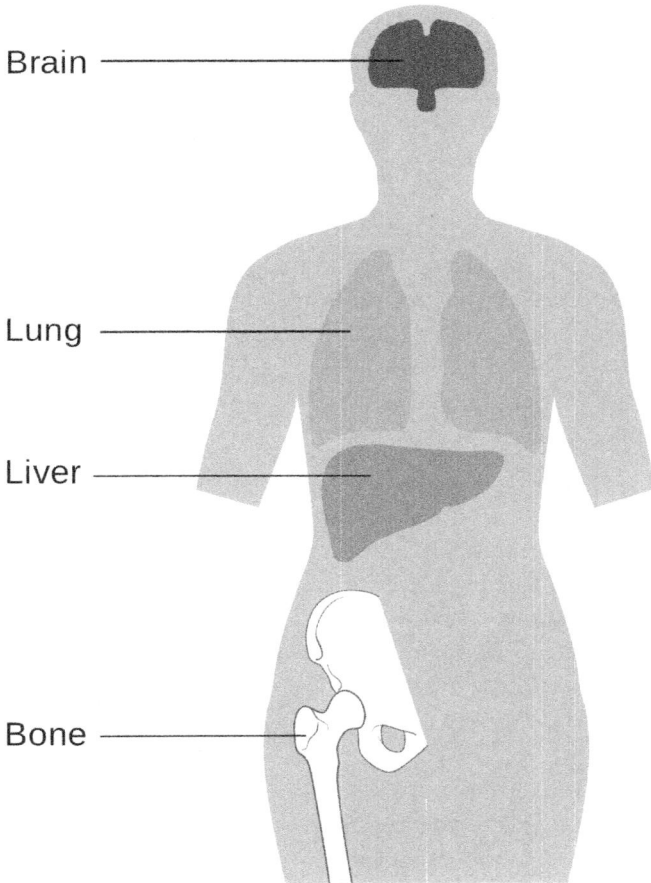

Brain

Lung

Liver

Bone

Predicting response

Metastases: Associated survival

Data from Helsinki (Finland) are illustrative, with researchers finding a **median breast cancer-specific survival time after recurrence of 2.7 years.** This means that fully half of patients will live beyond that number. Survival odds appeared better for those who had Stage I disease initially, compared to those with more advanced stages.

Predicting response

Two of the most important predictors of response to treatment include receptor status (estrogen receptor (ER), progesterone receptor (PR), and HER2). Having a breast cancer that is ER-positive is associated with a response to anti-estrogen (endocrine) treatment, while HER2 overexpression is linked to a potential response to anti-HER2 strategies such as trastazumab (Herceptin), pertuzumab (Perjeta), lapatinib, and ado-trastuzumab emtansine (Kadcyla).

Chemotherapy

You may have a lower probability of a response to chemotherapy if you have had progression after prior chemotherapy for metastatic breast cancer. Other predictors of a lower response chance include: 1) a greater number of metastatic sites; 2) involvement of so-called visceral structures (for example, the liver or lung); 3) you have great challenges in your day-to-day life (poor performance status).

Markers suggesting a higher rate of cancer cell division (high proliferation) portend a favorable response to chemotherapy. These features include a high S-phase fraction and/or a high Ki-67 proliferation index.

Clinical trials

Participation in a clinical trial of new management approaches for triple-negative breast cancer can be an excellent option, sometimes offering access to drugs not available for standard treatment while helping future individuals with the disease.

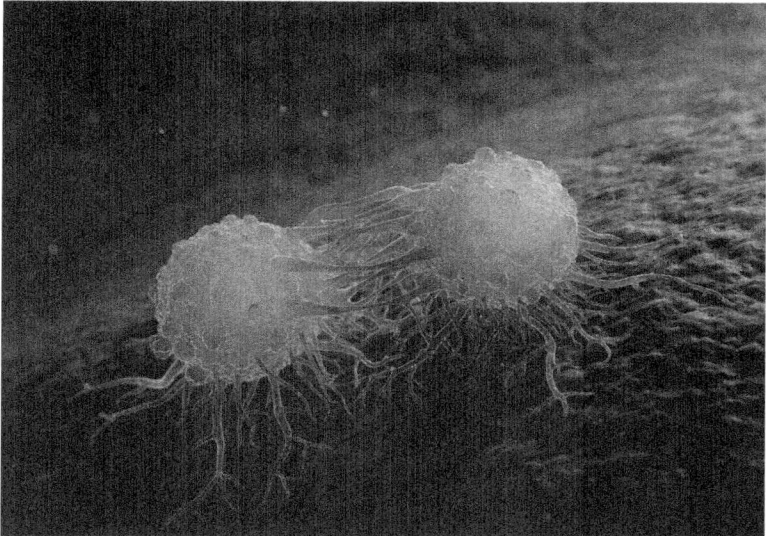

Metastasis: Summary
HER2-positive and postmenopausal*

For those with HER2-positive and postmenopausal (or premenopausal receiving ovarian ablation or suppression), recommended systemic therapy options include the following:

- Aromatase inhibitor, with or without Herceptin (trastuzumab)
- Aromatase inhibitor, with or without lapatinib
- Aromatase inhibitor, with or without lapatinib + Herceptin
- Fulvestrant, with or without Herceptin (trastuzumab)
- Tamoxifen, with or without Herceptin (trastuzumab)

Biosimilars; alternative routes of drug administration

A US Food and Drug Administration (FDA)-approved biosimilar is an appropriate substitute for trastuzumab. In addition, trastuzumab and hyaluronidase-oysk may be substituted for trastuzumab. The dose for this approach is different that for intravenous trastuzumab.

If treatment was initiated with chemotherapy and Herceptin (trastuzumab) + pertuzumab (Perjeta), and the chemotherapy was stopped, endocrine therapy may be added to the trastuzumab + pertuzumab.

The National Comprehensive Cancer Network (www.nccn.org) believes that the best management of any patient with cancer is in a clinical trial. Participation in clinical trials is especially encouraged.

---

*or premenopausal receiving ovarian ablation or suppression

Metastasis: Summary
HER2-positive and hormone receptor-negative

For those with recurrent unresectable (local or regional) or metastatic disease that is estrogen- and/or progesterone receptor-negative, HER2 positive disease, the National Comprehensive Cancer Network (www.nccn.org) recommends systemic therapy plus a HER2-targeted treatment.

Treatment should continue until there is unacceptable toxicity or progression of disease. Then, an alternate systemic therapy plus HER2-directed therapy is recommended.

HER2-targeted therapy - Optimal duration

HER2-targeted therapy is continued following progression on first-line HER2-targeted chemotherapy for metastatic disease. The optimal duration of trastuzumab (Herceptin in patients with long-term control of disease is unknown.

Shared decision-making

Most patients are candidates for several lines of systemic therapy for advanced disease. At each reassessment, clinicians should assess the value of ongoing treatment, the risks and benefits of an additional line of systemic therapy, patient performance status, and patient preferences through a shared decision-making process. If HER2-targeted therapy stops, supportive care continues.

Metastasis: Summary
ER or PR positive, HER2 negative

Visceral crisis

Consider initial systemic therapy.

No visceral crisis and prior endocrine therapy within one year

- Premenopausal: Ovarian ablation or suppression plus systemic therapy.

- Postmenopausal: Systemic therapy

No visceral crisis and no prior endocrine therapy within one year

- Premenopausal: Ovarian ablation or suppression plus systemic therapy versus selective estrogen receptor modulators

- Postmenopausal: Systemic therapy

For all of these approaches, treatment continues until there is progression or unacceptable toxicity.

ER and/or PR-positive, HER2-negative metastases

	Systemic therapy
No visceral crisis and prior endocrine therapy within one year	Premenopausal women should have ovarian ablation (or suppression) plus systemic therapy:
	Postmenopausal women should have systemic therapy.
No visceral crisis and no prior endocrine therapy within one year	Premenopausal women should have ovarian ablation (or suppression) plus systemic therapy: or Selective estrogen receptor modulators
	Postmenopausal women should have systemic therapy

Preferred first-line regimens include"

- An aromatase inhibitor plus a CDK4/6 inhibitor (abemaciclib, palbociclib, or ribociclib).

- An non-steroidal aromatase inhibitor (anastrazole, letrozole) plus a selective estrogen receptor downregulator (fulvestrant)

- Fulvestrant plus a CDK 4/6 inhibitor (abemaciclib, palbociclib, or ribociclib).

Metastasis: Summary

ER or PR negative, HER2 negative ("triple-negative")

"Triple-negative" metastatic breast cancer

For those with hormone receptor-negative, HER2-negative metastatic breast cancer, the National Comprehensive Cancer Network (www.nccn.org) recommends systemic therapy. Treatment is continued until there is progression or unacceptable toxicity.

Preferred regimes include:

- Anthracycline chemotherapy (doxorubicin/Adriamycin or liposomal doxorubicin/Abraxane)
- Taxanes (paclitaxel/Taxol)
- Anti-metabolites (capecitabine/Xeloda oral chemotherapy or gemcitabine)
- Microtubule inhibitors (vinorelbine or eribulin)
- Sacituzumab goveitecan-hziy

For those with HER2 score 1+ or 2+ , fam-trastuzumab deruxtecan-nxki is recommended, based on high-level evidence.

For those with a germline BRCA1/2 mutation, targeted therapies such as olaparib are endorsed. Alternatively, carboplatin or cisplatin may be offered.

Patients with PD-L1-positive triple-negative breast cancer should consider additional targeted therapy options (such as immunotherapy plus chemotherapy.). The preferred first-line therapy for those with PD-L1 TNBC is pembrolizumab (Keytruda) plus chemotherapy (Abraxane, paclitaxel, or gemcitabine and carboplatin).

Metastasis: Summary
Biomarker-directed therapy

Breast cancer type	Biomarker	Drugs
BRCA mutation	BRCA mutation	Olaparib Talazoparib
Hormone receptor-positive, HER2-negative	PIK3CA activating mutation	Alpelisib* + fulvestrant
Triple-negative (ER/PR/HER2-negative)	PD-L1 expression with combined positive score 10 or higher	Pembrolizumab (Keytruda) immunotherapy** plus chemotherapy (Abraxane, paclitaxel, or gemcitabine plus carboplatin)
Any	NTRK fusion	Larotrectinib*** Entrectinib**
Any	MSI-H/dMMR	Pembrolizumab (Keytruda) Dostarlimab-gxly
Any	TMB-H (10 or more mutations per mb)	Pembrolizumab (Keytruda) immunotherapy

* Alpelisib: The safety of this drug in patients with Type 1 (or uncontrolled Type 2 diabetes diabetes has not been established.

** For those progressing on immunotherapy, there is no data to support an additional line of therapy with another PD-1/PD-L1 immunotherapy agent.

** Larotrectinib and entrectinib are indicated for those with an NTRK gene fusion without a known acquired resistance mutation and have no satisfactory alternative treatments or that have progressed following treatment.

Metastases

Distant spread of cancer

Brain metastases

The chances of developing spread of cancer to the brain varies by initial cancer stage and subtype. For example, if you have *early* breast cancer, the odds of brain metastases may be 3 percent. On the other hand, if you already have metastases, the risk of symptomatic brain metastases may be up to 16 percent. Here are the 10-year risks of brain metastases by breast cancer subtype:

Luminal A	0.7 percent
Luminal B	12 percent
HER2 positive	12 percent
Triple negative	7 percent

The brain is increasingly reported as the first site of relapse among women with HER-2 positive breast cancer treated with trastazumab (Herceptin).

Management: Favorable prognosis

If you have a "favorable" prognosis (that is, you have a Karnofsky Performance Status of 70 or higher*; have a controlled primary cancer, controlled (or absent) metastases outside of the brain, and are under 65 year old), aggressive management is typically offered.

For example, if you have only a single site of spread in the brain, you may have the metastasis removed surgically, followed by radiation therapy (often highly focused, high-dose rather than whole brain) versus highly focused radiation therapy (radiosurgery) alone. Let's look in more detail at the management for those with a limited number (for example, 1 to 3) of metastases in the brain.

Limited volume brain metastases

For those who are in the "favorable" prognosis group, and who have a limited number/volume of brain metastases, here are some of your management options:

- **Surgery**

  If you have a single, large metastases in an area of the brain that is accessible to a neurosurgeon, surgery may offer the best chance for rapid symptom relief and control of the cancer in that particular area. You may also be offered surgery if you have more than one metastasis in the brain, but there is one that is dominant and causing you distressing symptoms. Finally, if cancer in the brain is blocking the fluid drainage system in and around the brain, a tube might be placed to bypass the blockage. We call this tube a shunt.

- **Stereotactic radiosurgery (SRS)**

  SRS (high doses of highly focused radiation therapy, given in as few as 1 to 3 treatments) can be a very effective alternative to surgery. You may be a candidate for this innovative form of radiation therapy if you metastasis is relatively small (say, smaller than 3 cm) and in a location that is suboptimal for surgery, or if you are not a candidate for surgery of the brain. SRS may still be an option even if you have more than 3 tumors in the brain.

- **Whole brain radiation therapy (WBRT)**

  Whole brain radiation therapy can be an important addition to surgery or stereotactic radiation therapy, as it can reduce the chances of a local recurrence or a recurrence elsewhere in the brain. However, WBRT can be associated with significant side effects involving your brain function, and so it must be used judiciously.

  Whole brain radiation therapy represents the gold standard management approach for those with more than 3 brain metastases, especially when the overall volume of cancer in the brain is large; stereotactic radiosurgery to multiple lesions may be offered even if you have more than 3 lesions, provided the volume of disease is limited.

Metastases

Distant spread of cancer

Brain metastases: In more detail

Surgery with or without whole brain radiation therapy

For solitary brain metastases, up front resection remains the standard of care. A randomized trial for 95 patients with a single brain metastasis compared a complete resection alone with surgery followed by radiation therapy to the whole brain. The addition of whole brain radiation therapy dropped the in-brain recurrence rate from 70 percent to 18 percent, and lowered the chances of a neurologic death from 44 percent to 14 percent. The addition of radiation therapy did not improve survival length, however. If you have multiple metastases to the brain, the role of surgery may be limited to obtaining biopsy samples or relieving mass effect when tumors are large. Resection may be offered to highly selected patients with up to three metastases to the brain.

Stereotactic radiosurgery (SRS) with or without whole brain radiation therapy

This innovative form of radiation therapy offers a minimally invasive alternative to surgery for selected individuals with a limited volume of metastases in the brain. We have growing evidence to suggest that the key determinant in whether you are a candidate for SRS is the volume (rather than the number) of metastases in the brain.

The Choosing Wisely campaign offers that we should *not* routinely add whole brain radiation therapy after stereotactic radiosurgery for limited brain metastases. The addition of whole brain radiation therapy to stereotactic radiosurgery is associated with diminished cognitive function and worse patient-reported fatigue and quality of life.

A Japanese randomized study of patients with 1 to 4 brain metastases (smaller than 3 cm) showed the addition of whole brain radiation therapy to SRS did *not* improve survival. However, the one year in-brain recurrence rate was lower (47%) with SRS plus whole brain radiation therapy, compared to SRS alone (76%). A meta-analysis (study of a collection of studies) found **no overall survival improvement with the addition of whole brain radiation therapy to stereotactic radiosurgery.**

Recurrence in brain after whole brain radiation therapy

Local control rates greater than 70% have been reported for individuals who receive stereotactic radiosurgery in the setting of recurrence following whole brain radiation therapy. SRS may be offered if you are otherwise doing reasonably well (good performance status), and have relatively stable cancer elsewhere.

Whole brain radiation therapy

Historically whole brain radiation represented the gold standard treatment for brain metastases. We still use it, particularly when surgery or stereotactic radiosurgery is not prudent. While we don't have randomized trials, case series point to up to 70% of patients deriving symptom relief from radiation therapy. Typically, a radiation therapy course for brain metastases is 2 to 3 weeks, Monday through Friday. This corresponds to 30 Gy ("gray") in 10 treatments or 37.5 Gy in 15 treatments. You will be in the radiation therapy department less than half an hour typically, and the treatment itself takes only minutes.

Systemic therapy

Chemotherapy is *not* typically offered as primary management of brain metastases, unless other reasonable options have been exhausted. Highly selected patients without symptoms may have systemic therapy, potentially delaying radiotherapy.

Surveillance

After whole brain radiation therapy or stereotactic radiosurgery patients should have a repeat MRI scan every 3 months for a year. If recurrence in the brain occurs and you have systemic (body) progression with limited systemic treatment options, you may choose palliative/best supportive care or re-irradiation. For those with stable systemic (body) disease, options may include surgery, re-irradiation, or chemotherapy.

Metastases

Distant spread of cancer

Brain metastases: Targeted drugs

Newer therapies are dramatically changing breast cancer management. An increase in the frequency of breast cancer metastasizing to the brain has created new challenges, however.

Recently, scientists have developed drugs that can get through the blood-brain barrier. Targeted therapies that are directed at human epidermal growth factor receptor type 2 (HER2) , vascular endothelial growth factor (VEGF), mammalian target of rapamycin (mTOR), epidermal growth factor receptor (EGFR), cyclin-dependent kinases 4 and 6 (CDK4/6), and poly(ADP-ribose) polymerase (PARP) for breast cancer patients with brain metastases are now available..

Generally, we reserve drugs as primary management of brain metastases for those who do not have symptoms and for whom the brain disease is not in a particularly critical location.

Drugs for HER2 positive brain metastases

About 30 to 50 percent of patients with HER2-positive breast cancer develop spread to the central nervous system.

Tucatinib as a pill that targets the HER-2 pathway. Fully approved for use in 2020 for use (in combination with Herceptin and Xeloda) for advanced HER2-positive breast cancer, patients with brain metastases are also potential candidates for the drug. Patients should have received at least one prior anti-HER2-based regimen in the metastatic setting. Researchers presented these findings at the American Society of Clinical Oncology Annual Meeting; June 4-8, 2021.

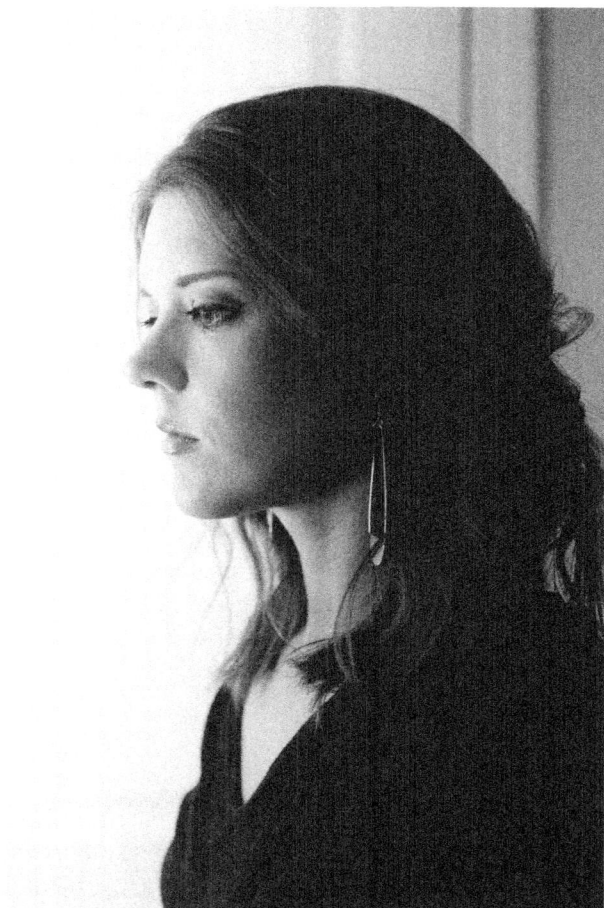

Progression-free survival	Herceptin and Xeloda	Herceptin, Xeloda, and tucatinib
	5.4 months	7.6 months

Metastases

Distant spread of cancer

Leptomeningeal metastases

This refers to multifocal spread of cancer to the membranes (meninges) surrounding the brain and spinal cord. We sometimes refer to it as leptomeningeal carcinomatosis or carcinomatous meningitis when the cancer has spread from a solid tumor such as is the case for breast cancer. The cancer cells gain access to the leptomeninges through the bloodstream, lymph system, or by direct extension. Once they enter the cerebrospinal fluid, they can disseminate throughout the central nervous system. Many patients develop problems with the nerves that supply the face and head (cranial nerves), headaches, mental changes, or motor weakness. Unfortunately, the median survival is measured in months.

Management

Treatment intervention is aimed at improving or stabilizing neurologic function, and to prolong survival. There is no standard approach, but radiation therapy may be offered for symptom relief, to shrink the tumor burden (for the select patient who will get chemotherapy), or to allow the cerebrospinal fluid to flow more normally. Surgery is limited primarily to placement of a catheter into the brain ventricles (reservoirs of spinal fluid in the central brain) for drug administration.

Chemotherapy may be offered, as it can reach the central nervous system. Alternatively, the direct of deliver of drugs (intrathecal therapy) may be offered either by a catheter placed in the spine region, or through a device your neurosurgeon can implant directly into your brain's ventricles (pools of spinal fluid in the central brain). Breast cancer may then respond to drugs such as methotrexate or trastazumab (Herceptin). At Memorial Sloan Kettering Cancer Center (USA), the half of patients lived beyond 3.5 months, with 20% surviving more than a year.

Brain metatases: Outcomes

	Median survival
ER negative, HER2 negative	27 months
HER2 positive	52 months
ER positive, HER2 negative, Ki-67 high	76 months
ER positive, HER2 negative, Ki-67 low	79 months

Brain metastases: Neuroprotective strategies

Unfortunately, whole brain radiation therapy can result in a decline in your brain function (neurocognitive changes). A a result, researchers are working hard to find ways of reducing risk. Here are some examples of these strategies:

Memantine (Namenda)

Memantine is a drug that is sometimes offered for Alzheimer's disease. It can delay the time to cognitive decline. More recently, we have begun to use it for patients receiving whole brain radiation therapy.

In a randomized trial compared memantine (beginning 3 days prior to radiation therapy, and continuing for 24 weeks) or a placebo. The time to cognitive decline appeared longer for the group on memantine. Recognizing the effectiveness of the drug, and its relatively favorable side effect profile, you may wish to consider this drug if you are to receive whole brain radiation therapy.

Hippocampal-sparing radiation therapy

Using a highly advanced form of radiation therapy known as intensity modulated radiation therapy (IMRT), one can attempt to avoid radiation injury to the hippocampus. This structure plays an important role in the formation of new memories about experienced events (episodic or autobiographical memory). This approach requires a great deal of treatment planning sophistication including robust physics team support. As it is relatively new, most patients do not have this approach.

431

Breast cancer may spread to brain by masquerading as nerve cells

City of Hope scientists wanted to explore how breast cancer cells cross the blood-brain barrier – a separation of the blood circulating in the body from fluid in the brain – without being destroyed by the immune system. If, by chance, a malignant breast cancer cell swimming in the bloodstream crossed into the brain, how would it survive in a completely new, foreign habitat?

Taking samples from brain tumors resulting from breast cancer, researchers found that the breast cancer cells were exploiting the brain's most abundant chemical as a fuel source. This chemical (GABA) is a neurotransmitter used for communication between neurons.

When compared to cells from non-metastatic breast cancer, the metastasized cells expressed a receptor for GABA, as well as for a protein that draws the transmitter into cells. This allowed the cancer cells to essentially masquerade as neurons."Breast cancer cells can be cellular chameleons (or masquerade as neurons) and spread to the brain," lead researcher Dr. Jandial offered. Jandial says that further study is required to better understand the mechanisms that allow the cancer cells to achieve this disguise. He hopes that ultimately, unmasking these disguised invaders will result in new therapies.

In-brain recurrence (after initial treatment of brain metastases)

If you have stable disease outside of the brain (and are in relatively good condition overall), potential options for re-treatment of brain metastases may include surgery and stereotactic radiosurgery.

Surgery: Results
Re-operation for recurrent brain metastases can sometimes help:

Symptom relief	75%
Median survival	1 year

Radiosurgery for recurrence in brain
A series of 111 patients who had previously received whole brain radiation therapy and were treated with radiosurgery after recurrence of their brain metastases. Of these, 25 percent recurred again after radiosurgery. The median survival after salvage radiosurgery was 10 months.

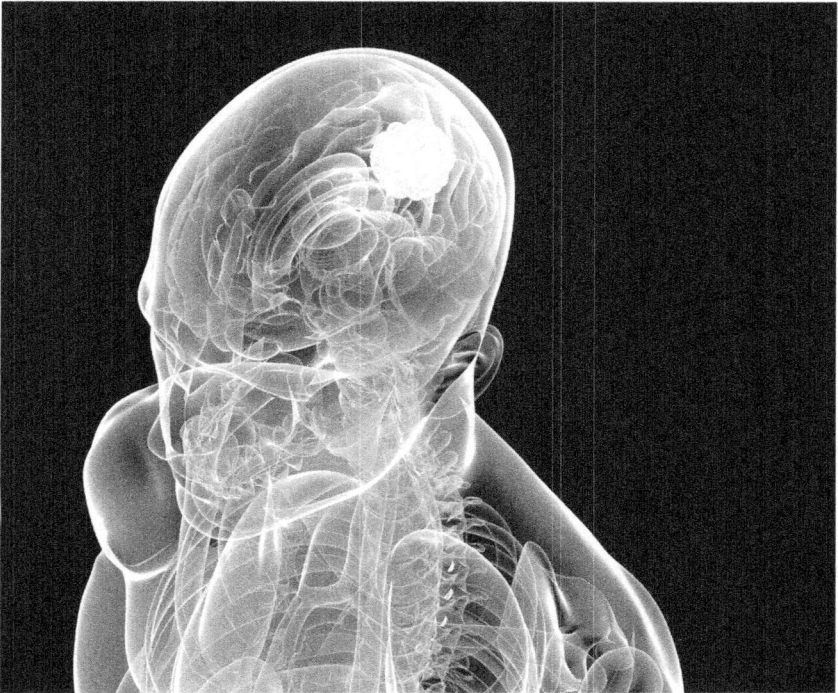

Metastases

Distant spread of cancer

Distant metastases: Any role for breast surgery?

Management for metastatic breast cancer is largely focused on symptom relief, improved quality of life, and prolongation of survival. Most patients with metastases will have a core biopsy of the tumor to confirm the diagnosis and will then proceed to systemic therapy (for example, anti-estrogen pills or chemotherapy, depending on the cancer "fingerprint," the location of the metastases, and other factors). Systemic therapy is a central component of management, but is there a role for local (breast) treatment?

Breast surgery for palliation (symptom relief)

If you have distressing symptoms such as bleeding or ulceration, resection of tumor may provide significant relief. However, as is discussed below, there does not appear to be a clear survival benefit associated with breast surgery in the setting of metastatic disease.

Breast surgery (in the presence of metastases): No clear survival advantage

Breast surgery in the presence of distant spread of cancer is not clearly associated with a lengthening in survival. To be honest, the data are relatively limited and conflicting. Here are the results of two prospective research studies:

India
Patients with new metastatic breast cancer who achieved at least a partial response to chemotherapy (anthracycline) were randomly assigned to either surgery (mastectomy or breast conserving) and postoperative radiation therapy versus no breast-directed treatment. While local treatment of the breast region improved local/regional control, there was no improvement in distant progression-free survival.

The researchers concluded that surgical removal of the primary tumor did *not* significantly improve the quality of life in women with metastatic breast cancer. Taken together with the survival results the data provides strong evidence that surgery for primary should *not* be routinely performed in women with metastatic breast cancer.

Turkey

The MF07-01 trial is a multicenter randomized trial of previously untreated patients with stage IV cancer. Researchers compared locoregional surgery followed by systemic therapy versus systemic therapy alone. The authors concluded that there was no improvement in 3-year survival with surgery. However, **longer follow up revealed a statistically significant improvement in median survival with surgery (46 versus 37 months)** at a median 40 months follow up. Additionally, patients with a more indolent form of metastatic breast cancer such as estrogen receptor-positive, HER2 negative, solitary bone metastasis, and patients under 55 years old have a significant survival benefit with initial surgery. Five-year overall survival was 42% with surgery, vs 25% with systemic therapy alone.

My take

Two studies presented at the 2016 ASCO Annual Meeting reached different conclusions about the benefit of surgical removal of the primary cancer for patients with stage IV (distant metastases at initial presentation) breast cancer. The prospective, randomized Turkish study showed a 9 month increase in median survival (46 months versus 37 months). Conversely, in a U.S.-based registry study of 112 women, the median overall survival was approximately 70 months, with no advantage conferred by surgery. A study from India showed no improvement in distant progression-free survival.

I think it is reasonable to consider surgery for *highly select* patients with a more favorable prognosis (for example, bone only metastases), but that surgery should not be routinely offered for those with distant metastases at diagnosis. One reasonable approach would be to first deliver systemic therapy, and then assess the response (before even considering breast region surgery).

Ongoing studies should provide some clearer answers.

Metastases

Oligometastases

Very limited distant spread

Are we broadening the path to cure? Many who are diagnosed with cancer either present with or will develop distant metastatic cancer. In general, metastatic disease is considered incurable, so there are two ways in which we may increase cancer cure rates: 1) improve our diagnose and management of cancer before it can spread; and 2) discover means to cure metastatic breast cancer.

Emerging data indicate that patients with metastasis to a **limited number of sites (termed oligometastatic disease)** may have improved outcomes with the use of locally ablative therapy (LAT). Historically, when the only management tool for cancer was surgery, the ground-breaking surgeon William Halstead offered a theory of cancer progression, first published in the early 1900s. According to his paradigm, cancer spreads in an orderly fashion initially through the lymphatic system. Therefore, once beyond the localized lymphatic drainage bed, cancer was a systemic disease for which there was no cure. For the most part, this perspective continues to hold true, with some exceptions including germ cell tumors and lymphomas.

Clinical experience, however, has shown that not all patients with metastases have widely disseminated disease. Hellman and Weichselbaum more recently proposed that cancer metastases fall on a continuum. Although some cancers feature either localized or disseminated characteristics, most fall between these extremes. Some tumors may metastasize to a limited number of sites, a condition we call oligometastatic cancer. In general, most studies of oligometastatic cancer have included patients with one to five distinct metastases. With a limited number of metastases, it becomes theoretically possible to treat all detectable tumors with curative intent using locally ablative therapy (LAT). With increasingly more advanced imaging techniques, we should improve our ability to find metastatic disease when it is early and limited, giving hope to many with metastases.

In fact, in 1999, Dr. Weichselbaum and his University of Chicago colleague Samuel Hellman, made the controversial suggestion that many patients with oligometastatic disease could be cured, depending on the extent of disease burden, with either surgery or targeted radiation therapy. We have a growing body of evidence that this may be true.

Hope

Some patients with breast cancer oligometastases treated with high-dose short course, and highly focused hypo-fractionated stereotactic radiation therapy can survive for more than ten years. Tumor burden (volume and number of tumors) appears to impact the risk of recurrence. Here are the findings from a small study from the University of Rochester (USA) of patients with oligometastases from breast cancer treated with stereotactic radiation therapy:

	5 year survival	10 year survival
Bone only (N = 12)	83%	75%
Non-bone only (n = 36)	31%	17%

Metastases

Distant spread of cancer

The Association of Community Cancer Centers (acc-cancer.org/Metastatic-BreastCancer) offers effective principles in metastatic cancer patient support. Let's take a look:

- **Empower**

Given the terminal nature of metastatic breast cancer, you may feel that the disease has stripped you of control. Life goals may start to feel less achievable, and because life expectancies are highly variable from person to person, you may not feel equipped to navigate conversations with family, friends, and co-workers. In order to try to empower you, oncology providers should communicate information to you in a way that does not rely on overly complex language. As a clinician, I try to strike a balance between honesty and hope - allowing you to understand the reality and then decide how to move forward.

- **Include**

Often, individuals with metastatic breast cancer feel excluded from the dominant breast cancer narrative. There seems to be a significant lack of understanding of the unique issues for those in this population. Unfortunately, many in the public rely on their understanding of early breast cancer to navigate conversations with patients who have metastatic breast cancer. In addition, some patients perceive the incurable nature of the disease as an immediate death sentence. As caregivers, we should aim to communicate clearly, yet also offer a source of hope.

- **Support**

Social support can be a key source of psychological and even physical relief. The dominant narrative of early detection and survivorship may lead you to feel that you are going through this process alone. How many of the general population really understand what you are going through when you have metastatic breast cancer? Social support can come in a variety of forms, including retreats, mentorship programs, in-person support groups, phone support groups, and online support groups. Optimally, given challenges in creating social spaces that include both those with metastatic disease and those without it, we need to do a better job of making appropriate spaces for those with metastases to share their experiences and needs.

• Help

The emotional stress of living with metastatic breast cancer produces additional difficulty for patients when they are faced with challenges that they are not "informationally" or emotionally equipped to handle. Logistical support needs may be in areas such as clinical trials and finances, and stress reduction. By getting help with logistics, you may be better able to focus on important facets of life, including family, extracurricular activities, and work.

• Connect

Your community may have additional resources, beyond those of your medical center. Ask your care providers about such resources.

Palliative care

Palliative care is an interdisciplinary medical specialty that focuses on preventing and relieving suffering. It aims at supporting the best possible quality of life for patients and those their support team members. Now the tricky part: While all care that is delivered by hospice is palliative care, not all palliative care delivered is in hospice. Indeed, palliative care can be appropriately offered to patients at any time along the trajectory of any form of serious life-threatening illness. In our center, many have palliative care while still receiving restorative, even life-extending therapies.

Despite the many benefits of palliative and hospice care, many patients in the terminal stages of a serious life-threatening illness die in settings where they do not receive care design to address suffering at the end of life. If you have advanced cancer, ask a valued member of your care team about the appropriateness of palliative care or hospice.

PHYLLODES

Phyllodes

Background

Phyllodes tumors represent only 0.5 percent of all breast cancers. While a genetic syndrome (Li-Fraumeni) is linked to the development of some phyllodes tumors, breast cancer, soft tissue sarcoma, bone sarcoma, brain tumors, adrenocortical, and Wilms' tumors, for most individuals, we don't know why the phyllodes tumor developed.

Most patients with phyllodes tumors present with breast mass or an abnormality on mammograms. Many describe a smooth, multinodular, and firm mass that is mobile and painless. While up to 20 percent will feel enlarged nodes in the axilla, spread to the nodes is uncommon.

Imaging

If a clinician suspects you may have a phyllodes tumor (based on a palpable mass, rapid growth, and a size more than three centimeters), you should have a physical exam, ultrasound, and (for those at least 30 years old) a mammogram.

A phyllodes tumor often appears on mammograms as a smooth, multi-lobulated mass. It can have a similar appearance to a benign fibroadenoma, although phyllodes tumors tend to be larger than three centimeters, are faster-growing, and are often painless. If you have a concerning mass on mammograms, the next step is typically an ultrasound: Phylloides tumors appear primarily solid and tend to be well-defined.

Diagnosis

A core needle biopsy of the mass is preferred, as getting a smaller sample with a fine needle aspiration is associated with low overall accuracy. Even a core biopsy is imperfect in rendering a diagnosis: A core biopsy can miss finding the phyllodes tumor 25 to 30 percent of the time. If you have a solid mass and the biopsy doesn't provide a definite diagnosis, you should have an excisional biopsy (lumpectomy).

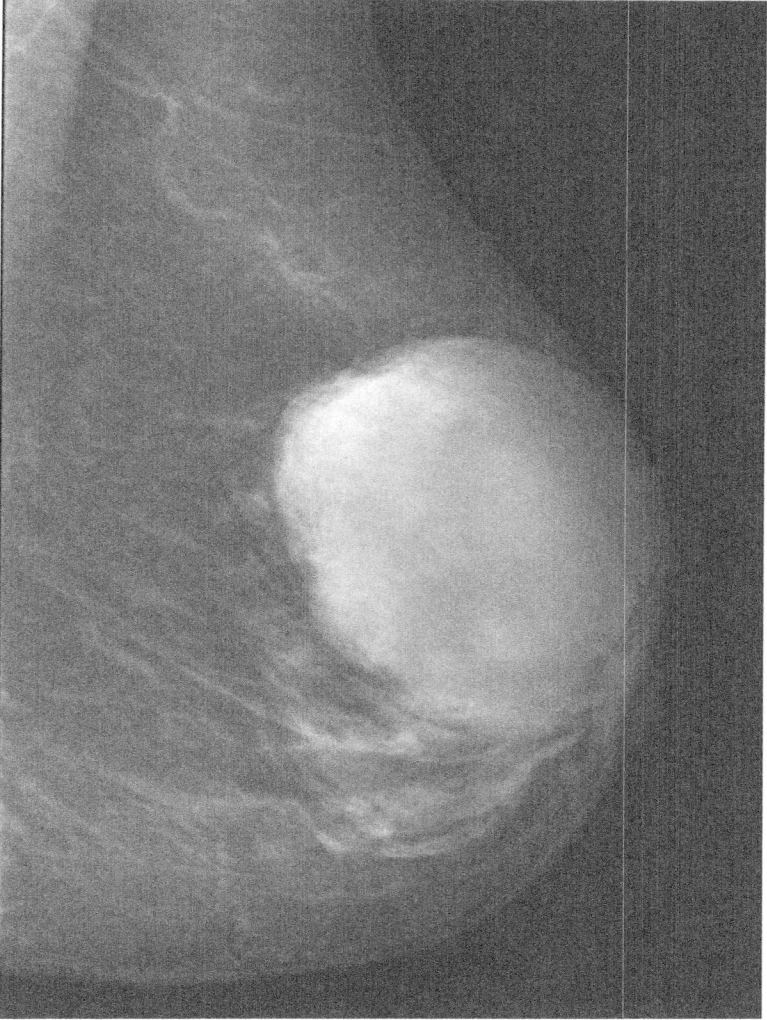

Phyllodes tumor

Phylloides

Management

Pathology

Some describe phyllodes tumors as resembling the head of a cauliflower but with a grayish-white appearance. Under the microscope, phyllodes tumors can appear in a variety of ways. We generally divide them into the following categories:

- Benign (50 percent)
- Borderline (25 percent)
- Malignant (25 percent)

These distinctions appear to have clinical value (if one sticks to specific criteria for defining the tumor), as benign tumors are associated with better in-breast (local) control and disease-free survival compared to their borderline and malignant counterparts. Finally, so-called stromal overgrowth is associated with a higher chance of spreading to distant sites (metastases).

Treatment

An excisional biopsy (lumpectomy) of the tumor is the gold standard of care for phyllodes tumors. A cancer-free zone (margin) around the tumor is critical, as an involved margin can raise your risk of an in-breast recurrence. There is no consensus on what amount of margin is adequate, with some studies suggesting at least 1 centimeter. If the margin is positive (involved with the tumor), the risk of recurrence, either in the breast or distantly, is 3.9 times higher. If your surgeon achieves adequate margins with a wide local excision (generous lumpectomy), you may not need to remove your breast (mastectomy). Fortunately, an axillary node dissection is not usually required since it is uncommon for cancer to spread to the axilla (underarm area).

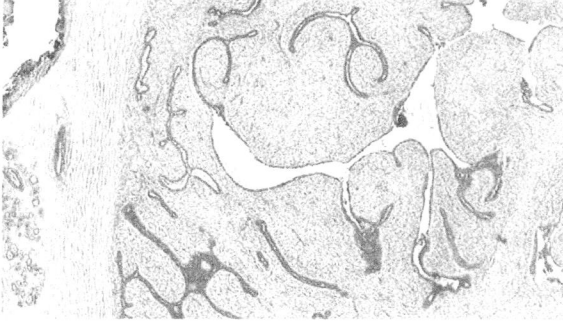

Phyllodes
("leaf-like")

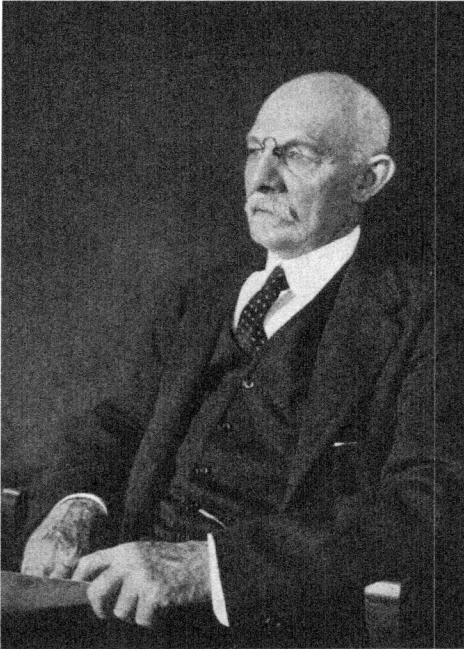

Phyllodes: Surgery
is a key

Phylloides

Management of the breast

The local (in-breast) recurrence rates following a wide excision are as follows:

Benign phyllodes	8 percent
Borderline/malignant phyllodes	21 to 36 percent

Radiation therapy: Benign phyllodes

If you have a benign phyllodes tumor, radiation therapy is unnecessary after a wide local excision that achieves adequate margins (cancer-free zone). However, if the phyllodes tumor is borderline or malignant, radiation therapy can lower the chances of it returning in the breast. A study of 443 patients showed radiation therapy to lead to a better local control rate at ten years, at least for borderline and malignant tumors:

	No radiation	**Radiation**
Local control (borderline/malignant)	**59%**	86%

After a mastectomy, there is no clear consensus about the use of radiation therapy, particularly if the margins are at least one centimeter.

Chemotherapy

The benefits of chemotherapy remain unclear. Unfortunately, we have no randomized trials to guide us. Chemotherapy may be offered for highly select patients with large tumors (over 5 cm) or high-risk or recurrent disease. The National Comprehensive Cancer Network Guidelines offer that it may be used according to the indications for soft tissue sarcoma (for example, metastatic disease).

Endocrine therapy

Endocrine (anti-estrogen) therapy does not appear effective for phyllodes tumors, even if hormone receptors are present.

Prognosis

Surgery is curative for most patients with benign or borderline phyllodes tumors. Here are the SArcoma and PHYllode Retrospective (SAPHYR) Study results. This retrospective study showed a three-year survival of 100 percent for benign and borderline tumors. This outcome compares to only 54 percent for malignant phyllodes tumors.

Follow-up

The National Comprehensive Cancer Network recommend clinical follow-up for three years for benign phyllodes. Those with a borderline or malignant phyllodes tumor should have a wide excision (without axillary surgery), then clinical follow-up for three years.

Local recurrence

Local recurrences typically occur within the first two years of the initial diagnosis, with malignant phyllodes typically recurring sooner than benign phyllodes tumors. Local only recurrences are optimally managed with resection (with wide margins without axillary node removal). Radiation therapy may be considered after surgery if there is no metastatic disease.

Metastatic disease (distant spread)

The lungs are the most common site of the distant spread of breast cancer. Following the development of metastases, the average survival is about 2.5 years, but as you can imagine, it is remarkably variable. Your team may offer surgery to remove the metastases if there is a limited-volume lung disease. Chemotherapy is often recommended for those for whom such surgery is not possible. In general, the management of the distant disease is not dissimilar to that of metastatic soft tissue sarcoma.

MEN

Male breast cancer

Invasive

Male breast cancer

In the USA, male breast cancer represents between 0.5 and 1 percent of all breast cancers. Risk factors include (but are not limited to) inherited genetics. The incidence of breast cancer gene (BRCA) mutations varies by ethnicity and family history; for example, in a population-based series of men with breast cancer not selected for family history, 0 to 4 percent have BRCA1 mutations, while between 5 and 15 percent have BRCA2 mutations. Looked at in reverse, if you have a BRCA2 gene mutation (defect), you may have a lifetime chance of 6 in 100 of getting breast cancer. If you have a BRCA1, the risk may be on the order of about 1 in 100.

Although mutations in the BRCA genes lead to an increased risk of breast cancer, other gene mutations can increase the risk. Examples include CHEK2 and PTEN gene mutations. Other risk factors for the development of male breast cancer:

- Estrogen treatment
- Obesity
- Testicular conditions
- Certain occupations (working in hot environments such as steel mills may affect the testicles, in turn changing hormone levels). Men with heavy exposure to gasoline fumes may also have an elevated risk.
- Klinefelter syndrome (a congenital condition)
- Radiation exposure (to the chest region)
- Heavy alcohol use
- Liver disease (severe liver disease can lead to low androgen and higher estrogen levels).

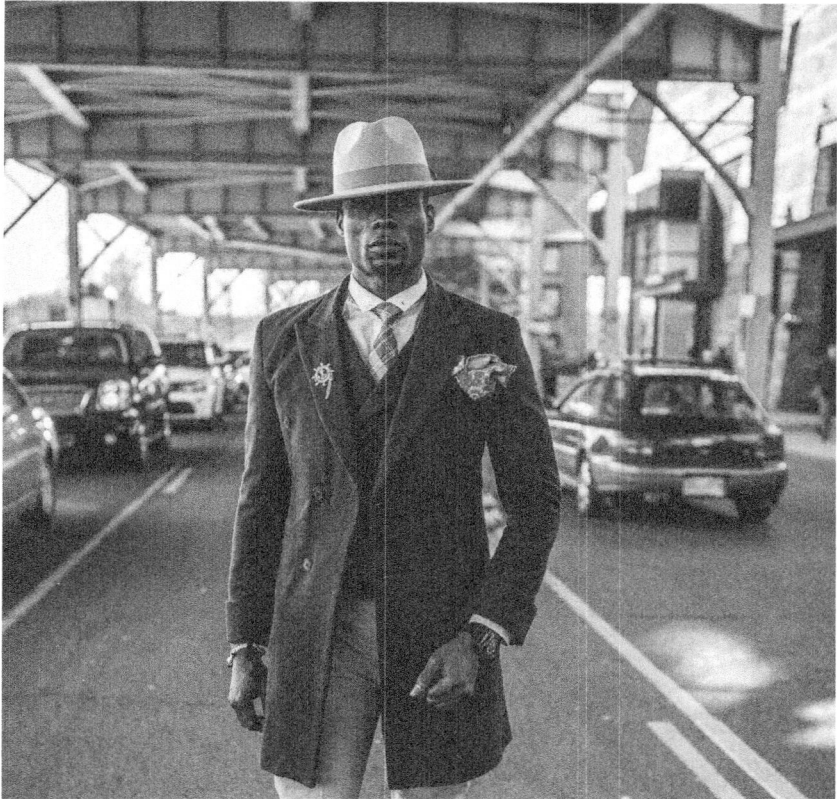

Genetic counseling and testing
All men with breast cancer should meet a genetic counselor.

Invasive

Male breast cancer

The National Comprehensive Cancer Network (www.nccn.org) recommendations include individuals of all sexual and gender identities to the greatest possible extent. Herein, the terms males and females refer to the sex assigned at birth. Unfortunately, few men participate in breast cancer clinical trials. We generally extrapolate evidence from clinical trials focusing on women. Despite biological and clinical differences between breast cancer in males and females, breast cancer management is similar.

Surgery: Typically, mastectomy

For early stage (T1-2, N0-1) disease. Most men will have a simple mastectomy (breast removal with the chest wall muscle left intact). This approach is based on the fact that: 1) more extensive surgery did not improve outcomes among women with early breast cancer, and 2) retrospective research suggests doing more extensive surgery, such as taking the chest wall/pectoralis muscle, improves outcomes.

We have limited data to suggest that breast-conserving surgery (followed by radiation therapy) is a reasonable alternative to mastectomy. Because most men have a small volume of breast tissue, most patients will have a mastectomy. Decisions about surgery type use the same criteria as for females.

Surgery: Nodes

Assessing the axillary (underarm) lymph nodes remains a vital component of early invasive breast cancer management, providing prognostic information and a potential regional control benefit.

We have limited experience with using a sentinel node procedure for men. Still, small series (including one from Italy) suggests it can work quite well as an alternative to taking out many nodes. The National Comprehensive Cancer Network offers that a sentinel lymph node biopsy should be performed in the setting of male breast cancer with clinically node-negative axilla (that is, there is no known involvement of axillary nodes).

A study analyzing 1,800 men found that while 56 percent had small primary cancers, only 4 percent had breast-conserving surgery. Most individuals had a breast removal (mastectomy), which significantly impacted the quality of life for many. While 56 percent had a diagnosis when the primary tumor was small, only four percent had breast-conserving surgery; most had a mastectomy.

Radiation therapy (RT) after surgery

The recommendations for radiation therapy are similar to those for women with breast cancer. RT is typically offered if:

- You had breast-conserving surgery
- You had a mastectomy for T3 or T4 disease
- You had a mastectomy and have a concerning surgical margin
- You had systemic therapy (such as chemotherapy) before surgery
- You have cancer involvement in your lymph nodes

Endocrine therapy

If your cancer is estrogen- or progesterone receptor-positive, your medical oncologist will likely recommend endocrine therapy. A large study of male breast cancer showed that 92 percent had estrogen receptor-positive cancer (ER+). This anti-estrogen approach is based on positive results for women with breast cancer. We also have retrospective reports suggesting that men with breast cancer who take drugs such as tamoxifen have better survival than those who did not take the pill.

An M.D. Anderson Cancer Center series looked at 156 men and found that men benefited from systemic therapy after surgery, with the greatest benefit from anti-estrogen (endocrine) therapy. Tamoxifen is the drug of choice, as we don't have as much data for using aromatase inhibitors for men. Decisions on whether to extend treatment beyond five years are individualized.

Chemotherapy

In general, recommendations for chemotherapy for males with breast cancer are based on the same principles and guidelines we use for females with breast cancer. We have limited data on molecular assays to predict chemotherapy benefits. Available data suggest that Oncotype DX provides prognostic information in males with breast cancer.

Invasive

Male breast cancer

Stage I

Surgery: Usually breast removal (mastectomy)

The primary management for stage I breast cancer is to remove it with surgery. Most men have a breast removal (mastectomy), but selected patients may be candidates for breast-conserving surgery. Because men typically have very little breast tissue, surgery usually includes the removal of the whole breast, including the nipple. For those who have breast-conserving surgery, radiation therapy usually follows.

Axillary node removal

Your surgeon will remove one or more axillary nodes to check for cancer spread, either with an axillary lymph node dissection (ALND) or a sentinel lymph node biopsy (SLNB). If the sentinel node contains cancer, a full ALND may be needed, depending on the number of nodes involved and whether another treatment, such as radiation therapy, is planned.

Systemic therapy

The oncology team may recommend endocrine ("anti-estrogen") therapy or chemotherapy. Recommendations depend on estrogen receptor status, primary cancer size, and proliferation measures such as grade and HER2 status. For example, endocrine therapy such as tamoxifen pills can be important treatment tools for those with estrogen receptor-positive cancers.

Chemotherapy may be an option if your primary cancer is larger than one centimeter (2.5 centimeters is one inch) and may also be an option if the cancer is smaller but more aggressive. Finally, men with HER2-positive tumors may have anti-HER2 drugs such as trastuzumab (Herceptin) and pertuzumab (Perjeta) added to chemotherapy. Herceptin is typically given for one year, continuing even after chemotherapy.

Stage II

Surgery

Stage II includes primary cancers that are 2.1 to 5 centimeters or have spread to a limited number of nearby lymph nodes. Surgery typically includes breast removal (mastectomy), with the removal of one or more axillary nodes to check for cancer spread, either with an axillary lymph node dissection (ALND) or sentinel lymph node biopsy. If the sentinel node contains cancer, radiation therapy typically follows.

Neoadjuvant (before surgery) chemotherapy

Sometimes, treatment begins with chemotherapy before surgery. This maneuver allows many patients to have cancer shrink before the operation. If the cancer is HER2-positive, anti-HER2 drugs such as trastuzumab (Herceptin) and pertuzumab (Perjeta) may be added to chemotherapy. Then, a mastectomy typically happens.

Radiation therapy may be given after surgery if the tumor is large, is found to have spread to several lymph nodes, or if the margins are concerning. Radiation therapy can lower the cancer recurrence risk.

Adjuvant endocrine ("anti-estrogen") therapy with tamoxifen is a standard treatment for estrogen- or progesterone receptor-positive tumors. If chemotherapy wasn't given before surgery, it might be offered after surgery, depending on your cancer characteristics, age, general health, and personal feelings about the treatment. If the cancer is HER2-positive, anti-HER2 drugs such as trastuzumab (Herceptin) and pertuzumab (Perjeta) may be added to chemotherapy.

Breast reconstruction: Uncommon

Breast reconstruction is not common in men but is sometimes possible (using tissue from your back, abdomen, or buttock). Breast implants are not used, as they are designed to recreate the appearance of a female breast. Nipple reconstruction may also be an option, rebuilding the nipple and the areola (the area around the nipple). Some have a tattoo to create a nipple, areola, or both. If you prefer no additional surgery, a nipple and areola tattoo can be done by itself. Finally, if you think breast reconstruction is something you might be interested in, please discuss it with your breast surgeon.

Invasive

Male breast cancer

Stage III

Neoadjuvant (before surgery) treatment
Stage III includes locally advanced cancer (large, growing into nearby skin or chest wall, or with a substantial burden of cancer in the regional nodes). Typically, patients are treated with chemotherapy before surgery, with anti-Her2 drugs added for those with HER2-overexpressing cancers. Alternatively, surgery can go first, followed by chemotherapy, radiation therapy, and (for estrogen receptor-positive cancer, tamoxifen pills). If the cancer is HER2 positive, anti-HER2 drugs such as trastuzumab (Herceptin) are used with chemotherapy, with the trastuzumab (Herceptin) continuing for a cumulative one year.

Surgery
Surgery (usually a breast removal) follows neoadjuvant chemotherapy. The surgeon may do a sentinel lymph node biopsy (SLNB) to check the lymph nodes for cancer if the nodes aren't known to contain cancer before surgery. Most patients require a full axillary lymph node dissection (ALND).

Radiation therapy (RT)
If recommended, radiation therapy (high-energy X-rays). Radiation therapy is daily and may last 5 to 6 weeks. The appointment times are about 15 minutes, with RT targeting the chest wall and regional lymph nodes.

Anti-estrogen pills
Adjuvant endocrine therapy with tamoxifen (pills) is given for at least five years after surgery if the tumor is hormone receptor-positive. Men with HER2-positive cancers will probably also receive trastuzumab to complete a year of that drug.

Stage IV

Systemic therapy

Management of advanced disease in males is similar to that in females. However, a GnRH inhibitor is also given if a male takes an aromatase inhibitor. While newer drugs (such as CDK4/6 inhibitors in combination with an aromatase inhibitor or fulvestrant, mTOR inhibitors, and PIK3CA inhibitors have not been well-studied in males but may be offered based on the criteria we use for females. Recommendations regarding HER2-targeted therapy, immunotherapy, and PARP inhibitors for advanced breast cancer in males are similar to those for advanced breast cancer in females.

Local therapy

On occasion, we offer surgery or radiation therapy. Here are some examples of occasions for which local therapy might be given (in the setting of distant spread of cancer or metastases):

- Cancer causes an open wound in the breast or chest wall
- Cancer is pressing on the spinal cord
- Cancer has spread to the brain
- Cancer causes pain or other bothersome symptoms
- Cancer causes the bone to be so weak that it may break
- Cancer causes a blockage in your liver
- You have a very limited amount of distant spread

Invasive

Male breast cancer

Recurrent cancer

Local (in-breast, skin or chest wall) recurrence

A cure may still be possible if you have a local recurrence and no evidence of distant metastases. Management depends on several factors, including the type of treatment you have already received. For example, if you initially had a mastectomy, recurrence is often treated by surgically removing recurrent cancer, if possible. Radiation therapy may then follow (for many patients, re-treatment of the chest wall with radiation therapy may be possible). Systemic therapy may include anti-estrogen approaches (for estrogen receptor-positive cancer), chemotherapy, and anti-HER2 tools (if your cancer over-expresses HER2).

Regional recurrence

If your cancer comes back in nearby lymph nodes (including those in the underarm area or around the collarbone), we refer to the disease as a regional recurrence, and a cure may still be possible. Care begins with surgical removal of the disease, if possible. Radiation therapy may follow surgery. Systemic therapy can include anti-estrogen approaches (for hormone receptor-positive cancer), chemotherapy, and anti-HER2 tools (if your cancer over-expresses HER2).

Distant recurrence

A distant recurrence is when cancer returns but in organs such as the bones, lungs, liver, or brain. Men with distant metastases are typically managed the same way as those with Stage IV breast cancer (spread to distant organs at the initial diagnosis). For the recurrent group, your care team must account for previous treatments.

Coping

It may be challenging for you to tell others about your diagnosis. Many find it helpful to start by informing family and close friends first, allowing you to become more familiar with the reactions to the news. Given the uncommonness of male breast cancer, some individuals may question you.

Unfortunately, the diagnosis can affect some friendships. This phenomenon is sometimes in the context of an inability to cope with the news. Friends may become more distant; conversely, some may become closer to you. There is no "right" way to respond, and you must navigate the course that works for you.

Lymphedema

While other side effects are possible, I want to talk about arm swelling. A surgeon removing lymph can restrict fluid flow from the breast region and arm. This restriction can sometimes result in swelling of the arm and hand, known as lymphedema. Fortunately, most men will not develop lymphedema. Still, it can occur at any time, even years after surgery. Ask a care team member if they can give you exercises to reduce risk.

If you develop any of these symptoms, please seek prompt advice from a medical team member.

- Arm or hand swelling (you may notice your shirt sleeves feel tight)
- Feelings of discomfort, heaviness, or fullness in the arm
- Aching, pain, or tension in the arm, shoulder, hand, or chest region

If you develop any of these symptoms, seek prompt advice from a member of your medical team.

Depression

In one study of over 160 men with breast cancer, psychological distress included significant depression (1%) and anxiety (6%). Psychological distress appeared higher among men who had a mastectomy, those who had side effects, and those who were not married. Cancer-related distress was associated with younger age, altered body image, and greater perceived stressfulness due to reduced physical ability, pain, fear, and uncertainty about the future.

RESTORE

Breast reconstruction

Restoration

Breast reconstruction: Basics

You may have had (or be about to have) a removal of your breast(s). Some will have a mastectomy as a part of treatment, while others do it because they are at a very high risk of developing breast cancer. Breast reconstruction, if performed, often takes place during the mastectomy procedure. Some patients elect delayed reconstruction months or years after the breast removal. Less commonly, patients desire reconstruction after a lumpectomy.

Losing a breast can be traumatic. Some patients feel sad, anxious, or mournful. Now, you may have the opportunity to reconstruct your breast. Some women choose not to reconstruct. Still, the option to undergo mastectomy alone with a surgically optimized closure should be offered to all as part of a comprehensive discussion of reconstructive options. So how do you decide? You may wish to consider the following:

- How important is your breast to you?
- Would you be comfortable with a prosthesis, a breast form that you take on and off?
- Will reconstruction help you to feel more whole?
- Are you comfortable with additional surgery and the potential associated complications?

Please note that even if you choose reconstruction, it doesn't restore sensation to the breast or the nipple. Now, if you decide to proceed with breast reconstruction, there are two major categories:

- Implant-based reconstruction (uses saline or saltwater versus a silicone implant to create a breast shape;
- Autologous (flap) reconstruction (uses tissue taken from another area of your body to create a breast form).

On occasion, a surgeon may combine the two approaches.

Reconstruction: Implants

A plastic surgeon may perform a reconstruction using prosthetic devices in one or two stages. For one-stage reconstruction, a permanent implant is inserted during your mastectomy. With two-stage reconstruction, a tissue expander is placed at the same time as your breast removal and gradually filled until you get to your desired size. A permanent implant replaces the tissue expander at a later date.

Reconstruction: Autologous

Here, you use your tissues to create a new breast. Donor sites may be from the abdomen, back, inner thigh, or buttocks.

Reconstruction: Following oncoplastic surgery

Oncoplastic surgery involves the creation of a wider resection of the breast cancer (as compared with traditional breast-conserving surgery), followed by immediate or delayed (but before radiation therapy) reconstruction of the breast deformity. There is tissue rearrangement to restore a more natural breast contour. Such surgery may allow for better margins than a traditional lumpectomy, decreasing the need for mastectomy (particularly for those with a larger breast cancer-to-breast size ratio).

Reconstruction: The nipple

After breast reconstruction, if the nipple was removed as a part of your cancer operation, you may desire a nipple-areolar reconstruction. This restoration is often done during the second stage of breast reconstruction. A plastic surgeon may use one of several techniques. A tattooing procedure for the areola (colored area around the nipple) may be added to optimize the cosmetic outcome. Some patients will create a 3-dimensional tattoo as an alternative to surgical reconstruction of the nipple.

Trouble? Tobacco, diabetes, obesity, COPD, and more

Tobacco users have a significantly higher risk of surgical complications, especially with reconstruction using their tissues. Obesity, insulin-dependent diabetes, chronic obstructive pulmonary disease, connective tissue disorders, and thrombophilia (an abnormality of blood coagulation that increases the risk of blood clots in blood vessels) can raise risk, too.

Restoration

Breast reconstruction: Skin-sparing mastectomy

A mastectomy typically removes the breast, overlying skin, nipple, and areola. With a skin-sparing mastectomy, much of the skin is preserved. Your surgeon will only use a skin-sparing approach when a breast reconstruction will begin during the same operation.

The surgeon removes the skin of your nipple and areola. She then removes the breast tissue through the same incision. A plastic surgeon then reconstructs the breast using your own tissue, with or without an implant. Then, the skin is sutured closed around it.

Are you a candidate?

Skin-sparing surgery may be an appropriate option for you if you desire immediate reconstruction after a mastectomy. Many women who a having a risk-reducing breast removal (prophylactic mastectomy) opt for this surgical approach.

The surgical margins should appear to be uninvolved; that is there should be no concerns about the cancer being very close to the skin or underlying chest wall. Finally, those with inflammatory breast cancer or multiple tumors may not be candidates for a skin-sparing mastectomy.

Reconstruction

Some women have an abdominal-based flap reconstruction (TRAM or DIEP flap). Your surgeon removes some skin, muscle, and fat from your abdomen, just below your belly button. This tissue is then transferred to your chest to create a soft, natural breast. The operation leaves a surgical scar on the belly. Alternatively, tissue may be transferred from your latissimus muscle.

Alternatively, a permanent or temporary saline implant might be used. If a temporary implant is placed, and you need to return for another operation to place a permanent one.

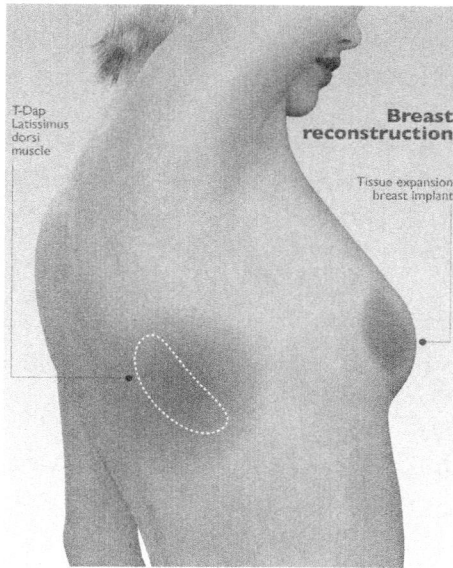

T-Dap
Latissimus
dorsi
muscle

**Breast
reconstruction**

Tissue expansion
breast implant

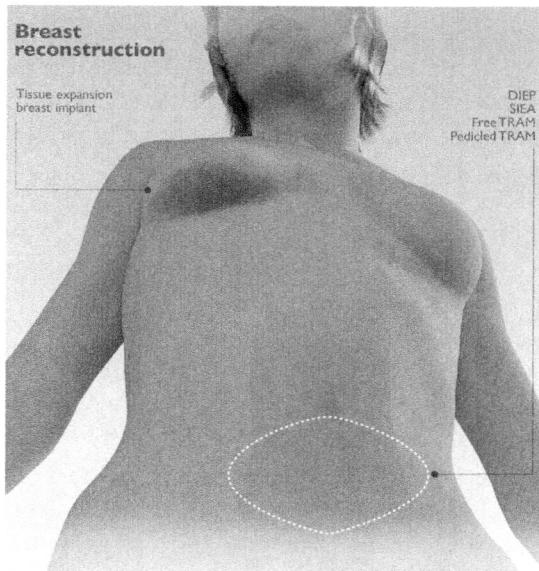

**Breast
reconstruction**

Tissue expansion
breast implant

DIEP
SIEA
Free TRAM
Pedicled TRAM

Restoration

Breast reconstruction: Timing

A plastic surgeon may perform reconstruction at the same operation as a mastectomy. Alternatively, a patient may have a delayed reconstruction. Let's look first at the timing of reconstruction:

- *Immediate*

Years ago, delayed reconstruction was preferred, but there has been an evolution over time: Today, we know that immediate reconstruction can be associated with significant psychological benefits. In addition, the surgery process is streamlined, as the breast removal and reconstruction can be done in one setting. Normal breast landmarks, including the junction of the breast and chest (infra-mammary fold), are preserved with immediate breast reconstruction.

Of course, there are potential downsides too. Immediate reconstruction prolongs the surgery time, adding an hour or more for implant-based reconstruction and even more for reconstructions using your tissue. Some patients will have a breakdown (necrosis) of the mastectomy skin flaps, negatively affecting the cosmetic outcome.

Finally, those with large cancers, direct skin or chest wall invasion, nodal involvement, or concerning margins (cancer-free zone around the removed breast) strongly recommend radiation therapy (RT). Radiation therapy can negatively impact your breast reconstruction.

- *Delayed*

Delayed reconstruction may be recommended if you have suboptimal blood flow to the skin flaps after mastectomy. Some patients who need radiation therapy, have significant other illnesses, or suboptimal social habits (obesity, poorly-controlled diabetes, tobacco usage) may need to delay reconstruction. Those with the locally advanced form of breast cancer known as inflammatory breast cancer should delay reconstruction, too.

Delayed reconstruction allows for assurance of clear margins prior to restoration. It can reduce the chances of having inadequate blood flow to the mastectomy skin flaps. Disadvantages include the need for surgery at a later date, often a less good cosmetic outcome (compared with immediate reconstruction), and limits on reconstruction options after radiotherapy.

The optimal timing of reconstruction, relative to radiation therapy, remains controversial. Some advocate looking at a removed sentinel node at the time of surgery and delaying reconstruction if the node is involved. An alternative for those getting implant-based reconstruction is to place a tissue expander at the time of the breast removal, preserving the shape of the breast envelope. After the final pathology report comes out several days to about a week later, those who don't need radiation therapy may proceed to early completion of their reconstruction process; those that need RT may delay the final reconstruction. Your radiation oncologist may (or may not) request a temporary deflation of one or both tissue expanders to optimize radiation therapy targeting.

Implants associated with a small risk of lymphoma

A study from 2018 found that one in 6,920 women with breast implants will develop an aggressive form of cancer known as anaplastic large-cell lymphoma (ALCL) in the breast before they reach age 75.

ALCL is a type of non-Hodgkin's lymphoma that can affect the skin, lymph nodes, or organs throughout the body. In a recent study, researchers examined the nationwide Dutch pathology registry to identify all cases of breast ALCL in the country from 1990 to 2016. Among the 43 cases found, 32 were in women with breast implants. So-called macro-textured implants were found in 23 of 28 patients (for whom the implant type was known) with lymphoma; micro-textured implants were found in the remaining five patients. ALCL patients had polyurethane-covered implants.

Saline versus silicone

Saline and silicone breast implants both have an outer silicone shell. The implants differ in material and consistency, however. Saline implants are filled with sterile salt water. They're inserted empty and then filled once they're in place. Silicone implants are pre-filled with silicone gel — a thick, sticky fluid that feels like human fat. Most women feel that silicone breast implants look and feel more like natural breast tissue.

Restoration

Breast reconstruction: Impact of radiation

A minority of patients with a mastectomy will need radiation therapy (RT) based on the involvement of the nodes with cancer, concerning margins, or locally advanced disease. Radiation therapy can be problematic, as it increases the chance of complications associated with reconstruction.

• *Radiation therapy (RT) and implant complications*

Radiation therapy complications are highest among women with expander/implant reconstruction, whether RT occurs before or after the surgery. Complications may include scar formation at the implant/tissue interface, contracture of the capsule, or skin healing problems. Some patients will experience implant rupture, have the implant rupture through the skin, or become badly positioned.

> In a study from Utah (USA), radiation therapy did *not* affect patient satisfaction. Still, radiation therapy led to a higher rate of breast implant removal. The **implant removal rates for non-radiation and radiation therapy patients were 4% and 22%,** respectively.

Implants placed in front of (instead of behind) the chest wall muscle may have a lower complication rate, but this is an evolving area.

• *Radiation therapy (RT) and autologous (flap) tissue complications*

Radiation therapy can result in flap shrinkage, necrosis (tissue death), or scarring. Still, flap-based reconstructions generally tolerate radiation therapy better than implant-based ones. Late complications may be lower when flap-based reconstruction is done after (instead of before) radiation therapy. Still, complications are not uncommon: One retrospective study found a complication rate of 32 percent for those who had radiation therapy first, compared to 44 percent for those who had breast reconstruction first.

Breast reconstruction: After

Walk

Your surgeon may ask you to begin gentle walking soon after the operation. Early activity can reduce the risk of forming clots, a condition known as deep vein thrombosis (DVTs), and improve lung function.

Drains

Following an implant-based reconstruction, a drain is usually placed in the implant space and will remain there for several days. By day 2 or 3 after surgery, most patients are allowed to shower. With a tissue expander process, expansion in the office or clinic is typically done at one- or two-week intervals until complete. For a reconstruction using your tissues, the drain duration is variable. Many patients are in the hospital for three to four days and often can shower on postoperative days 2 or 3.

Discomfort

Many experience pain at the incision site and may experience spasms of local muscles. Perhaps not surprisingly, you will likely have to avoid strenuous activities for about six weeks after the surgery. As physicians, we are working hard to reduce the use of narcotic medications for pain. Enhanced recovery after surgery (ERAS) protocols include preoperative counseling, optimization of nutrition, standardized analgesic and anesthetic regimens, and early mobilization. Ask your surgeon about what you can do to reduce your probability of having long-term problems with narcotics.

Don't forget to 1) make the narcotic pain medications in your home inaccessible to others; 2) watch for constipation; 3) not operate heavy machinery (including automobiles); and 4) get the narcotics out of your home as soon as reasonable (for example, select pharmacies have boxes for trashing them).

Surveillance after breast reconstruction

Mastectomy is not a guarantee that there will not be a local recurrence. In that context, follow-up is important. The vast majority of local and regional recurrences are palpable; you can feel them. Thus, a physical exam is central to detecting recurrent breast cancer. Most feel mammograms after reconstruction (following breast removal) are unnecessary.

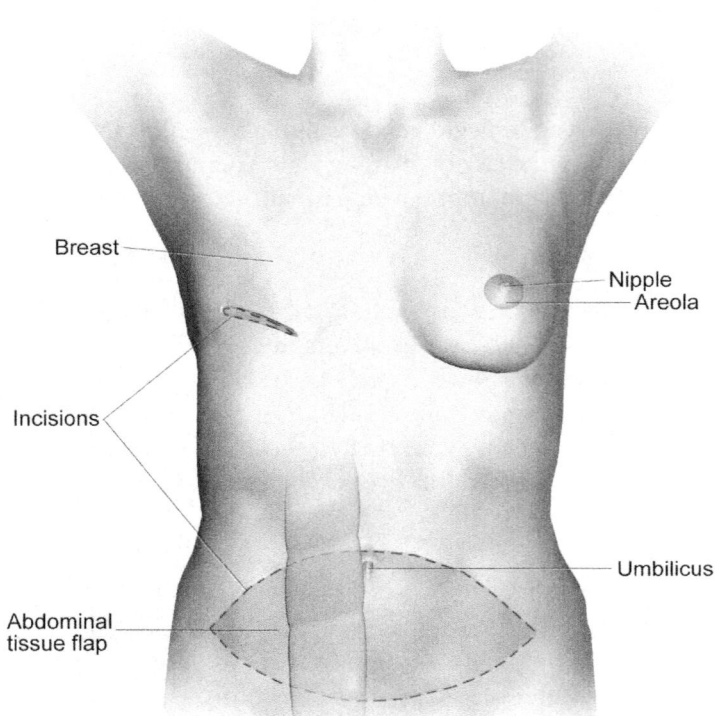

TRAM (transverse rectus abdominis) is a muscle in your lower abdomen between your waist and your pubic bone. A flap of this skin, fat, and all or part of the underlying rectus abdominus ("6-pack") muscle are used to reconstruct the breast in a TRAM flap procedure.

A DIEP flap is similar to a muscle-sparing free TRAM flap, except that no muscle is used to rebuild the breast. (A muscle-sparing free TRAM flap uses a small amount of muscle.) A DIEP flap is considered a muscle-sparing type of flap. DIEP stands for the deep inferior epigastric perforator artery, which runs through the abdomen.

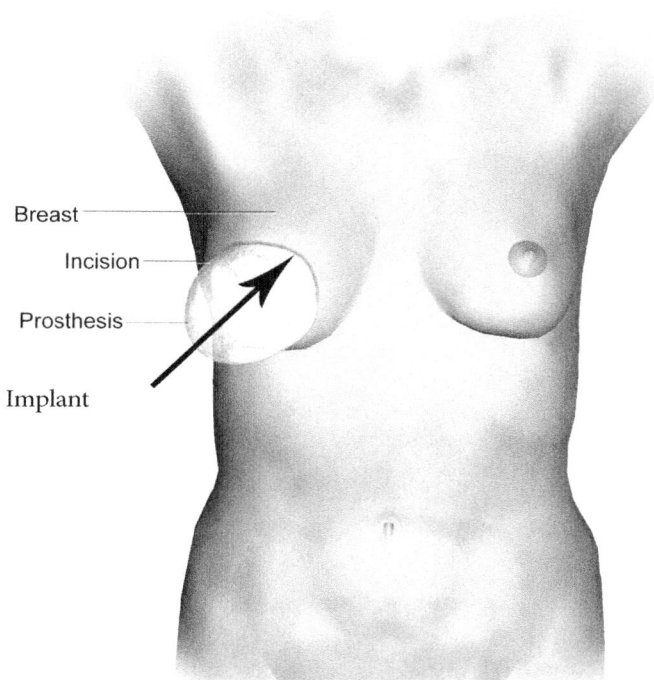

Breast

Incision

Prosthesis

Implant

Implant-based reconstruction typically requires less extensive surgery than flap reconstruction, as it only involves the chest area and not tissue donor sites. Still, you may need additional surgery in the future, as implants can wear out (often within 10 to 20 years) or develop other issues (e.g., scar tissue forming around the implant).

Implants may be filled with saline (salt water), silicone gel, or a combination. The plastic surgeon often places the implant behind the chest muscle. The device itself may be round or tear-shaped, and the surface may be smooth or have a slightly rough texture.

Restoration

Summary

Types

- *Devices-based reconstruction*
Tissue expanders; salt water-filled implants; silicone-filled implants

- *Oncoplastic reconstruction*
Volume displacement or replacement techniques)

- *Autologous reconstruction*
Involves the transfer of a flap of tissue from a donor site (for example, the abdomen or belly) to the front chest wall.

The choice of reconstruction depends on body shape, other medical problems (diabetes; smoking; obesity), the size and shape of the other breast, prior surgical procedures, the quality of the chest skin, and patient preference.

Timing

Breast reconstruction is often performed immediately after breast removal; it may be done during the same operating room time. Immediate reconstruction allows for reduced costs, often better cosmetic outcomes, psychological benefits, and more streamlined care. Immediate reconstruction may be especially appealing for those with a prophylactic (preventative or risk-reducing) breast removal or a mastectomy for ductal carcinoma in situ or for invasive breast cancers that are 5 centimeters or less and are not known to be associated with spread to regional lymph nodes.

For those needing radiation therapy after a mastectomy, delayed or delayed-immediate reconstruction may be considered. Many surgeons don't like to irradiate a flap reconstruction, as long-term complications can occur. Still, autologous (your tissues) reconstruction is often preferred (as compared to an implant) following radiation therapy since there are fewer complications following radiation therapy.

Breast implant

Breast implant

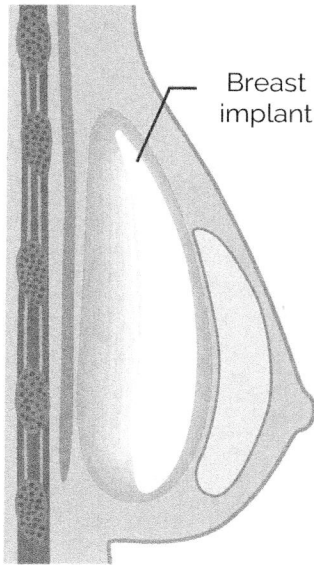

Subglandular insertion

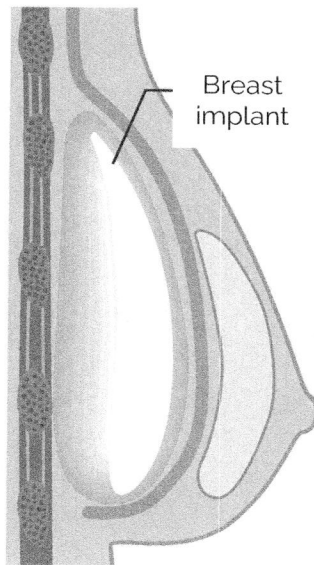

Submuscular insertion

SPECIAL

Inflammatory; Pregnancy; Unknown primary
Paget's; Lymphoma; Young

Inflammatory

Inflammatory breast cancer

Inflammatory breast cancer (IBC) is an uncommon form of breast cancer that accounts for 0.5 to two percent of all breast cancers in the USA but may be higher elsewhere. It is especially **aggressive**, with a median survival of 57 months for those without metastases. The 20-year disease-specific survival is 20 percent, a marked improvement from 1995. For those with a distant spread of cancer, the median survival is about 21 months.

Rapid onset

Those with IBC typically present with breast pain or a rapidly growing breast lump. They may also report a tender, firm, or enlarged breast, with or without breast itchiness. Almost all women have lymph node involvement, and about one-third will have a distant spread of cancer or metastases. The onset of symptoms is usually rapid, from weeks to months. Many patients initially receive antibiotics for presumed mastitis.

On physical exam, the breast skin is often thickened and warm to the touch, with a peau d'orange (skin of an orange) appearance. The skin may appear pink, red, or purplish over at least one-third of its area. The nipple may be red, crusty, or have other changes, and a breast lump may or may not be present.

Prompt diagnosis and staging are critical to optimizing outcomes. A multidisciplinary approach typically includes systemic therapy (for example, chemotherapy), breast removal, and radiation therapy. But we first begin with proper diagnosis and determining the extent of cancer (staging).

Mammograms

Patients with suspected inflammatory breast cancer should have diagnostic mammograms. Breast swelling and tenderness sometimes make imaging with mammograms challenging. Mammograms may demonstrate a mass, a large area of calcifications or breast tissue distortion, and skin thickening. Mastitis and inflammatory breast cancer with no underlying mass may appear similar on mammograms. If a week or so of antibiotics don't improve symptoms, you should have a biopsy promptly.

Before any intervention (including biopsies), a photograph can visually document your degree of redness and swelling. Later, your doctor can compare the current exam to the original photo to help assess your response to treatment.

Ultrasound

After diagnostic mammograms, an ultrasound may be offered. Ultrasound can help determine if your axillary/underarm lymph nodes are enlarged and may find breast mass(es) if they are present. Finally, ultrasound can help determine the optimal location for a needle biopsy.

Diagnosis

While we use the term "inflammatory," the characteristic features of inflammatory breast cancer are due to the blockage (by small bits of cancer or tumor emboli) of small lymph channels in the skin. Although you will need a biopsy to evaluate for cancer in breast tissue and the dermal lymphatics, a diagnosis of inflammatory breast cancer depends on a physical exam (and imaging support). Skin lymphatic involvement is neither required nor sufficient to assign a diagnosis.

Workup

Typical tests include a complete history and physical examination, and blood work. Imaging studies typically include diagnostic mammograms of both breasts, with ultrasound added as needed. While a breast MRI scan is optional, we routinely get one in my institution.

Evaluations for the presence of **distant spread of cancer** often include liver function blood work, bone scan or sodium fluoride PET/CT scan, and diagnostic CT imaging of the chest and abdomen (with or without the pelvis).

Before you move to chemotherapy, your care team will determine whether the hormones estrogen or progesterone and the status of the HER2 receptor drive cancer. HER2 predicts which patients will likely benefit from HER2-targeted therapy. You should have genetic counseling if you are at high risk for hereditary breast cancer.

Inflammatory

Inflammatory breast cancer

Management

Inflammatory breast cancer is a very aggressive form of locally advanced breast cancer. While inflammatory breast cancer is managed similarly to other locally advanced breast cancers, those with inflammatory breast cancer are not potential candidates for breast-conserving management, even those who respond well to treatment (such as chemotherapy) before surgery.

Begin with chemotherapy

Treatment begins with chemotherapy. The preferred approach is anthracyclines (doxorubicin (Adriamycin) or epirubicin) plus a taxane. Those with human epidermal growth receptor 2 (HER2) overexpression should also receive HER2-directed therapy. Treatment after initial chemotherapy depends on the response:

- For those with cancer that can be removed should have a breast removal (mastectomy) with an axillary dissection; a sentinel lymph node biopsy is not recommended; immediate reconstruction is not generally done, given the high risk for a local recurrence. Radiation therapy is given, most commonly over approximately six weeks.

  Patients then complete planned chemotherapy (if not finished before surgery). Those with ER- or PR-positive have endocrine therapy.

  The anti-HER2 agent trastuzumab (Herceptin) continues for a cumulative one year.

- For those who do not have operable cancer following chemotherapy before surgery, second-line systemic may be offered. Radiation therapy may be offered to shrink the disease for those who still cannot have a mastectomy.

Management is individualized for those for whom chemotherapy does not elicit a response. Finally, metastatic (distant spread) cancer is managed similarly to metastatic non-inflammatory breast cancer.

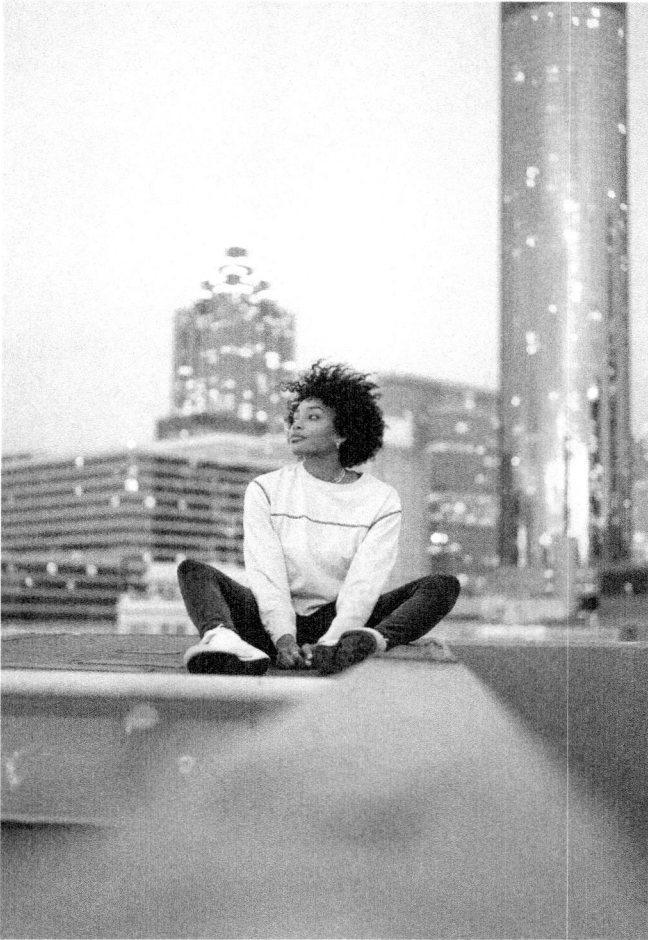

Premenopausal women should have fertility counseling. Those at risk for hereditary breast cancer should have genetic counseling.

Pregnancy

Breast cancer during pregnancy

Breast cancer occurring with pregnancy is infrequent: A California study showed 1.3 breast cancers diagnosed per 10,000 live births. Alas, many such cancers are associated with spread to regional nodes and often present with a larger cancer in the breast, more aggressive cancer cell characteristics. They are more likely to over-express HER2 or be estrogen- and progesterone receptor-negative.

Initial evaluation

The natural tenderness and engorgement of the breasts of pregnant and lactating women may make the early diagnosis of breast cancer a challenge. Often, pregnancy-related cancers are detected at a later stage than in a non-pregnant, age-matched population.

Physical exams and imaging come first. The National Comprehensive Cancer Network Guidelines (www.nccn.org) call for a chest X-ray (with abdominal shielding). If there is a concern for liver metastases, a woman may have an abdominal ultrasound. Finally, if there is a concern for bone metastases, you and your doctors may consider a non-contrast MRI of the spine.

Ultrasound An ultrasound of the breasts and regional lymph nodes allows for assessing the disease extent.

Biopsy

While fine needle aspiration biopsies may be done, a core needle biopsy is preferred. It allows for assessing the status of estrogen- and progesterone receptors (ER, PR) and HER2. Breast cancer pathology is similar in age-matched pregnant and non-pregnant women. However, elevated estrogen levels associated with pregnancy may lead to a higher incidence of ER detection with an immunohistochemistry test than radiolabeled ligand-binding testing. Ask your doctor how your cancer was checked for estrogen receptors, as the radiolabeled ligand-binding test has a higher chance of finding estrogen receptors, which is important for prognosis and management.

Management

Pregnancy assessment should include a maternal-fetal medicine consultation and review of current maternal risks such as hypertension, diabetes, and complications with prior pregnancies. It would be best if you had an assessment of fetal growth and development and fetal age with an ultrasound exam. Estimation of the date of the delivery can help with systemic chemotherapy planning if this treatment is indicated. Maternal-fetal medicine consultation should include counseling regarding maintaining or terminating the pregnancy, although most women can maintain it despite the need for cancer treatment.

Your care team may discuss pregnancy termination if you are in your first trimester. For those continuing the pregnancy in the first trimester, mastectomy and axillary staging is usually the first step. For those in the second trimester or early third trimester, initial options include a mastectomy or breast-conserving surgery (either approach with axillary staging) versus preoperative chemotherapy followed by surgery.

For women in their late third trimester, treatment is typically surgery with a mastectomy or breast-conserving surgery (either approach with axillary staging).

In general, we manage early breast cancer in the same way as we do non-pregnant women. Of course, there can be some modifications to protect the fetus. Breast cancer surgery appears to be safe during pregnancy. Although the anesthesia used during surgery can cross the placenta to the fetus, fortunately, it doesn't appear to cause congenital disabilities or serious pregnancy problems.

Surgery options for early breast cancer may include mastectomy versus breast-conserving surgery ad radiation. We cannot give radiation therapy to a pregnant woman. Still, suppose she is towards the end of her pregnancy or needs chemotherapy before radiation therapy is given. In that case, breast conservation followed by delivery of the baby by radiation therapy may be an excellent option for select individuals. Alas, I am unaware of high-level evidence suggesting that a sentinel node procedure is safe for pregnant women, so a more thorough nodal removal may be necessary for invasive breast cancer.

Chemotherapy may be delivered, but only after the first trimester. The indications for systemic chemotherapy are the same for a pregnant patient as for a non-pregnant breast cancer patient.

The largest pregnancy experience is with anthracyclines (for example, doxo-rubicin/Adriamycin) and alkylating chemotherapy drugs. Fetal malformation risks in the second and third trimesters are about 1.3 percent, not different than that of fetuses not exposed to chemotherapy during pregnancy. We have fewer data regarding the use of taxanes. If a pregnant woman has chemothera-py, there should be fetal monitoring before each chemotherapy cycle.

Chemotherapy during pregnancy should not be given after week 35 of preg-nancy or within three weeks of the planned delivery to avoid the chance of blood-related complications during delivery. Women receiving chemotherapy should not breastfeed their children.

If **trastuzumab (Herceptin)** is recommended, it should be administered after the baby is delivered; the National Comprehensive Cancer Network, a group of some of the top cancer-treating facilities in the world (www.nccn.org), recom-mends against its use during pregnancy. We have limited data regarding other anti-HER2 drugs, including lapatinib.

Endocrine therapy (such as tamoxifen or aromatase inhibitors) and radiation therapy are contraindicated during pregnancy. If indicated, endocrine and radiation therapy should thus not be initiated until the postpartum period.

Advanced breast cancer

There is no standard management approach for patients with advanced (stage III or stage IV) breast cancer during pregnancy; treatment is individualized. Some of the same principles as early breast cancer apply: Chemotherapy during the first trimester should be avoided; radiation therapy should not be received during pregnancy. While some patients may consider an abortion, therapeutic abortion does not improve prognosis. Many studies point to a 5-year survival chance of about 10 percent among pregnant patients with stage III or IV breast cancer.

Pregnancy after breast cancer treatment: Appears safe

While we do not have high-level evidence, the available clinical literature sug-gests that women who have a pregnancy after having been managed for breast cancer do not compromise their survival chances. In addition, there appear to be no harmful effects on the fetus. Still, given the recurrence risk is highest in the first couple of years after a breast cancer diagnosis, many prefer to wait for some time (for example, two years) before attempting to conceive.

Research shows no damaging effects on the fetus from maternal breast cancer, and there are no reported cases of maternal-fetal transfer of breast cancer cells.

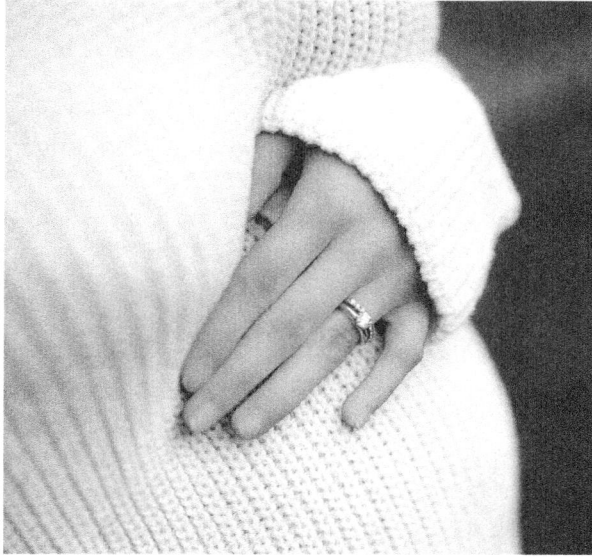

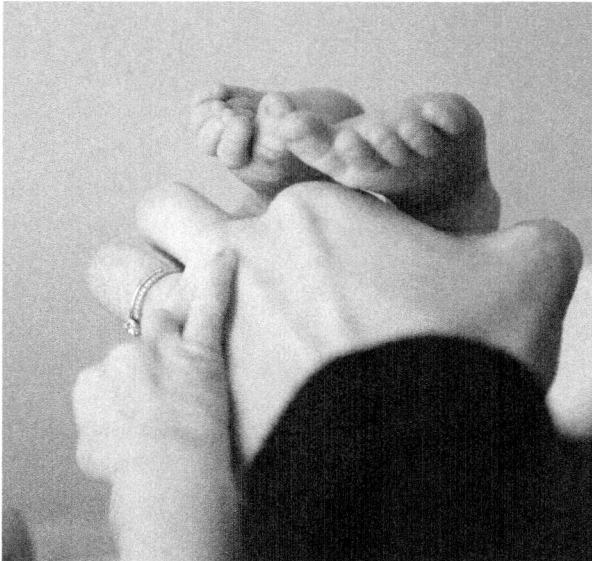

Unknown primary site

Axillary cancer with no identifiable origin site

Occult breast cancer that presents as a disease in the axillary nodes (with no identifiable cancer in the breast) is uncommon, accounting for under one percent of all breast malignancies. A core needle biopsy of axillary nodes is preferred. The pathologist will determine if the available biopsy material is adequate or if additional biopsies are necessary to provide an accurate and complete diagnosis.

While treating women with occult breast cancer typically involves mastectomy and axillary node dissection, axillary nodal dissection followed by radiation therapy has been successful for many.

Looking for the primary site

Testing for cancer markers, including estrogen receptors (ER), progesterone receptors (PR), and HER2, is recommended. Elevated ER/PR levels point to a breast cancer diagnosis. Breast MRI can be useful in identifying the primary site for about 70 percent of patients with occult primary breast cancer and may also facilitate breast conservation for selected women. Additional evaluation may include chest and abdominal CT scans to look for distant metastases.

Treatment

The clinical stage is central to treatment recommendations. Nodal status informs treatment recommendations for those with breast MRI-negative disease. For those with no known breast primary site (who, in addition, have limited spread to the axillary nodes - clinical stage T0, N1, M0), options include mastectomy plus axillary lymph node dissection or axillary lymph node dissection followed by whole breast radiation therapy (typically with RT also targeting nodes). A series from Roswell Park Cancer Center (USA) found no recurrences among ten patients, with only one patient managed with mastectomy.

Chemotherapy, endocrine therapy, or trastuzumab is given according to standard recommendations for stage II or III disease. Drugs (such as chemotherapy) should be considered for more advanced nodal disease, as for patients with locally advanced disease.

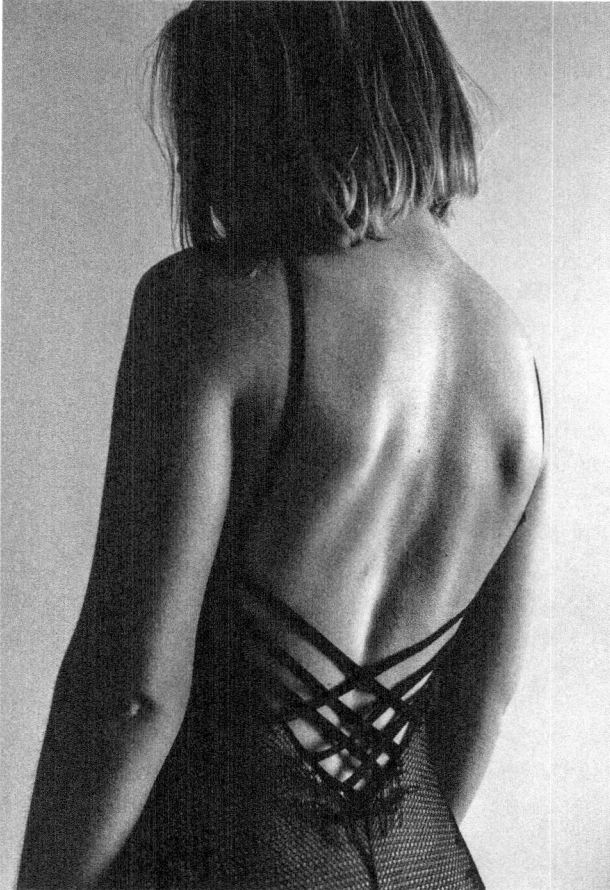

Breast lymphoma

Primary breast lymphoma

Primary breast lymphoma (PBL) is a rare disease accounting for 0.4-0.5% of all breast malignancies. Non-Hodgkin lymphoma is a cancer that starts in cells called lymphocytes, which are a part of the body's immune system. Diffuse large B-cell lymphoma (DLBCL) is the most common type of breast lymphoma (representing about half of all breast lymphomas). There are many other types of lymphoma.

Rare

We often use the term "primary breast lymphoma" (PBL) to define a lymphoma primarily occurring in the breast without previously detected lymphoma. The median age of patients ranges from 60 to 65 years. The disease occurs almost exclusively in women. Bilateral breast involvement accounts for 11% of all breast lymphomas. This rare situation is especially observed during pregnancy or postpartum, suggesting that hormonal stimulation influences tumor growth. Primary breast lymphoma comprises only tumors in stage I (lymphoma limited to the breast) and stage II (lymphoma limited to the breast and axillary lymph nodes), not tumors originating from non-breast sites.

We believe breast lymphomas arise from lymphocytes that live in lymph nodes within the breast or the breast lymphatic system. Lymphocytes in the breast are a part of so-called mucosa-associated lymphoid tissue (MALT). T-cell lymphoma tends to behave more aggressively than its more common B-cell counterpart. We are increasingly aware that women with a *textured* type breast implant may have a very small increased risk of developing anaplastic large cell lymphoma.

Symptoms

A painless mass is the most common presenting sign in primary breast lymphoma, occurring in approximately 61 percent of cases. Twelve percent will present with localized pain, 11 percent with local inflammation, 25 percent with palpable nodes, and as an incidental finding on mammograms for another 12 percent.

Evaluation: Excisional biopsy preferred

While a core biopsy may be adequate to diagnose a breast lymphoma, an excisional biopsy is preferred when possible. We stage primary breast lymphomas according to the Lugano revisions to the Ann Arbor staging system.

Stage	Involvement
Limited	
I	1 (or a group of adjacent) node(s)
II	2+ nodal groups on the same side of the diaphragm

Prognosis: Breast lymphoma

Prognosis depends on the stage of cancer, as well as the cancer cell type. Poor prognostic indicators include age over 60, an elevation in the blood level of lactate dehydrogenase (LDH), Stage II (rather than Stage I) disease, and your general day-to-day condition (performance status).

A British Columbia (Canada) study of 50 patients with limited-stage primary breast lymphoma included 16 patients with indolent cell types and 34 with more aggressive cell types. Most patients with the less aggressive cell types got radiation therapy (75 percent) or observation (13 percent). The five-year disease-specific survival rates (not dying of lymphoma) were 91 percent. Most of those with Stage I or II aggressive lymphomas got chemotherapy plus radiation therapy or chemotherapy alone. The estimated five-year lymphoma-specific survival rates were 71 percent.

Meta-analysis (collection of studies)

A meta-analysis of 465 PBL cases from 3 decades (1972-2005) had an average follow-up of 48 months and a mean age of 54. Diffuse large B-cell lymphoma was the most common subtype (53%). This study found that mastectomy offered no benefit.

Treatment that included radiation therapy in stage I patients (node negative) showed benefits in survival and recurrence rates. Treatment that included chemotherapy for stage II (nodes involved) patients showed benefits in survival and recurrence rates. Data regarding combined radiation and chemotherapy were equivocal due to small sample sizes. However, they probably had the same survival and recurrence advantages as single treatment options in appropriate node status groups. The authors emphasized the importance of node status for patients with PBL.

Paget

Paget disease of the breast

Paget disease is uncommon, representing no more than 1 to 3 percent of new cases of female breast cancer. It is extremely rare among men. Paget disease has a scaly or ulcerated lesion that starts on the nipple and then spreads to the areola. On occasion, a bloody nipple discharge may be present. Some patients will have associated pain, burning sensation, or itchiness.

Underlying breast cancer is present in 85 to 88 percent of cases, with a palpable mass associated in about half of cases. For 20 percent of patients, a non-palpable mammogram abnormality is present. In comparison, up to 15 percent of cases will not be linked to a palpable mass, mammogram abnormality, or any disease in the underlying breast tissue.

Initial evaluation

Your health care provider should obtain a detailed history, documenting the length of time the lesions have been present and associated symptoms. There should be an examination of both breasts.

What else could it be? Possibilities include benign causes such as eczema, a skin reaction to something, or nipple adenoma. Other cancer possibilities may include skin cancer. Given this range of diagnoses, a short course of steroids applied to the nipple, and surrounding skin may be an initial option. Unfortunately, we sometimes see temporary improvement of the nipple and skin changes with such treatment, even if Paget disease is present. In this context, any persistent nipple abnormality should lead to a biopsy (tissue sampling).

Biopsy and imaging

Nipple scraping can diagnose Paget's disease accurately, but a punch biopsy is usually done. The pathologist checks for estrogen and progesterone receptors, but about half of Paget disease cases will not have an expression of these hormone receptors.

You need mammograms of both breasts, and consideration may be given to adding an ultrasound to evaluate and guide biopsies of any mammogram-defined lesion. A breast MRI may be added.

There are two theories to explain Paget disease of the nipple:

- Epidermotropic theory (most accepted): The Paget cell arises from underlying breast cancer, with cells migrating through the ductal system into the nipple's outer layer (epidermis).

- Transformation theory: The outer layer of cells of the nipple transform into malignant Paget cells; the Paget disease of the nipple is independent of any underlying breast ductal cancer.

Management: Is there underlying cancer?

The limited evidence suggests that a central lumpectomy or complete resection of the nipple-areolar complex followed by whole breast radiation therapy is reasonable for women with no palpable mass or mammogram abnormality. The surgical margins and cosmetic outcome should both be acceptable. A simple mastectomy is an alternative.

But what if you have Paget disease and there is underlying cancer in the breast, too? Many patients will require a mastectomy, but if breast-conserving surgery of the nipple-areolar complex and underlying cancer can be achieved with acceptable margins and cosmetic outcome, breast-conserving surgery followed by whole breast radiation therapy may be offered. Those with cancer in several areas of the underlying breast (multicentric disease) or diffuse calcifications should have a mastectomy.

Axillary nodes

Those with pure ductal carcinoma in situ (DCIS or intraductal carcinoma) do not need an evaluation of the nodes. However, a limited (sentinel) sampling is routinely done if you have a mastectomy. On the other hand, anyone with invasive cancer should have the removal of a limited number of axillary nodes, irrespective of the surgery type.

The cancer stage informs the use of chemotherapy. Women with Paget's disease treated with breast conservation (and radiation therapy), without associated cancer, or those with associated estrogen receptor-positive DCIS should consider endocrine therapy such as tamoxifen. Those with an associated invasive cancer should receive systemic therapy (some may need chemotherapy, for example) based on their risk of distant spread.

Young

Most breast cancers occur in women 50 or older, but breast cancer affects younger women, too. About 11 percent of all new breast cancer cases in the United States are among women younger than 45. While breast cancer diagnosis and treatment are difficult for women of any age, young survivors may find it particularly overwhelming.

Breast cancer in young women is —

- More likely to be hereditary than breast cancer in older women.
- More likely to be found later and is often more aggressive and difficult to treat.
- Often coupled with unique issues, including concerns about body image, fertility, finances, and feelings of isolation.
- All women are at risk for getting breast cancer, but some things can raise a woman's risk of getting breast cancer before age 45.

If you are under the age of 45, you may have a higher risk for breast cancer if—

- You have close relatives diagnosed with breast cancer before age 45 or ovarian cancer at any age, especially if more than one relative was diagnosed or a male relative had breast cancer.
- You have changes in certain breast cancer genes (BRCA1 and BRCA2) or have close relatives with these changes but have not been tested yourself.
- You have Ashkenazi Jewish heritage.
- You received radiation therapy to the breast or chest during childhood or early adulthood.
- You have had breast cancer or other breast health problems, such as lobular carcinoma in situ (LCIS), ductal carcinoma in situ (DCIS), atypical ductal hyperplasia, or atypical lobular hyperplasia.
- You have been told that you have dense breasts on a mammogram.
- Do any of these characteristics describe you? If so, talk to your doctor about your family history and other risk factors you might have.

• Inform: All premenopausal patients should be informed about the potential impact of chemotherapy on fertility and asked about their desire for potential future pregnancies. Those who may desire future pregnancies should be referred to fertility specialists before chemotherapy or endocrine therapy to discuss the options based on patient specifics, disease stage, and biology (which determine the urgency, type, and treatment sequence).

• Although lack of menstrual periods frequently occurs during or after chemotherapy, most women younger than 35 resume menses within two years of finishing adjuvant chemotherapy.

• Menses and fertility are not necessarily linked. The absence of regular menses, particularly if the patient takes tamoxifen, does not necessarily imply a lack of fertility. Conversely, the presence of menses does not guarantee fertility. There are limited data regarding continued fertility after chemotherapy.

• **Patients should not become pregnant during treatment** with radiation therapy, chemotherapy, or endocrine therapy.

• **Hormone-based birth control is discouraged** regardless of the hormone receptor status of the patient's cancer, although data is limited.

• **Alternative birth control methods** include intrauterine devices (IUDs), barrier methods, or, for patients with no intent of future pregnancies, tubal ligation or vasectomy for the partner.

• **Ovarian suppression:** Randomized trials have shown that ovarian suppression with GnRH agonist therapy administered during adjuvant chemotherapy in premenopausal women with breast tumors (regardless of hormone receptor status) may preserve ovarian function and diminish the likelihood of chemotherapy-induced amenorrhea.

• **Breastfeeding** following breast-conserving cancer treatment is not contraindicated. However, the quantity and quality of breast milk produced by the breast conserved may not be sufficient or may be lacking some of the nutrients needed. Breastfeeding during active treatment with chemotherapy, endocrine therapy, or HER2-targeted drugs, and other systemic therapies is not recommended.

Wait to conceive

Many experts recommend waiting two years after diagnosis before attempting conception to avoid pregnancy at the highest relapse risk. Still, some evidence suggests that pregnancy may be safe: A study from Ontario (Canada) and one from Eskilstuna (Sweden) did not find adverse effects on survival.

A subsequent **pregnancy does not appear to compromise survival** for women with a history of breast cancer. A 2012 study presented at the European Breast Cancer Conference suggests that pregnancy after breast cancer is safe, regardless of the estrogen receptor status. In addition, an analysis of a collection of 14 studies found that, compared with women who did not become pregnant, those who became pregnant had a 40 percent reduction in the risk of death. This advantage is probably the product of the "healthy mother effect": Only healthy survivors can conceive and carry a pregnancy.

Those who have received Herceptin should use effective contraception for at least seven months after stopping the drug before attempting pregnancy. The drug is associated with fetal complications and even death.

Younger women may have chemotherapy-related infertility. Still, others cannot try to conceive, as they are on endocrine therapy (for example, tamoxifen). We do not yet know the implications of interrupting endocrine therapy while attempting to conceive. We may get answers from the ongoing POSITIVE trial, a research study examining the feasibility of stopping endocrine therapy from having a child.

Interrupting endocrine therapy for pregnancy

Can endocrine therapy be safely interrupted for women with breast cancer who wish to become pregnant? Researchers provided some answers at the 2022 San Antonia Breast Cancer Symposium.

The study enrolled over 500 women for whom endocrine therapy had been stopped as the women tried to become pregnant. Almost all (94 percent) had stage I/II hormone receptor-positive breast cancer. The primary objective was to determine the risk of breast cancer relapse associated with interrupting therapy for about two years. Seventy-four percent had at least one pregnancy, and 64 percent had at least one live birth. At a median follow-up of 41 months, the three-year recurrence rate was 8.9 percent, similar to the 9.2 percent rate in an external control cohort. In addition, 76 percent of patients resumed endocrine therapy; 15 percent had not yet resumed therapy.

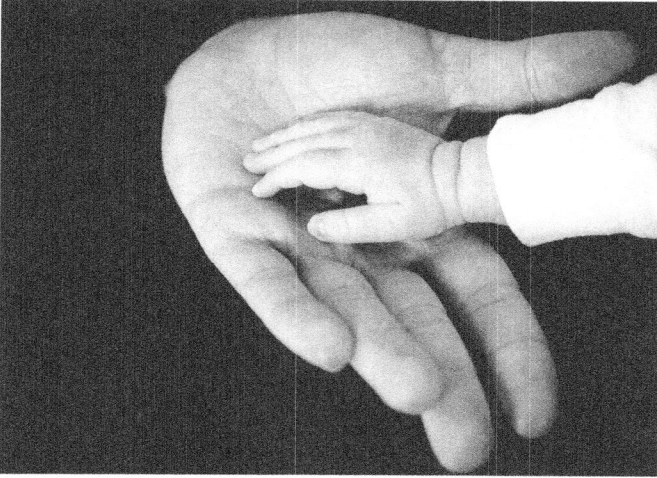

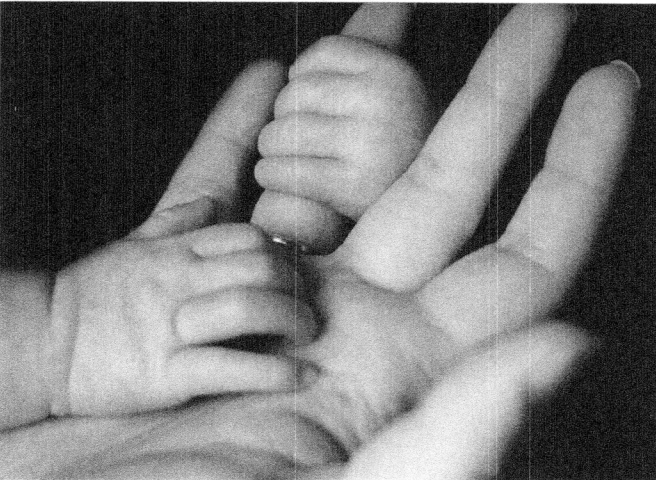

GnRH agonists (such as goserelin)

Treatment for breast cancer, especially with chemotherapy, can impair fertility. Moreover, endocrine therapy can impact the ability to conceive during its use.

GnRH agonists are substances that keep the testicles (in males) and ovaries (in women) from making sex hormones by blocking other hormones that are needed to make them. In men, GnRH agonists cause the testes to stop making testosterone. In women, the drugs cause the ovaries to stop making estrogen and progesterone.

These medicines are also called GnRHa, gonadotropin-releasing hormone agonist, LHRH agonist, and luteinizing hormone-releasing hormone agonist.

Randomized trials show that GnRH agonists (such as goserelin) given before and during chemotherapy improves the chances of pregnancy from 11 to 21 percent in patients with hormone receptor-negative early-stage breast cancer. The clinical literature is less clear for those with hormone receptor-positive breast cancer regarding the protective effects of GnRH agonists in fertility preservation.

A fertility specialist can discuss the specifics of fertility preservation options, including stimulation of the ovaries, embryo or oocyte cryopreservation, and other approaches.

It is important that patients actively avoid becoming pregnant during cancer treatment.

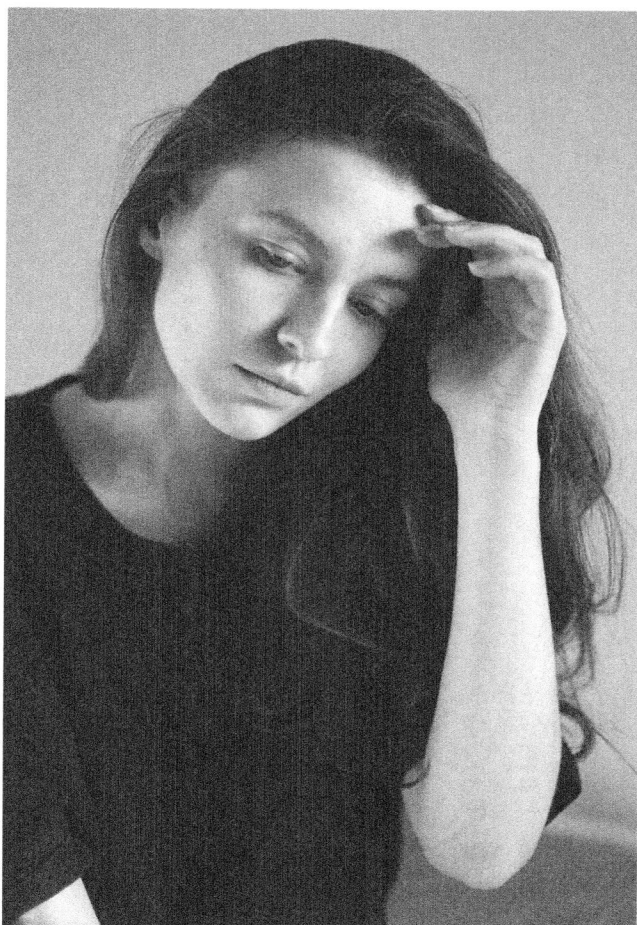

AFTER

Survivorship

Survivorship

A survivor is defined by me as any person with cancer, starting from the moment of diagnosis. There are 14 million breast cancer survivors in the USA alone and as many as 29 million worldwide. Long-term follow-up is important: A recent study in Denmark informs us that breast cancer recurrence risk extends past 30 years. The cumulative incidence of recurrence was 8.5% at 15 years; 12.5% at 20 years; 15.2% at 25 years, and 16.6% at 32 years. The recurrence risk was greatest early on.

Follow-up

I use the National Comprehensive Cancer Network (NCCN) Guidelines. For **invasive** breast cancer, the pathway is as follows:

- History and physical exam one to four times per year as clinically appropriate for five years, then annually.

- Periodic screening for changes in family history and referral to genetic counseling as indicated

- Educate, monitor, and refer for lymphedema management

- Mammograms every 12 months

- In the absence of clinical signs and symptoms suggestive of recurrent cancer, there is no indication for ab or imaging studies for metastases (distant spread of cancer) screening

- For women on tamoxifen, annual gynecologic assessment (if uterus present)

- For women on an aromatase inhibitor (or who enter menopause because of treatment), there should be monitoring of bone health with a bone mineral density (DEXA) test at baseline and then periodically.

- Encouragement of adherence to endocrine therapy (such as tamoxifen or aromatase inhibitor pills)

We do not have a lot of data to inform optimal follow-up for males with breast cancer and typically apply the guidelines above.

Cancer surveillance

History and physical examination remain the principal means for detecting breast cancer recurrence. For patients who have had breast-conserving management, breast imaging is indicated:

- Mammograms

While data is limited, surveillance mammograms for residual breast tissue after breast-conserving treatment or the contralateral breast (after a mastectomy for one side) appears to lower breast cancer mortality. There is indirect evidence from retrospective series that supports a benefit for mammograms of the opposite (contralateral) breast. Some advocate no imaging for those with a life expectancy of under 5 to 10 years.

- Breast MRI

Breast magnetic resonance imaging is not routinely recommended for breast cancer survivors. Still, breast MRI can be of value for patients suspected of having a breast cancer recurrence or when the mammogram is inconclusive.

- Ultrasound

Routine use of ultrasound is not recommended.

- Reconstructed breasts

Surveillance is primarily via physical examination for those who have had a breast removal or mastectomy. Routine mammograms are not done for those with prosthetic implants. While mammograms are technically possible after a TRAM flap reconstruction, there is no consensus on whether to do them, as we do not have much evidence to guide us. Still, physical examination can be invaluable in detecting a local recurrence.

Bone density

Women with a history of breast cancer can have a higher risk of developing bone loss, including osteoporosis, due to cancer treatment. In this context, the American Society of Clinical Oncology (ASCO) recommends a baseline screening evaluation (typically with a dual-energy X-ray absorptiometry, or DEXA scan) for those over 65 years of age, for those 60 to 64 who have a family history of osteoporosis, body weight under 154 pounds (70 kg), a history of a non-traumatic fracture, or other risk factors (such as smoking, alcohol use, or a sedentary lifestyle).

Blood work and imaging

Routine laboratory surveillance (or imaging) is not recommended for breast cancer survivors without symptoms should not have routine laboratory surveillance, according to the National Comprehensive Cancer Network. We have high-level evidence: A 2005 meta-analysis of two randomized trials that compared routine follow-up (physical exam and mammograms) versus intensive surveillance (including imaging and blood tests) showed no differences between the groups in overall or disease-free survival odds.

Routine tumor marker testing

The 2012 American Society of Clinical Oncology (ASCO) Guidelines offer the following: CA 15-3 or CA 27.29 is not recommended for routine surveillance of patients following primary management for breast cancer. CEA is also not recommended.

Circulating tumor cells (CTCs)

The current evidence does not support the use of circulating tumor cells to evaluate for recurrence after treatment for primary breast cancer. While the presence of CTCs is linked with a poorer prognosis, we have limited data.

DCIS

The National Comprehensive Cancer Network (NCCN) guidelines for **ductal carcinoma *in situ* (DCIS)** call for:

- History and physical exam every six to 12 months for five years, then annually.

- Mammograms should be done every 12 months (with the first one six to 12 months after breast-conserving therapy).

Women on tamoxifen should have an annual gynecologic assessment (if the uterus is present). Women on an aromatase inhibitor (or who enter menopause because of treatment) should have monitoring of bone health with a bone mineral density (DEXA) test at baseline and then periodically. I also encourage adherence to endocrine therapy (such as tamoxifen or aromatase inhibitor pills).

The standard dose of tamoxifen is 20 milligrams daily for five years. Low-dose tamoxifen (five milligrams daily for three years) is an option for those who are symptomatic on the 20-milligram dose or if the patient is unwilling or unable to take standard-dose tamoxifen.

Lifestyle

My patients frequently ask what they can do to optimize their prognosis from breast cancer. Lifestyle modification can be an effective and empowering way to not only help with physical and psychological well-being but may improve your disease-free and overall survival opportunities.

Soy: Okay to eat

I am unaware of evidence to suggest that dietary soy (which contains phytoestrogens) affects breast cancer recurrence rates.

Alcohol: Increases risk

We do not have many studies linking alcohol consumption and recurrence. Still, the largest study showed that those who drank the equivalent of at least 3 to 4 standard drinks (more than 6 grams) of alcohol per week had a 1.35-fold higher risk of recurrence and a 1.5-fold increase in breast cancer death compared to those who consumed less than 0.5 grams daily. In this Life After Cancer Epidemiology (LACE) study, the risk among overweight and postmenopausal women appeared highest.

Complementary

A comprehensive overview of this topic is beyond the scope of this book. The Society for Integrative Oncology (SIO) produced an evidence-based guideline on integrative therapies for managing symptoms such as anxiety and stress, mood disorders, fatigue, chemotherapy-induced nausea and vomiting, lymphedema, chemotherapy-induced neuropathy, pain, and sleep disturbance.

The American Society of Clinical Oncology (ASCO) expert panel endorsed the guideline. Key recommendations include music therapy, meditation, stress management, and yoga for anxiety and stress reduction. Meditation, relaxation, yoga, massage, and music therapy are recommended for depression/mood disorders. Meditation and yoga are recommended to improve the quality of life. Acupressure and acupuncture are recommended for reducing chemotherapy-induced nausea and vomiting. No strong evidence supports using ingested dietary supplements to manage breast cancer treatment-related side effects.

Physical activity, body weight, and diet

Observational studies show an association between survival and physical activity, with most data involving breast, colon, or prostate cancer patients.

Physical activity: Drops death rates

A meta-analysis of 16 prospective observational trials showed a near halving (48 percent reduction) in overall mortality and a 28 percent drop in breast cancer mortality in the most versus least active breast cancer survivors. Breast cancer survivors who increased their activity after diagnosis (relative to pre-diagnosis levels) dropped their mortality by more than a third (39 percent relative risk reduction).

Exercise can also help improve aerobic fitness, quality of life, strength, anxiety and depression, fatigue, body image, and body size and composition. While the optimal exercise program remains unclear, I counsel my patients to get moderate physical activity (e.g. a brisk walk for 30 minutes five days per week).

Weight loss

Two large trials have examined the benefits of weight loss among women with breast cancer. The Lifestyle Intervention Study for Adjuvant Treatment of Early Breast Cancer (LISA) randomly assigned 338 post-menopausal women with hormone receptor-positive breast cancer to a two-year telephone-based weight loss intervention or usual care. The telephone group lost 5.4 percent weight in one year and 3.7 percent in two years. The control group lost less (0.7 and 0.4 percent, respectively). In addition, those in the intervention group significantly improved their physical functioning. The Exercise and Nutrition to Enhance Recovery and Good Health for You (ENERGY) trial confirmed these results. We look forward to determining whether such weight loss improves breast cancer outcomes, as several trials look at that.

Hot flashes

We generally avoid estrogen and progesterone for those with a history of breast cancer. Some patients with severe symptoms may benefit from non-hormonal drugs such as gabapentin in the evening or so-called serotonin reuptake inhibitors (SSRIs)/serotonin-norepinephrine reuptake inhibitors (SNRIs). Some have concerns about interactions with tamoxifen, however. In this context, many avoid paroxetine or fluoxetine but may use other drugs such as citalopram or venlafaxine.

Acupuncture has shown promising results in some clinical trials, with one study showing it works better than gabapentin. A Wake Forest Baptist Medical Center (USA) study found that acupuncture reduced hot flashes and night sweats by over a third, with this benefit lasting for at least six months.

Depression and libido

Depression is a common result of breast cancer management, and can in turn affect sexuality. If you are depressed, please let your care team know. Many patients turn to therapists or group support. Antidepressant medications are sometimes offered, but this needs to be done in consultation with your medical oncologist; some medicines may affect drugs such as tamoxifen. For example, paroxetin (Paxil), buproprion (Wellbutrin), Prozac, duloxetine (Cymbalta) and Zoloft may challenge your body's ability to convert tamoxifen into its active form, potentially reducing the full benefits of tamoxifen.

If loss of libido is an issue, you may be a candidate for testosterone (the primary hormone in men). However, if your testosterone levels are within normal limits, more testosterone will not likely provide a benefit to you. Finally, treatment-induced nausea can understandably take away your interest in sex.

Vaginal dryness

Menopause, whether natural or treatment-caused, may result in thinning and shortening of your vaginal walls. There can be associated dryness, or lack of lubrication which can lead to pain associated with sex. Some find relief with topical lidocaine. The American Society of Clinical Oncology recommends the use of non-hormonal treatments, including water- or silicone based lubricants of moisturizers as first line treatment for vaginal dryness and pain associated with sex. Vaginal moisturizers include products containing gelatins, gums, polycarbophil, or hyaluronic acid.

Lymphedema (arm swelling)

Lymphedema (edema) is defined as the collection of protein-rich fluid in the spaces within a tissue, due disruption of the flow of lymph fluid. Lymphedema is an overflow problem: The lymph load exceeds the transport capacity of the lymphatic system. Unfortunately, this swelling (for example of the arm) can be associated with surgery or radiation therapy. It can manifest as slowly progressive swelling of the arm, and can also include the breast or upper chest wall.

In a systematic review of 72 studies, the overall incidence of arm edema among survivors of breast cancer was 17 percent. Risk factors for breast cancer-associated lymphedema (arm swelling) include the following:

Axillary node dissection
The surgical removal of nodes is the primary cause of breast and arm swelling, with the incidence increasing with the number of axillary

nodes removed or disrupted. The risk is around 20 percent for those who have an axillary node dissection (removal of several nodes from a geographic zone), compared to 5.6 percent for those having a sentinel node biopsy.

Radiation therapy

Lymphedema risk appears is much higher if you have had axillary dissection *and* radiation therapy, as compared with axillary dissection alone. In one systematic review, the risk of edema was 41 percent with both, compared to 17 percent with surgery alone. Radiation therapy field design affects risk, too: More comprehensive radiotherapy volumes covering more of the axilla, nodes around the collarbone, and nodes next to the breast bone can further increase risk, compared to more limited radiation therapy.

Other

Excessive body weight (body mass index) can increase edema risk, as can infections after surgery, blood or fluid collections after surgery, and possibly medications such as chemotherapy. Weight gain can put you at additional risk, as it may impair lymphatic function.

The breast cancer management type may affect the timing of the development of lymphedema. It appears that early-onset edema (less than one year after surgery) may be more associated with surgery, while late-onset lymphedema seems more associated with radiation therapy to regional lymph nodes (note: most patients who get radiation therapy have more limited targets).

Lymphedema risk reduction

Primary prevention

The judicious use of a sentinel node sampling)rather than a more thorough axillary node dissection) is a primary means of reducing risk, but may not be appropriate for all patients. Sophisticated radiotherapy techniques may lower risk, too, as may surgical techniques such as reverse mapping or lymphatic bypass.

Secondary prevention

Here, the goal is to control arm swelling. We often monitor arm circumference. I ask patients to maintain excellent skin and nail care, as infection can lead to skin inflammation (cellulitis). A good skin moisturizer may help, as can protection of your hands with gloves when you are participating in activities that may lead to skin injury. If you have any signs of infection, report them.

Many patients benefit from arm elevation, particularly in the early stages of edema. Properly fitted compression sleeves may lower the amount of edema. In addition, try to avoid procedures that puncture the skin of the arm (for example, blood draws or vaccinations). It is generally best to do blood pressure measurements using the opposite arm. Finally, maintain good body weight, preferably with a body mass index of 20 to 25.

Travel

Given the lower atmospheric pressure at altitude, the risk from air travel or precipitating or worsening edema is present but, fortunately, is low. Some patients use compression sleeves during air travel, but there is no consensus on whether this is required, particularly with flights under 4.5 hours.

Exercise

We typically offer our patients (who have had any surgery of nodes) range of motion exercises for the affected arms. After you have healed appropriately following surgery, exercise (including weight training) appears safe and beneficial. Early physiotherapy, such as manual lymphatic drainage, can provide benefits. If you have had reconstruction, please check with your plastic surgeon about restrictions.

Surgery

Surgery may aid highly select patients with lymphedema, and may help with pain. It appears to work best for those with early-stage lymphedema. Left untreated, the degree of lymphedema typically increases over time. Conservative management may include:

Compression therapy

Often combined with physiotherapy, your physical therapist may offer compression therapy may be offered for early lymphedema. Limb compression and fitted compression garments may play roles, as can appropriately fitted compression hand pieces (such as gloves).

Manual lymphatic drainage

Manual lymphatic drainage may provide additional benefits (although this is controversial) when added to compression therapy. A specially trained physical therapist may offer this massage-like technique. A systematic review of six trials concluded that the approach is safe and may offer additional benefits to compression.

Those with mild-to-moderate lymphedema are the ones who benefit from adding manual lymphatic drainage to an intensive course of compression bandaging.

Intermittent pneumatic compression

Intermittent pneumatic compression is another method of compression therapy. It is most typically offered to those with severe lymphedema. Unfortunately, we do not have high-level evidence regarding its effectiveness, but some are concerned about pressures exceeding 60 millimeters of mercury.

Complete decongestive therapy (CDT)

This technique may be recommended if you have moderate-to-severe lymphedema. A small trial randomized patients to CDT (including lymph drainage, multilayer compression bandaging, elevation, remedial exercise, and skin care versus standard physiotherapy (elevation, bandages, head-neck and shoulder exercises, and skin care)) found a greater improvement in lymphedema with the more intense approach. However, a second similar study found no such benefit.

Pregnancy

Having a child after breast cancer treatment does not worsen survival. Women diagnosed with breast cancer who want a child after treatment should talk to a fertility specialist as early as possible, ideally before treatment begins. Even if you choose not to take one of the steps available, exploring all of your options may help you feel more comfortable with your choices later in life.

Imaging

Breast imaging after surgery can be confusing. Sometimes, calcifications, masses, and architectural distortion can mimic cancer. Adding to the diagnostic challenge is that the most common area for those with a local recurrence is right where cancer used to be. In general, indeterminate or suspicious findings may require a biopsy to exclude malignancy.

In the weeks to months after surgery, acute mammogram changes can include retraction, scar formation, pockets of fluid, and swelling. Chronic changes can last for years. One can see scarring, retraction, and calcifications due to tissue damage (dystrophic calcifications), tissue asymmetry (secondary to tissue removal), fat necrosis, or architectural distortion.

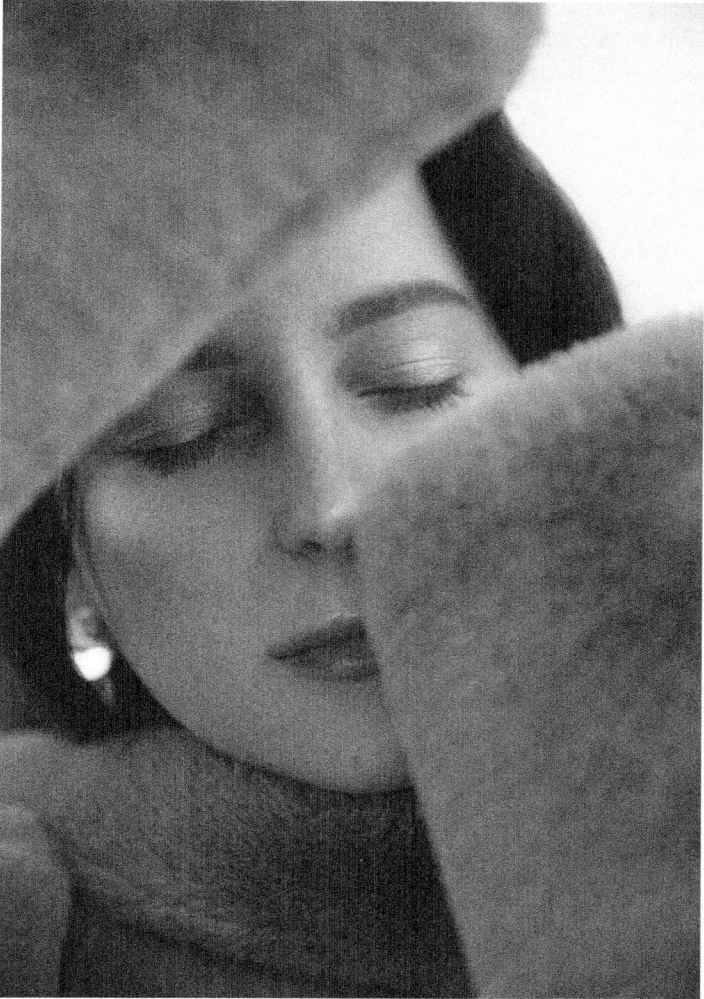

Final thoughts

by Michael Hunter MD

Thank you for allowing me to enter your life with this book. I hope that it has been valuable to you. Herein, I have tried to be clear in presenting information critical to you. Before we end, I should chat a bit about clinical trials.

- *Clinical trials*

A clinical trial is a research study that tries to find new ways to improve health. In phase 1 (I) trials, doctors check the safety of a new treatment. They learn how to administer a medicine, what dose is safe, and what the side effects are. In phase 2 (II) trials, doctors give a new treatment to a group of people with a certain disease. The doctors check the treatment's side effects and how it works to treat the disease. In phase 3 (III) trials, researchers compare a new treatment with the usual treatment for the disease or a placebo. This way, researchers can learn how the new treatment compares to the current treatment or placebo.

To search for clinical trials in the USA and elsewhere, go to www.cancer.gov/clinicaltrials. To see videos answering common clinical trial questions, please go to www.cancer.net/pre-act.

As we close, I ask that you pursue, wherever possible, evidence-based management strategies. This way, you optimize the chances of having the best care while reducing your chances of potential harm. Now that we have addressed management, what can you do that may reduce your chances for a return (or progression) of cancer?

- Have a balanced diet
- Optimize your body to mass index (BMI)
- Be prudent with alcohol consumption
- Try to comply with endocrine therapy recommendations.
- Avoid tobacco
- Get some physical activity

I wish you all the best and feel privileged to communicate with you through this book. You may also find me at www.newcancerinfo.com. Thank you.

508

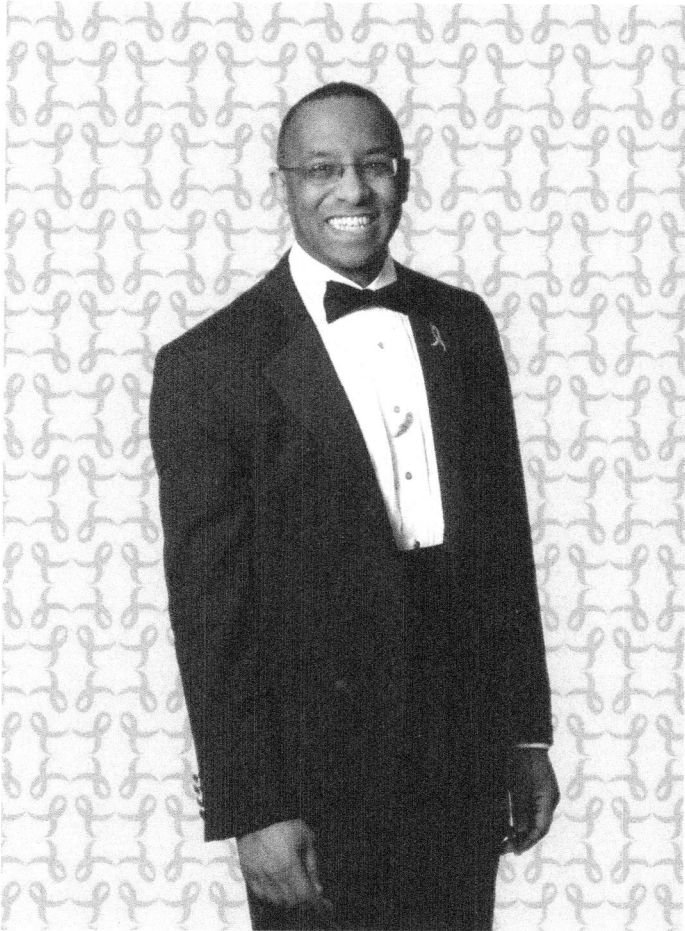

Thank you!

EDITING

Maya Hunter (lead editor); Lauren Pederson

NOTES

1. BASICS

1. American Cancer Society. How Common Is Breast Cancer? Available at: https://www.cancer.org/cancer/breast-cancer/about/how-common-is-breast-cancer.html.
2. American Cancer Society. Key Statistics for Breast Cancer in Men. Jan. 2021. Available at: https://www.cancer.org/cancer/breast-cancer-in-men/about/key-statistics.html.
3. American Cancer Society. Cancer Facts & Figures 2022. Available at: https://www.cancer.org/content/dam/cancer-org/research/cancer-facts-and-statistics/annual-cancer-facts-and-figures/2021/cancer-facts-and-figures-2022.pdf.
4. http://www.cancer.org/acs/groups/content/@editorial/documents/document/acspc-044552.pdf
5. http://globocan.iarc.fr/Pages/fact_sheets_cancer.aspx, 2020.
6. statecancerprofiles.cancer.gov
7. wcrf.org (World Cancer Research Dund International)
8. Stanford, J, Herrinton, L., Schwartz, S., & Weiss, N. (1995). Breast cancer incidence in Asian migrants to the United States and their descendants. Epidemiology, 6, 181–183.
9. Hemminki, K., & Li, X. (2002). Cancer risks in second-generation immigrants to Sweden. Int J Cancer, 99, 229–237.
10. Beiki, O, Hall, P, Ekbom, A, et al. (2012). Breast cancer incidence and case fatality among 4.7 million women in relation to social and ethnic background: a population-based cohort study. Breast Cancer Res, 14(1), R5.

Age
11. American Cancer Society, Inc., Surveillance Research, 2017
12. http://www.targetedonc.com/news/expert-examines-impact-of-age-on-prognosis-molecular-subtype-in-breast-cancer

Race
13. CA: A Cancer Journal for Clinicians. doi: 10.3322/caac.21320. Online at cacancerjournal.com.
14. Keenan T, Moy B, Mroz EA, et al. Comparison of the Genomic Landscape Between Primary Breast Cancer in African American Versus White Women and the Association of Racial Differences With Tumor Recurrence. Presented at the 37th Annual San Antonio Breast Cancer Symposium, San Antonio, TX, December 9-13, 2014, and the 51st Annual Meeting of the

American Society of Clinical Oncology, Chicago, IL, May 29-June 2, 2015.

15. American Cancer Society. Cancer Prevention & Early Detection Facts & Figures, 2015-2016.

Genes

16. http://www.cancer.gov/cancertopics/pdq/genetics/breast-and-ovarian/HealthProfessional#sthash.f98eeZ90.dpuf
17. Cancer (2015; doi: 10.1002/cncr.29645)
18. CA Cancer J Clin 2015
19. Walsh T, King MC. Ten genes for inherited breast cancer. Cancer Cell 2007; 11:103-5.
20. Hwang SJ, Lozano G, Amos CI et al. Germline p53 mutations ina cohort with childhood sarcoma: sex differences in cancer risk. Am J Hum Genet 2003; 72(4):975-83.
21. Mouchawar J, Korch C, Byers T et al. Population-based estimate of the contribution of TP53 mutations to subgroups of early-onset breast cancer: Australian Breast Cancer Family Study. Cancer Res 2010; 70(12): 4705-800.
22. Melhem-Bertrandt A, Bojadzieva J, Ready KJ, et al. Early onset HER2-positive breast cancer is associated with germline TP53 mutations. Cancer 2012; 118(4): 908-13.
23. Min-Han T, Mester JL, Ngeow J, et al. Lifetime cancer risks in individuals with germline PTEN mutations. Clin Cancer Res 2012; 18(2): 400-7.
24. Walsh T, King MC. Ten genes for inherited breast cancer. Cancer Cell 2007; 11:103-5.

Radiation exposure

25. Land CE, Tokunaga M, Koyama K et al. Incidence of female breast cancer among atomic bomb survivors. Hiroshima and Nagasaki, 1950-1990. Radiat Res 2003;160: 707-717.
26. Preston DL, Mattsson A, Holmberg E et al. Radiation effects on breast cancer risk for young women treated for Hodgkin lymphoma. J Natl Cancer Inst 2005; 97:1428-37.

Family

27. Collaborative Group on Hormonal Factors in Breast Cancer: Familial breast cancer collaborative reanalysis of individual data from 52 epidemiological studies including 58,209 women with breast cancer and 101,986 women without the disease. Lancet 358: 1389-99, 2001.

Breast density

28. McCormack VA, dos Santos Silva I. Breast density and parenchymal patterns as markers of breast cancer risk: a meta-analysis. Cancer Epidemiol Biomarkers Prev. 2006;15:1159-1569
29. Katavic N, et al "Association of breast density with breast cancer risk in screening mammography" RSNA Meeting 2015; Abstract BR-5A-01.

Menarche, menopause, height, and obesity

30. Ritte R, et al. Height, age at menarche and risk of hormone receptor-positive and =negative breast cancer as a cohort study. Int J Cancer 2013; 132:2619.
31. Hsieh CC, et al. Age at menarche, age at menopause, height and obesity as risk factors for breast cancer: associations and interactions in an international case-control study. Int J Cancer 1990; 46:796.
32. Collaborative Group on Hormonal Factors in Breast Cancer. Menarche, menopause, and breast cancer risk: individual participant meta-analysis, including 118 964 women with breast cancer from 117 epidemiological studies. Lancet Oncol. 13(11):1141-51, 2012.
33. Colditz GA, et al. Cumulative risk of breast cancer to age 70 years according to risk factor status: data from the Nurses' Health Study. Am J Epidemiol 200; 152:950.

Childbearing; breast-feeding

34. Kelsey JL, et al. Reproductive factors and breast cancer. Epidemiol Rev 1993; 15:36.

35. Rosner B, et al. Reproductive risk factors in a prospective study of breast cancer: the Nurses' Health Study. Am J Epidemiol 1994; 139:814.

36. Annals of Oncology 00: 1–10, 2015 doi:10.1093/annonc/mdv379

Immigrants

37. John EM, Phipps AI, Davis A, Koo J. Migration history, acculturation, and breast cancer risk in Hispanic women. Cancer Epidemiol Biomarkers Prev 2005; 14:2905-13.

Alcohol

38. Alcohol drinking. IARC Working Group, Lyon, 13-20 October 1987. IARC Mongr Eal Carcinog Risks Hum. 1988; 44:1-378.

39. Roswall N, Weiderpass E. Alcohol as a risk factor for cancer: existing evidence in a global perspective. J Prev Med Public Health. 2015; 48:1-9.

40. Schütze M et al. Alcohol attributable burden of incidence of cancer in eight European countries based on results from prospective cohort study. BMJ. 2011 Apr 7;342:d1584.

41. https://www.pennmedicine.org/news/news-releases/2014/july/new-study-shows-drinking-alcohol

Weight gain

42. Newhouser ML et al. JAMA Oncol. 2015;doi:10.1001/jamaoncol.2015.1546.

Risk: Putting it all together (table)

43. Clemons M, et al. N Engl J Med 2001; 344: 276.

Diet

44. Estefania T, Salas-Salvado J, Donat-Vargas C, et al. Mediterranean diet and invasive breast cancer risk among women at high cardiovascular risk in the PREDIMED 10.1001.jamainternmed.2015.4838

45. Nutr Rev. 2014 Jan;72(1):1-17. doi: 10.1111/nure.12083. Epub 2013 Dec 13.

46. ASCO Abstract 520. "Low-fat dietary pattern and long-term breast cancer incidence and mortality. The Women's Health Initiative randomized clinical trial. 2019.

Exposure to light (especially blue light)

47. http://www.health.harvard.edu/staying-healthy/blue-light-has-a-dark-side

Diabetes

48. A. S. Glicksman and R. W. Rawson, "Diabetes and altered carbohydrate metabolism in patients with cancer.," Cancer, vol. 9, no. 6, pp. 1127–34.

49. Giovannucci E, Harlan D, Archer M, et al. "Diabetes and cancer: a consensus report.," Diabetes Care, vol. 33, no. 7, pp. 1674–85, Jul. 2010.

50. P. J. Hardefeldt, S. Edirimanne, and G. D. Eslick, "Diabetes increases the risk of breast cancer: a meta-analysis.," Endocr. Relat. Cancer, vol. 19, no. 6, pp. 793–803, Dec. 2012.

51. P. Boyle, M. Boniol, A. Koechlin, C. Robertson, F. Valentini, K. Coppens, L.-L. Fairley, T. Zheng, Y. Zhang, M. Pasterk, M. Smans, M. P. Curado, P. Mullie, S. Gandini, M. Bota, G. B. Bolli, J. Rosenstock, and P. Autier, "Diabetes and breast cancer risk: a meta-analysis.," Br. J. Cancer, vol. 107, no. 9, pp. 1608–17, Oct. 2012.

52. Centers for Disease Control and Prevention, "National diabetes fact sheet," 2011.

Thyroid cancer and breast cancer link

53. Hyun JA, Yul, H, Young AH, et al. A possible association between thyroid cancer and breast cancer. Thyroid. Dec 2015, 25(12):1330-1338.

Triple negative breast cancer

54. Swain S. Triple-Negative Breast Cancer: Metastatic risk and role of platinum agents 2008 ASCO Clinical Science Symposium 2008. June 3, 2008.

55. Trivers KF, Lund MJ, Porter PL et al. The epidemiology of triple-negative breast cancer, including race. Cancer Causes Control 2009; 20: 1071.

Risk Calculators

56. http://ccge.medschl.cam.ac.uk/boadicea/ Centre for Cancer Genetic Epidemiology. BOADICEA. Accessed March 14, 2017.

57. http://www.ems-trials.org/riskevaluation/ Accessed March 14, 2017.

58. https://www.cancer.gov/bcrisktool/ Accessed March 14, 2017.

59. http://www.yourdiseaserisk.wustl.edu/ Siteman Cancer Center. Accessed March 14, 2017.

Implementing risk reduction

60. Goss PR, Ingle JN, Pritchard K, et al: Extending aromatase-inhibitor therapy to 10 years. N Engl J Med 375:209-219, 2016.

61. Chlebowski R. Improving Breast Cancer Risk Assessment Versus Implementing Breast Cancer Prevention. J Clin Oncol, 35(7), 2017: 702-704.

62. Newman L and Petrelli N, eds. Breast cancer. Surgical Oncology Clinics of North America 23 (3): 424-425, 2014.

Oral contraceptives

63. Collaborative Group on Hormonal Factors in Breast Cancer. Breast cancer and hormonal contraceptives: collaborative reanalysis of individual data on 53,297 women with breast cancer and 100,239 women without breast cancer from 54 epidemiological studies. Collaborative Group on Hormonal Factors in Breast Cancer. Lancet. 347:1713-27, 1996.

64. Gierisch JM, Coeytaux RR, Urrutia RP, et al. Oral contraceptive use and risk of breast, cervical, colorectal, and endometrial cancers: a systematic review. Cancer Epidemiol Biomarkers Prev. 22(11):1931-43, 2013.

Breast feeding

65. Collaborative Group on Hormonal Factors in Breast Cancer. Breast cancer and breast feeding: collaborative reanalysis of individual data from 47 epidemiological studies in 30 countries, including 50,302 women with breast cancer and 96,973 women without the disease. Lancet 20:187-95, 2002. - See more at: http://ww5.komen.org/BreastCancer/LowerYourRiskReferences.html#sthash.XMUSDrLo.dpuf

Hormone replacement therapy

66. Goss PE, Ingle JN, Alés-Martínez JE, et al. for the NCIC CTG MAP.3 Study Investigators. Exemestane for breast-cancer prevention in postmenopausal women. N Engl J Med. 364(25):2381-91, 2011.

67. U.S. Food and Drug Administration. Menopause and hormones: Common questions. http://www.fda.gov/ForConsumers/ByAudience/ForWomen/ucm118624.htm, 2014.

68. Holmberg L, Iverson OE, Rudenstam CM, et al., for the HABITS Study Group. Increased risk of recurrence after hormone replacement therapy in breast cancer survivors. J Natl Cancer Inst. 100(7):475-82, 2008.

69. Colditz GA, Hankinson SE, Hunter DJ, et al. The use of estrogens and progestins and the risk of breast cancer in postmenopausal women. N Engl J Med. 332: 1589-93, 1995.

70. Cancer Epidemiol Biomarkers Prev. 2005 Dec;14(12):2905-13. Migration history, acculturation, and breast cancer risk in Hispanic women.
71. John EM, Phipps AI, Davis A, Koo J. Cancer Epidemiol Biomarkers Prev. 2005 Dec;14(12):2905-13. Migration history, acculturation, and breast cancer risk in Hispanic women.

Worldwide - Incidence
72. https://www.wcrf.org/dietandcancer/cancer-trends/breast-cancer-statistics

2. IMAGE

Mammograms
1. U.S. Preventive Services Task Force. Ann Intern Med. 151(10):716-726, 2009.
2. http://www.cancer.org/cancer/breastcancer/moreinformation/breastcancerearlydetection/breast-cancer-early-detection-acs-rec
3. http://www.nccn.org/professionals/physician_gls/pdf/breast-screening.pdf

Age
4. NCI-funded Breast Cancer Surveillance Consortium (HHSN26121000031C) http://breas screening.cancer.gov/ (Accessed on November 09, 2015).
5. Fletcher SW, Elmore JG. Clinical practice. Mammographic screening for breast cancer. N Engl J Med. 2003;348:1672-1680.
6. Schonberg MA, McCarthy EP, Davis RB, et al. Breast cancer screening in women aged 80 and older: results from a national survey. J Am Geriatr Soc. 2004;52:1688-1695.
7. Schonberg MA, Ramanan RA, McCarthy EP, Marcantonio ER. Decision making and counseling around mammography screening for women aged 80 or older. J Gen Intern Med. 2006;21:979-985.
Breast Tumor Prognostic Characteristics and Biennial vs Annual Mammography, Age, and Menopausal Status
8. Miglioretti DL, Zhu W, Kerlikowske K. Breast tumor prognostic characteristics and biennial vs annual mammography, age, and menopausal status. JAMA Oncol. 2015;1(8):1069-1077.

Mammograms: Cons
9. U.S. Preventive Services Task Force. Screening for breast cancer: U.S. Preventive Services Task Force recommendation statement. Ann Intern Med. 151(10):716-726, 2009.
10. Ronckers CM, Erdmann CA, Land CE: Radiation and breast cancer: a review of current evidence. Breast Cancer Res 7 (1): 21-32, 2005.

11. Goss PE, Sierra S: Current perspectives on radiation-induced breast cancer. J Clin Oncol 16 (1): 338-47, 1998.
12. Radiology 241 (1): 55-66, 2006.
13. Bleyer A, Welch HG: N Engl J Med 367 (21): 1998-2005, 2012.
14. Jørgensen KJ, Gøtzsche PC: BMJ 339: b2587, 2009.
15. Kalager M, Zelen M, Langmark F, et al.: N Engl J Med 363 (13): 1203-10, 2010.

Breast MRI
16. American College of Radiology. ACR Practice Parameter for the Performance of Contrast-Enhanced Magnetic Resonance Imaging (MRI) of the Breast. http://www.acr.org/~/media/2a0eb 28eb59041e2825179afb72ef624.pdf. Accessed June 15, 2015.

17. Dontchos BN, DeMartini WB, Rahbar H, Peacock S, Lehman CD. Influence of Menstrual Cycle Timing on Screening Breast MRI Performance in Pre-Menopausal Women. Presented at: Radiological Society of North America (RSNA) Annual Meeting; November 25-30, 2012; Chicago, IL.

18. Saslow D et al. CA Cancer J Clin 2007;57:75-89

Ultrasound

19. Berg WA, Zhang Z, Lehrer D, et al. for the ACRIN 6666 Investigators. Detection of breast cancer with addition of annual screening ultrasound or a single screening MRI to mammography in women with elevated breast cancer risk. JAMA. 307(13):1394-404, 2012.

20. Scheel JR, Lee JM, Sprague BL, Lee CI, Lehman CD. Screening ultrasound as an adjunct to mammography in women with mammographically dense breasts. Am J Obstet Gynecol. 212(1):9-17. 2015.

Tomosynthesis

21. Skaane P, Bandos AI, Gullien R, et al. Comparison of digital mammography alone and digital mammography plus tomosynthesis in a population-based screening program. Radiology. 267(1):47-56, 2013.

22. Ciatto S, Houssami N, Bernardi D, et al. Integration of 3-D digital mammography with tomosynthesis for population breast-cancer screening (STORM): a prospective comparison study. Lancet Oncol. S1470-2045(13)70134-7, 2013.

23. Friedewald SM, Rafferty EA, Rose SL, et al. Breast cancer screening using tomosynthesis in combination with digital mammography. JAMA. 311(24):2499-2507, 2014.

24. http://www.cancer.org/cancer/news/news/breast-cancer-screening-with-3-d-technology-finds-more-cancers

25. http://www.massgeneral.org/imaging/services/3D_mammography_tomosynthesis.aspx High-risk: Screening

26. American Cancer Society. Mammogram reports – BI-RADS.

27. U.S. Preventive Services Task Force. Screening for breast cancer: U.S. Preventive Services Task Force recommendation statement. Ann Intern Med. 151(10):716-726, 2009.

28. http://www.facingourrisk.org/understanding-brca-and-hboc/publications/documents/Surveillance%20Flyer%207.16.14.pdf

Molecular imaging

29. Hendrick RE. Radiation doses and cancer risks from breast imaging studies. Radiology. 257(1):246-53, 2010.

Clinical breast exam

30. Fenton JJ, Rolnick SJ, Harris EL, et al.: Specificity of clinical breast examination in community practice. J Gen Intern Med 22 (3): 332-7, 2007.

Thermography

31. Lee CI and Elmore JC. Chap 11. Breast Cancer Screening, in Harris JR, Lippman ME, Morrow M, Osborne CK. Diseases of the Breast, 5th edition. Lippincott Williams and Wilkins, 2014.

32. http://www.fda.gov/NewsEvents/Newsroom/PressAnnouncements/ucm257633.htm

MRI

33. Berg WA, Zhang Z, Lehrer D, et al. for the ACRIN 6666 Investigators. Detection of breast cancer with addition of annual screening ultrasound or a single screening MRI to mammography

in women with elevated breast cancer risk. JAMA. 307(13):1394-404, 2012.

34. Pinsky RW, Helvie MA. Mammographic breast density: effect on imaging and breast cancer risk. J Natl Compr Canc Netw. 8(10):1157-64, 2010.

35. O'Flynn EA, Ledger AE, deSouza NM. Alternative screening for dense breasts: MRI. AJR Am J Roentgenol. 204(2):W141-9, 2015.

36. Tagliafico AS, et al. Adjuvant screening with tomosynthesis or ultrasound in women with mammography-negative dense breasts: Interim report of a prospective comparative trial. J Clin Oncol 34: 1883-88 (16), 2016.

37. http://www.medscape.com/viewarticle/810492

38. Pilewskie M, Olcese C, BS,Eaton A et al. Perioperative Breast MRI Is Not Associated with Lower Locoregional Recurrence Rates in DCIS Patients Treated With or Without Radiation. Ann Surg Oncol. 2014 May; 21(5): 1552–1560.

Self-exam

39. Thomas DB, Gao DL, Ray RM, et al.: Randomized trial of breast self-examination in Shanghai: final results. J Natl Cancer Inst 94 (19): 1445-57, 2002.

40. Semiglazov VF, Manikhas AG, Moiseenko VM, et al.: [Results of a prospective randomized investigation [Russia (St.Petersburg)/WHO] to evaluate the significance of self-examination for the early detection of breast cancer]. Vopr Onkol 49 (4): 434-41, 2003.

Breast density; high risk imaging

41. Gierach GL, Ichikawa L, Kerlikowske K, et al. Relationship between mammographic density and breast cancer death in the Breast Cancer Surveillance Consortium. J Natl Cancer Inst 2012; 104(16):1218-27.

42. https://www.breastcancer.org/symptoms/testing/types/mri/screening

Fact box

43. Gøtzsche PC, Jørgensen KJ (2013). Cochrane Database of Systematic Reviews (6): CD001877.pub5.

44. https://www.harding-cancer.mpg.de/en/health-information/facts-boxes/mammography

Inflammatory breast cancer

45. http://www.cancer.net/cancer-types/breast-cancer-inflammatory/statistics

46. Chow CK. Imaging in inflammatory breast carcinoma. Breast Dis 2005-2006;22:45–54.

47. Tardivon AA, Viala J, Corvellec Rudelli A, Guinebretiere JM, Vanel D. Mammographic patterns of inflammatory breast carcinoma: a retrospective study of 92 cases. Eur J Radiol 1997;24(2):124–130.

DCIS: Imaging

48. http://www.medscape.com/viewarticle/810492

49. Pilewskie M, et al. Ann Surg Oncol. 2014 May; 21(5): 1552–1560.

Mammograms

50. Gold RH, Bassett LW, Widoff BE. Highlights from the history of mammography. Radiographics 1990; 10(6):1111.

51. Muir BB, Kirkpatrick AE, Roberts MM et al. Oblique-view mammography: adequacy for screening. Work in progress. Radiology 1984;151(1);39.

52. Wald NJ, Murphy P, Major P et al. UKCCCR multicentre randomised controlled trial of one and two view mammography in breast cancer screening. BMJ 1995;311(7014):1189.

53. Ikeda DM, Andersson I. Radiology 1989;172(3):661.

54. Friedewald SM, Rafferty EA, Rose SL, et al. Breast cancer screening using tomosynthesis in combination with digital mammography. JAMA 2014;311(24):2499.

Biopsy
55. Brennan ME, Turner RM, Clatto S et al. Ductal carcinoma in situ at core-needle biopsy: meta-analysis of underestimation and predictors of invasive breast cancer. Radiology 2011;260:119-128.
56. https://en.wikipedia.org/wiki/Paget%27s_disease_of_the_breast#/media/

3. BIOPSY

DCIS
1. Bestill WL Jr., Rosen PP, Lieberman PH, Robbins GF. Intraductal carcinoma: long-term follow-up after treatment by biopsy alone. JAMA 1978;239(18):1863-1867.
CrossRefMedlineWeb of ScienceGoogle Scholar
2. Eusebi V, Feudale E, Foschini MP, et al. Long-term follow-up of in situ carcinoma of the breast. Sem Diag Pathol 1994;11:223-235.
3. Page DL, Dupont WD, Rogers LW, Landenberger M. Intraductal carcinoma of the breast: follow-up after biopsy only. Cancer 1982;49(4):751-758.
4. Rosen PP, Braun DW Jr., Kinne DE. The clinical significance of preinvasive breast carcinomas. Cancer 1980;46:919-925.
5. Semin Diagn Pathol 1994;11:208–14.
6. http://www.breastcancer.org/symptoms/testing/types/biopsy
7. Wellings RR, Jensen HM. On the origin and progression of ductal carcinoma in the human breast. J Natl Cancer Inst 1973;50(5):1111-1118.
8. Cheatle GL, Cutler M. Malignant epithelial neoplasia. Carcinoma. The precancerous or potentially carcinomatous state. In: Cheatle GL, Cutler M, editors. Tumours of the Breast. 1st ed. Philadelphia, PA: Lippincott; 1926. p. 161-332.
9. Foote FW, Stewart FW. Comparative studies of cancerous versus noncancerous breasts. Ann Surg 1945;121(1):6-53. 197–222.
10. Page DL, Rogers LW. Carcinoma in situ (CIS). In: Page DL, Anderson TJ, editors. Diagnostic Histopathology of the Breast. 1st ed. New York, NY: Churchill Livingston; 1987. p. 157-174.
11. Wellings SR, Jensen HM, Marcum RG. An atlas of subgross pathology of the human breast with special reference to possible precancerous lesions. J Natl Cancer Inst 1975;55(2):231-273.
12. Muir R. The evolution of carcinoma of the mamma. J Pathol Bacteriol 1941;LII(2):155-172.
13. Fechner RE. History of ductal carcinoma in situ. In: Silverstein ML, editor. Ductal Carcinoma In Situ of the Breast. 2nd ed. Philadelphia, PA: Lippincott Williams and Wilkins; 2002. p. 3-16.
14. Rose RE, Paulson EC, Sharma A, et al. HER-2/neu overexpression as a predictor for the transition from in situ to invasive breast cancer. Cancer Epidemiol Biomarkers Prev 2009;18:1386-1389.

Benign breast disases
15. Hartmann LC, Degnim AC, Santen RJ, et al. N Engl J Med. 2015;372:78-89.
16. Hartmann LC, Radisky DC, Frost MH, et al. Cancer Prev Res (Phila). 2014;7:211-217.
17. Page DL, Schuyler PA, Dupont WD, et al. Lancet. 2003;361:125-12918. Sabel MS. Overview of benign breast disease. In: Chagpar AB, ed. UpToDate. Waltham, MA, UpToDate, 2015.
18. https://en.wikipedia.org/wiki/Atypical_ductal_hyperplasia#/media/File:Atypical_ductal_hyperplasia_-_high_mag.jpg

DCIS versus LCIS
19. Mommers ER, et al. J Pathol 194:327-333.
20. Warnberg et al. Br J Cancer 85:869-874.
21. JAMA. 2015;313(11):1122-1132.

DCIS and HER2
22. Latta EK, Tain S, Parkes RK, O'Malley FP. The role of HER2/neu overexpression in the progression of ductal carcinoma in situ to invasive carcinoma of the breast. Mod Pathol 2002 Dec; 15(12):1318-25.

Microinvasion
23. Sue GR, Lannin DR. Killelea B, Chagpar AB. Predictors of microinvasion and its prognostic role in ductal carcinoma *in situ*. Am J Surg 2013; 206(4):478.
24. Vierira CC, Mercado CL, Cangiarella JF, et al. Microinvasive ductal carcinoma in situ: clinical presentation, imaging features, pathologic findings, and outcome. Eur J Radiol. 2010 Jan;73(1):102-7.
25. Chen CY, Sun LM, Anderson BO. Paget disease of the breast: changing patterns of incidence, clinical presentation, and treatment in the U.S. Cancer 2006; 107(7):1448.
26. Ashikari R, Park K, Huvos AG, et al. Paget's disease of the breast. Cancer. 1970; 26(3):680.
27. Nance FC, DeLoach DH, Welsh RA, et al. Paget's disease of the breast. Ann Surg 1970; 171(6):864.
28. https://en.wikipedia.org/wiki/Paget%27s_disease_of_the_breast#/media/ File:Extramammary_Paget_disease_-_high_mag.jpg

Fat necrosis
29. https://en.wikipedia.org/wiki/Fat_necrosis#/media/File:Breast_tissue_showing_fat_ necrosis_4X.jpg

Margins
30. Monica Morrow, Kimberly J. Van Zee, Lawrence J. Solin, Nehmat Houssami, Mariana Chavez-MacGregor, Jay R. Harris, Janet Horton, Shelley Hwang, Peggy L. Johnson, M. Luke Marinovich, Stuart J. Schnitt, Irene Wapnir, and Meena S. Moran Journal of Clinical Oncology 2016 34:33, 4040-4046.
31. Moran MS, Stuart Schnitt J, Giuliano AE, et al. Society of Surgical Oncology–American Society for Radiation Oncology Consensus Guideline on Margins for Breast-Conserving Surgery With Whole-Breast Irradiation in Stages I and II Invasive Breast Cancer. Annals of Surgical Oncology; March 2014, Volume 21, Issue 3, pp 704-716.

Invasive ductal cancer
32. Li CI, Uribe DJ, Daling JR. Clinical characteristics of different histologic types of breast cancer. Br J Cancer 2005; 93: 1046.

HER2
33. Slamon DJ, Godolphin W, Jones LA, et al. Science. 1989;244:707-712.
34. Sliwkowski MX. In: Harris JR, Lippman ME, Morrow M, Osborne CK, eds. Diseases of the Breast. 3rd ed. Philadelphia, PA: Lippincott Williams & Wilkins; 2004:415-426.
35. Ménard S, Tagliabue E, Campiglio M, Pupa SM. J Cell Physiol. 2000;182:150-162.
36. Sergina NV, Rausch M, Wang D, et al. Nature. 2007;445:437-441.

Paget's disease of the nipple

37. Photomicrograph: https://en.wikipedia.org/wiki/Paget%27s_disease_of_the_breast

38. Thin G. On the connection between disease of the nipple and areola and tumors of the breast. Trans Pathol Soc Lond 1881; 32:218.

39. Morrow M, Harris JR. Ductal carcinoma in situ and microinvasive carcinoma. In: Harris JR, Lippman ME, Morrow M, Osborne CK, editors. Diseases of the Breast. 3rd ed. Philadelphia, PA: Lippincott Williams and Wilkins; 2004. p. 521-537.

40. http://jncimono.oxfordjournals.org/content/2010/41/134.long#ref-3

41. Semin Diagn Pathol 1994;11:208–14.

42. Lewis GD, Lofgren JA, McMurtrey AE, et al. Cancer Res. 1996;56:1457-1465.

43. http://www.gene.com/patients/disease-education/her2-disease-in-breast-cancer

44. http://ww5.komen.org/BreastCancer/SubtypesofBreastCancer.html#sthash.qOuPw8j5.dpuf

45. Moran MS, Stuart Schnitt J, Giuliano AE, et al. Society of Surgical Oncology–American Society for Radiation Oncology Consensus Guideline on Margins for Breast-Conserving Surgery With Whole-Breast Irradiation in Stages I and II Invasive Breast Cancer. Annals of Surgical Oncology 2014;21 (3): 704-716.

Hamartoma

46. Hu H, Zhang M, Liu Y, Li XR, Liu G, Wang Z. Mammary hamartoma: is ultrasound-guided vacuum-assisted breast biopsy sufficient for its treatment? Gland Surg. 2020;9:1278–1285. [PMC free article] [PubMed] [Google Scholar]

47. Herbert M, Sandbank J, Liokumovich P. Breast hamartomas: clinicopathological and immunohistochemical studies of 24 cases. Histopathology. 2002;41:30–34

Phylloides

48. https://en.wikipedia.org/wiki/Phyllodes_tumor#/media/File:Phylloidestumor_der_Mamma_-_Mammographie.jpg

Intraductal papilloma; PASH

49. Sydnor MK et al. Underestimation of the presence of breast carcinoma in papillary lesions initially diagnosed at core-needle biopsy. Radiology 242 (1) 2007: 58-62. https://en.wikipedia.org/wiki/Pseudoangiomatous_stromal_hyperplasia

Metaplastic

50. Joneja U, Vranic S, Swensen J et al. Comprehensive profiling of metaplastic breast carcinomas reveals frequent overexpression of programmed death-ligand 1. J Clin Pathol 2017;70(3):255-259.

51. Chen DS, Mellman I. Oncology meets immunology: the cancer-immunity cycle. Immunity. 2013;39:1-10.

52. Chen DS, et al. Molecular pathways: next-generation immunotherapy-inhibiting programmed death-ligand 1 and programmed death-1. Ciln Cancer Res. 2012;18:6580-6587.

Invasive ductal cancer

53. Li CI, Uribe DJ, Daling JR. Clinical characteristics of different histologic types of breast cancer. Br J Cancer 2005; 93: 1046.

HER2

54. Slamon DJ, Godolphin W, Jones LA, et al. Science. 1989;244:707-712.

55. Sliwkowski MX. In: Harris JR, Lippman ME, Morrow M, Osborne CK, eds. Diseases of the Breast. 3rd ed. Philadelphia, PA: Lippincott Williams & Wilkins; 2004:415-426.

56. Ménard S, Tagliabue E, Campiglio M, Pupa SM. J Cell Physiol. 2000;182:150-162.
57. Sergina NV, Rausch M, Wang D, et al. Nature. 2007;445:437-441.
58. Lewis GD, Lofgren JA, McMurtrey AE, et al. Cancer Res. 1996;56:1457-1465.
59. http://www.gene.com/patients/disease-education/her2-disease-in-breast-cancer
60. http://ww5.komen.org/BreastCancer/SubtypesofBreastCancer.html#sthash.qOuPw8j5.dpuf
61. Moran MS, Stuart Schnitt J, Giuliano AE, et al. Society of Surgical Oncology–American Society for Radiation Oncology Consensus Guideline on Margins for Breast-Conserving Surgery With Whole-Breast Irradiation in Stages I and II Invasive Breast Cancer. Annals of Surgical Oncology 2014;21 (3): 704-716.

Phylloides
62. https://en.wikipedia.org/wiki/Phyllodes_tumor#/media/File:Phylloidestumor_der_Mamma_-_Mammographie.jpg

Invasive ductal cancer
63. http://www.choosingwisely.org/societies/american-society-of-clinical-oncology/
64. https://cancerstaging.org/references-tools/quickreferences/Documents/BreastMedium.pdf

7. PROGNOSIS - DCIS

1. http://media.jamanetwork.com/news-item/study-examines-breast-cancer-mortality-after-ductal-carcinoma-in-situ-diagnosis/
2. National Comprehensive Cancer Network (NCCN). NCCN Clinical practice guidelines in oncology: Breast cancer v.3.2014, http://www.nccn.org/, 2014.
3. Wapnir IL, Dignam JJ, Fisher B, et al. Long-term outcomes of invasive ipsilateral breast tumor recurrences after lumpectomy in NSABP B-17 and B-24 randomized trials for DCIS. J Natl Cancer Inst 2011; 103:478.
4. Van Zee KJ,White J, Morrow M, Harris JR. Chapter 23: Ductal carcinoma in situ and microinvasive carcinoma. In Harris JR, Lippman ME, Morrow M, Osborne CK. Diseases of the Breast. 5th edition. Lippincott Williams and Wilkins, 2014.
5. Recht, A. Are the Randomized Trials of Radiation Therapy for Ductal Carcinoma in Situ Still Relevant? J Clin Oncol 32 (32), 2014.

Tamoxifen
6. Kane RL, Virnig BA, Shamliyan T, et al. The impact of surgery, radiation, and systemic treatment on outcomes in patients with ductal carcinoma in situ: a study based on NSABP protocol B-24. J Clin Oncol. 30(12):1268-73, 2012.
7. D. Craig Allred, Stewart J. Anderson, Soonmyung Paik, et al. Adjuvant tamoxifen reduces subsequent breast cancer in women with estrogen receptor-positive ductal carcinoma in situ: A study based on NSABP protocol B-24. J Clin Oncol. 2012 Apr 20; 30(12); 1268-73.
8. Wapnir IL, Dignam JJ, Fisher B, et al. Long-term outcomes of invasive ipsilateral breast tumor recurrences after lumpectomy in NSABP B-17 and B-24 randomized clinical trials for DCIS. J Natl Cancer Inst 2011;103:478-488.

Review of randomized trials
9. Goodwin A, Parker S, Ghersi D, Wilcken N. Post-operative radiotherapy for ductal carcinoma in situ of the breast - a systematic review of the randomised trials. Breast 2009; 18:143.
HER2 status
10. G. Curigliano, D. Disalvatore, A. Esposito et al. Risk of subseuqent in situ and invasive breast

cancer in human epidermal growth factor receptor 2-positive ductal carcinoma in situ. Ann Oncol 2015;26(4):682-687.

11. Michael D Alvarado, Mitchell T Hayes, Rajni Sethi, Elissa Ozanne. NSABP B-43 is unlikely to produce a cost-effective treatment strategy for HER2+ DCIS [abstract]. In: Proceedings of the Thirty-Seventh Annual CTRC-AACR San Antonio Breast Cancer Symposium: 2014 Dec 9-13; San Antonio, TX. Philadelphia (PA): AACR; Cancer Res 2015;75(9 Suppl):Abstract nr P1-10-03.

Microinvasive carcinoma

12. Vieira CC, Mercado CL, Cangiarella JF et al. Microinvasive ductal carcinoma in sity: clinical presentation imaging features, pathologic findings, and outcome. Eur J Radiol 2010; 73(1): 102-107.

13. Padmore RF, Fowble B Hoffman J et al. Microinvasive breast carcinoma: clinicopathologic analysis of a single institution experience. Cancer 2000; 88(6): 1403-1409.carcinoma-in-situ-diagnosis/

14. National Comprehensive Cancer Network (NCCN). NCCN Clinical practice guidelines in oncology: Breast cancer v.3.2014, http://www.nccn.org/, 2014.

15. Wapnir IL, Dignam JJ, Fisher B, et al. Long-term outcomes of invasive ipsilateral breast tumor recurrences after lumpectomy in NSABP B-17 and B-24 randomized trials for DCIS. J Natl Cancer Inst 2011; 103:478.

16. Van Zee KJ,White J, Morrow M, Harris JR. Chapter 23: Ductal carcinoma in situ and microinvasive carcinoma. In Harris JR, Lippman ME, Morrow M, Osborne CK. Diseases of the Breast. 5th edition. Lippincott Williams and Wilkins, 2014.

17. Recht, A. Are the Randomized Trials of Radiation Therapy for Ductal Carcinoma in Situ Still Relevant? J Clin Oncol 32 (32), 2014.

Margins

18. Dunne C, Burke JP, Morrow M, Kell MR. Effect of margin status on local recurrence after breast conservation and radiation therapy for ductal carcinoma in situ. J Clin Oncol 2009; 19:1615-1620.

20. Groot G, Rees H, Pahwa P, et al. Predicting local recurrence following breast-consering therapy for early stage breast cancer: the significance of a narrow (</= 2mm) surgical resection margin. J Surg Oncol 2011; 103:212-216.

21. http://www.nccn.org

22. 2014 San Antonio Breast Cancer Symposium validated this gene test in a diverse population of women with DCIS (Abstract S5-04).

23. Moran MS, Stuart Schnitt J, Giuliano AE, et al. Society of Surgical Oncology–American Society for Radiation Oncology Consensus Guideline on Margins for Breast-Conserving Surgery With Whole-Breast Irradiation in Stages I and II Invasive Breast Cancer. Annals of Surgical Oncology; 2014, Volume 21, Issue 3, pp 704-716.

Molecular profiling

24. Hughes LL, Wang M, Page DL, et al. Local excision alone without irradiation for ductal carcinoma in situ of the breast: a trial of the Eastern Cooperative Oncology Group. J Clin Oncol 2009;27:5319-24.

25. JAMA Oncol. 2015 Oct;1(7):888-96. doi: 10.1001/jamaoncol.2015.2510. Breast Cancer Mortality After a Diagnosis of Ductal Carcinoma In Situ.

Age

26. Fredholm H, Eaker S, Frisell J et al. PLosS One 2009, 4:e7695.

27. Partridge AG, Hughes ME, Warner ET, et al. Subtype-dependent relationship between young age at diagnosis and breast cancer survival. [Published online ahead of print August 1, 2016]. J Clin Oncol. doi:10.1200/JCO.2015.65.8013.
28. Pan H, Gray R, Braybrooke J, et al. EBCTCG. 20-year risks of breast-cancer recurrence after stopping endocrine therapy at 5 years. N Engl J Med. 2017;377(19):1836–1846.

7. PROGNOSIS - INVASIVE

Metastases and prognosis

1. Swenerton KD, Legha SS, Smith T, et al. Prognostic factors in metastatic breast cancer treated with combination chemotherapy. Cancer Res 1979; 39: 1552.
2. Hortobagyi GN, Smilty TL, Legha SS, et al. Multivariate analysis of prognostic factors in metastatic breast cancer. J Clin Oncol 1983; 1: 776.
3. Robertson JF, Dixon AR, Nicholson RI, et al. Confirmation of a prognostic index for patients with metastatic breast cancer treated by endocrine therapy. Breast Cancer Res Treat 1992; 22:221.
4. Stuart-Harris R, Shadbolt B, Palmqvist C, Chaudri Ross HA. The prognostic significance of single hormone receptor positive metastatic breast cancer: an analysis of three randomized phase III trials of aromatase inhibitors. Breast 1009; 18: 351.

First recurrence

5. Clark GM, Sledge GW Jr, Osborne CK, McGuire WL. Survival from first recurrence: relative importance of prognostic factors in 1,015 breast cancer patients. J Clin Oncol 1987; 5:55.

Survival curve

6. Harris JR, Hellman S. Observations on survival curve analysis with particular reference to breast cancer treatment. Cancer 1986; 57: 925.

Prognostic and predictive factors: Using for management

7. Rampaul RS, Pinder SE, Elston CW, Ellis IO: Prognostic and predictive factors in primary breast cancer and their role in patient management: The Nottingham Breast Team. Eur J Surg Oncol 2001, 27:229–238.
8. Cianfrocca M, Goldstein LJ: Prognostic and predictive factors in early-stage breast cancer. Oncologist 2004, 9:606–616.

Lymphvascular invasion (LVI)

9. Mohammed RA, Martin SG, Gill MS, et al: Improved methods of detection of lymphovascular invasion demonstrate that it is the predominant method of vascular invasion in breast cancer and has important clinical consequences. Am J Surg Pathol 2007, 31:1825–1833.
10. Mohammed RA, Martin SG, Mahmmod AM, et al.: Objective assessment of lymphatic and blood vascular invasion in lymph node-negative breast carcinoma: findings from a large case series with long-term follow-up. J Pathol 2011, 223:358–365.
11. Pinder SE, Ellis IO, Galea M, O'Rouke S, Blamey RW, Elston CW: Pathological prognostic factors in breast cancer. III. Vascular invasion: relationship with recurrence and survival in a large study with long-term follow-up. Histopathology 1994, 24:41–47.
12. Rakha EA, Martin S, Lee AH, et al.: The prognostic significance of lymphovascular invasion in invasive breast carcinoma. Cancer 2012, 118:3670–3680.

13. Goldhirsch A, Glick JH, Gelber RD, Coates AS, Thürlimann B, Senn HJ: Meeting highlights: international expert consensus on the primary therapy of early breast cancer 2005. Ann Oncol 2005, 16:1569–1583.

14. Lee AH, Pinder SE, Macmillan RD, et al.: Prognostic value of lymphovascular invasion in women with lymph node negative invasive breast carcinoma. Eur J Cancer 2006, 42:357–362.

16. Rampaul RS, Pinder SE, Elston CW, Ellis IO: Prognostic and predictive factors in primary breast cancer and their role in patient management: The Nottingham Breast Team. Eur J Surg Oncol 2001, 27:229–238.

17. Cianfrocca M, Goldstein LJ: Prognostic and predictive factors in early-stage breast cancer. Oncologist 2004, 9:606–616.

18. Ejertsen B, et al. Population-based study of peritumoral lymphvascular invasion and outcome among patients with operable breast cancer. J Natl Cancer Inst 2009; 101:729.

Disparities

19. Eaker S. Dickman PW, et al. Differences in management of older women influence breast cancer survival: results from a population-based database in Sweden. PLoS Med 2006; 3:e25.

20. Siegel R, Ward E, Brawley O et al. Cancer statistics, 2011: the impact of eliminating socioeconomic and racial disparities on premature cancer deaths. CA Cancer J Clin 2011; 61:212.

21. Silber JH, Rosenbaum PR, Clark AS et al. Characteristics associated with differences in survival among black and white women with breast cancer. JAMA 2013; 310:389.

22. Park JH, Anderson WF, Gail MH. Improvements in US breast cancer survival and proportion explained by tumor size and estrogen-receptor status. J Clin Oncol 33: 2870-2876, 2015.

23. Elkin EB, Hudis CA. Parsing progress in breast cancer. J Clin Oncol 33:2837-2838, 2015.

24. American Cancer Society: Breast Cancer Facts and Figures 2013-2014. Atlanta, GA. American Cancer Society, 2015.

25. Kohler BA, Sherman RL, Howlader N, et al. Annual Report to the Nation on the Status of Cancer. 1976-2011, featuring incidence of breast cancer subtypes by race/ethnicity, poverty, and state. J Natl Cancer Inst 107:djv048, 2015.

26. Newman LA: Parsing the etiology of breast cancer disparities. J Clin Oncol 34:1013-1014, 2016.

27. DeSantis CE, Fedewa SA, Goding Sauer a, et al. Breast cancer statistics. 2015. Convergence of incidence rates between black and white women. CA Cancer J Clin doi: 10.3322/caac.21320 [epub ahead of print on October 29,2015]

28. Menashe I, Anderson WF, Jatoi I, et al. Underlying causes of the black-white racial disparity in breast cancer mortality. A population-based analysis. J Natl Cancer Inst 101:993-1000, 2009.

Size, nodes, and survival

29. Carter CL, Allen C, Hensen DE. Relation of tumor size, lymph node status, and survival in 740 breast cancer cases. Cancer 1989; 63:181

30. de Boer M, van Dijck JA, Bult P et al. Breast cancer prognosis and occult lymph node metastases, isolated tumor cells, and micrometastases. J Natl Cancer Inst 2010; 102:410.

31. Fisher B, Redmond C, Fisher ER, Caplan R. Relative worth of estrogen or progesterone receptor and pathologic characteristics of differentiation as indicators of prognosis in node-negative breast cancer patients: Findings from National Surgical Adjuvant Breast and Bowel Project Protocol B-06. J Clin Oncol. 6(7):1076-87, 1988.

32. Ries LAG and Eisner MP. Chapter 13 - Cancer of the female breast. In: Ries LAG, Young JL, Keel GE, et al. (eds). SEER Survival Monograph: Cancer survival among adults: U.S. SEER Program, 1988-2001, patient and tumor characteristics. National Cancer Institute, SEER Program, NIH Pub. No. 07-6215, Bethesda, MD, 2007.

Estrogen receptors

33. Bentzon N, Düring M, Rasmussen BB, Mouridsen H, Kroman N. Prognostic effect of estrogen receptor status across age in primary breast cancer. Int J Cancer. 122(5):1089-94, 2008.
34. Fisher B, Redmond C, Fisher ER, Caplan R. Relative worth of estrogen or progesterone receptor and pathologic characteristics of differentiation as indicators of prognosis in node-negative breast cancer patients: Findings from National Surgical Adjuvant Breast and Bowel Project Protocol B-06. J Clin Oncol. 6(7):1076-87, 1988.
35. Bentzon N, Düring M, Rasmussen BB, Mouridsen H, Kroman N. Prognostic effect of estrogen receptor status across age in primary breast cancer. Int J Cancer. 122(5):1089-94, 2008.

Stage migration

36. Wishart GC, Greenberg DC, Britton PD et al. Screen-detected versus symptomatic breast cancer: is improved survival due to stage migration? Br J Cancer 2008; 98: 1741.

Multifocal or multicentric cancer

37. Weissenbacher TM, Zschage M, Janni W et al. Multicentric and multifocal versus unifocal breast caner: is the tumor-node-metastasis classification justified? Breast Cancer Res Treat 2010;122:27.
38. Lynch SP, Lei X, Chavez-MacGregot M et al. Multifocality and multicentricity in breast cancer and survival outcomes. Ann Oncol 2012; 23:3063.

Predictive factors

39. de Duenas EN, Hernandez AL, Zotano AG, et al. Prospective evaluation of the conversion rate in the receptor status between primary breast cancer and metastasis: results from the GEI-CAM 2009-03 ConvertHER study. Breast Cancer Res Treat 2014; 143: 507.
40. Amir E, Clemons M, Purdie CA, et al. Tissue confirmation of disease recurrence in breast cancer patients: pooled analysis of multi-centre, multi-disciplinary prospective studies. Cancer Treat Rev 2012; 38: 708.

Smoking

41. http://www.ajmc.com/newsroom/smoking-can-reduce-survival-in-breast-cancer-patients-?utm_source=Informz&utm_medium=AJMC&utm_campaign=MC%5FMinute%5F1%2D28%2D16
42. Passarelli MN, Newcomb PA, Hampton JM, et al. Cigarette Smoking Before and After Breast Cancer Diagnosis: Mortality From Breast Cancer and Smoking-Related Diseases. Presented at the 38th Annual Meeting of the American Society of Preventive Oncology, Arlington, VA, March 8-11, 2014.

Tumor infiltrating lymphocytes (TILs)

43. Demaria S, Pilones KA, Adams S: Cross-talk of breast cancer cells with the immune system, in Gunduz M, Gunduz E (eds): Breast Cancer: Carcinogenesis, Cell Growth and Signalling Pathways. Rijeka, Croatia, InTech, 2011, pp 457-482
44. Aaltomaa S, Lipponen P, Eskelinen M, et al: Lymphocyte infiltrates as a prognostic variable in female breast cancer. Eur J Cancer 28A:859-864, 1992
45. Denkert C, Loibl S, Noske A, et al: Tumor- associated lymphocytes as an independent predictor of response to neoadjuvant chemotherapy in breast cancer. J Clin Oncol 28:105-113, 2010
46. Loi S, Sirtaine N, Piette F, et al: Prognostic and predictive value of tumor-infiltrating lymphocytes in a phase III randomized adjuvant breast cancer trial in node-positive breast cancer comparing the addition of docetaxel to doxorubicin with doxorubicin-based chemotherapy:

BIG 02-98. J Clin Oncol 31:860-867, 2013

47. West NR, Milne K, Truong PT, et al: Tumor- infiltrating lymphocytes predict response to anthracycline-based chemotherapy in estrogen receptor-negative breast cancer. Breast Cancer Res 13:R126, 2011

48. Barrios CH, Sampaio C, Vinholes J, Caponero R. What is the role of chemotherapy in estrogen receptor-positive, advanced breast cancer? Ann Oncol. 2009;20(7):1157–1162.

49. Smith NZ. Treating metastatic breast cancer with systemic chemotherapies: current trends and future perspectives. Clin J Oncol Nurs. 2012;16(2):E33–E43.

50. Pritchard KI, et al. Endocrine therapy for postmenopausal women with hormone receptor-positive her2-negative advanced breast cancer after progression or recurrence on nonsteroidal aromatase inhibitor therapy: a Canadian consensus statement. Curr Oncol. 2013;20(1):48–61.

51. Janicke F, Prechtl A, Thomssen C, et al. Randomized adjuvant chemotherapy trial in high-risk, lymph node-negative breast cancer patients identified by urokinase-type plasminogen activator and plasminogen activator inhibitor type 1. J Natl Cancer Inst 2001; 93:913.

Circulating Tumor Cells (CTCs)

52. Lucci A, Hall CS, Lodhi AK, et al. Circulating tumour cells in non-metastatic breast cancer: a prospective study. Lancet Oncol 2012; 13:688.

53. Rack B, Schindlbeck C, Juckstock J et al. Circulating tumor cells predict survival in early average-to-high risk breast cancer patients. J Natl Cancer Inst 2014; 106.http://seer.cancer.gov/statfacts/html/breast.html

54. Giuliano AE, Hawes D, Ballman KV et al. Association of occult metastases in sentinel lymph nodes and bone marrow with survival among women with early-stage invasive breast cancer. JAMA. 2011; 306:385-393.

Special topics

55. Andersson Y, Frisell J, Sylvan M, et al. Breast cancer survival in relation to the metastatic tumor burden in axillary lymph nodes. J Clin Oncol [early online publication]. May 10, 2010.

56. Carter BA, Page DL. Sentinel lymph node histopathology in breast cancer: minimal disease versus artifact. J Clin Oncol 2006;24(13);1978.

57. Youngson BJ, Liberman L, Rosen PP. Displacement of carcinomatous epithelium in surgical breast specimens following stereotaxic core biopsy. Am J Clin Pathol 1995; 103(5):598.

58. Douglas-Jones AG, Verghese A. Diagnostic difficulty arising from displaced epithelium after core biopsy in intracystic papillary lesions of the breast. J Clin Pathol 2002;55(10):780.

59. Moore KH, Thaler HT, Tan LK, et al. Immunohistochemically detected tumor cells in the sentinel lymph nodes of patients with breast carcinoma: biologic metastasis or procedural artifact? Cancer 2004; 100(5):929.

Gene expression profiles

60. http://breast-cancer.oncotypedx.com/en-US/Patient-Invasive/WhatIsTheOncotypeDXCancerTest.aspx

61. Paik S, Shak S, Tang G, et al. A multigene assay to predict recurrence of tamoxifen-treated, node-negative breast cancer. N Engl J Med. 2004;351:2817-2826.

62. Paik S, Tang G, Shak S, et al. Gene expression and benefit of chemotherapy in women with node-negative, estrogen receptor–positive breast cancer. J Clin Oncol. 2006;24:3726-3734.

63. Albain KS, Barlow WE, Shak S, et al. Prognostic and predictive value of the 21-gene recurrence score assay in a randomized trial of chemotherapy for post-menopausal, node-positive, estrogen receptor-positive breast cancer. Lancet Oncol. 2010; 11:55-65.

64. Mook S, Schmidt MK, Viale G, et al. The 7--gene prognosis-signature predicts disease outcome in breast cancer patients with 1-3 positive lymph nodes in an independent validation study. Breast Cancer Res Treat 2009;116:295-302.

65. Mook S, Schmidt MK, Viale G, et al. The 7--gene prognosis-signature predicts disease outcome in breast cancer patients with 1-3 positive lymph nodes in an independent validation study. Breast Cancer Res Treat 2009;116:295-302.

66. NCCN clinical practice guidelines in oncology: breast cancer. Available at https://www.nccn.org/professionals/physician_gls/pdf/breast.pdf. Accessed March 19, 2017.

Measures of proliferation

67. Gnant M, Filipits M, Greil R, et al. Ann Oncol 2014; 25:339.

68. Viale F, Giobbe-Hirder A, Gusterson BA, et al. Adverse prognostic value of peritumoral vascular invasion: is it abrogated by adequate endocrine adjuvant therapy? Results from two International Breast Cancer Study Group randomized trials. Ann Oncol 2010; 21:245.

69. Colzani E,Liljegren A, Johansson AL et al. Prognosis of patients with breast cancer: causes of death and effects of time since diagnosis, age, and tumor characteristics. J Clin Oncol 2007; 25:5287.

70. http://www.agendia.com/healthcare-professionals/breast-cancer/mammaprint/

71. King TA, Lyman JO, Gonen M, et al. Prognostic impact of 21-gene recurrence score in patients with stage IV breast cancer: TBCRC 013. J Clin Oncol 2016 Mar 21. pii: JCO631860 [Epub ahead of print]

Neoadjuvant treatment and HER-2

72. Mieog JSD, van der Hage JA, van de Velde CJH. Neoadjuvant chemotherapy for operable breast cancer. Br J Surg. 94(10):1189-1200, 2007.

73. J Clin Oncol 32, 2015 (suppl 26; abstr 61).

Breast density and prognosis

74. Davies C, Godwin J, Gray R, et al: Relevance of breast cancer hormone receptors and other factors to the efficacy of adjuvant tamoxifen. Lancet 378:771-784, 2011

75. Jordan VC: New insights into the metabolism of tamoxifen and its role in the treatment and prevention of breast cancer. Steroids 72:829-842, 2007

76. Boyd NF, Martin LJ, Yaffe MJ, et al: Mammographic density and breast cancer risk: Current understanding and future prospects. Breast Cancer Res 13: 223, 2011

77. Huo CW,Chew GL,Britt KL,et al: Mammographic density - A review on the current understanding of its association with breast cancer. Breast Cancer Res Treat 144:479-502, 2014

79. Kim J, Han W, et al: Breast density change as a predictive surrogate for response to adjuvant endocrine therapy in hormone receptor positive breast cancer. Breast Cancer Res 14:R102, 2012

80. Ko KL, Shin IS, You JY, et al: Adjuvant tamoxifen-induced mammographic breast density reduction as a predictor for recurrence in estrogen receptor-positive premenopausal breast cancer patients. Breast Cancer Res Treat 142:559-567, 2013

81. Li J, Humphreys K, Eriksson L, et al: Mammographic density reduction is a prognostic marker of response to adjuvant tamoxifen therapy in postmenopausal patients with breast cancer. J Clin Oncol 31:2249-2256, 2013

80. Nyante SJ, Sherman ME, Pfeiffer RM, et al: Prognostic significance of mammographic density change after initiation of tamoxifen for ER-positive breast cancer. JNCI 107:dju425, 2015

82. Hance KW, Anderson WF, Devesa SS, Young HA, Levine PH. Trends in inflammatory breast carcinoma incidence and survival: the surveillance, epidemiology, and end results program at the National Cancer Institute. J Natl Cancer Inst. 97(13):966-75, 2005.

83. Untch M, Möbus V, Kuhn W, et al. Intensive dose-dense compared with conventionally scheduled preoperative chemotherapy for high-risk primary breast cancer. J Clin Oncol. 27(18):2938-45, 2009.

84. Yang R, Cheung MC, Hurley J, et al. A comprehensive evaluation of outcomes for inflamma-

tory breast cancer. Breast Cancer Res Treat. 117(3):631-41, 2009.

85. Ellis GK, Barlow WE, Gralow JR, et al. Phase III comparison of standard doxorubicin and cyclophosphamide versus weekly doxorubicin and daily oral cyclophosphamide plus granulocyte colony-stimulating factor as neoadjuvant therapy for inflammatory and locally advanced breast cancer: SWOG 0012. J Clin Oncol. 29(8):1014-21, 2011.

86. Matro JM, Li T, Cristofanilli M, et al. Inflammatory breast cancer management in the National Comprehensive Cancer Network: the disease, recurrence pattern, and outcome. Clin Breast

87. Loi S, Drubay D, Adams S et al. Tumor-Infiltrating Lymphocytes and Prognosis: A Pooled Individual Patient Analysis of Early-Stage Triple-Negative Breast Cancers. J Clin Onc 2019 37:7, 559-569.

Locoregional Relapse

88. Aebi S, Gelber S, Anderson SJ, et al. Chemotherapy for isolated locoregional recurrence of breast cancer (CALOR): a randomised trial. Lancet Oncol 2014;15:156-163.

89. Mamounas EP, Anderson SJ, Dignam JJ, et al. Predictors of locoregional recurrence after neoadjuvant chemotherapy: results from combined analysis of national surgical adjuvant breast and bowel project B-18 and B-27. J Clin Oncol. 30(32):3960-6, 2012.

90. Hind D, Wyld L, Beverley CB, Reed MW. Surgery versus primary endocrine therapy for operable primary breast cancer in elderly women (70 years plus) Cochrane Database Syst Rev. 2006:CD004272.

91. www.cancer.org/research/cancerfactsstatistics/breast-cancer-facts-figures

92. Eleanor E. R. Harris, M.D. et al. Prognosis after Regional Lymph Node Recurrence in Patients with Stage I–II Breast Carcinoma Treated with Breast Conservation Therapy. Presented in part at the 44th Annual Meeting of the American Society for Therapeutic Radiology and Oncology, New Orleans, Louisiana, October 6–10, 2002.

93. Pedersena AN, Møllerb S, Steffensenc D. Supraclavicular recurrence after early breast cancer: A curable condition? Breast Cancer Research and Treatment 125(3):815-22 · April 2010.

94. Halverson KJ, Perez CA, Kuske RR, et al. Survival following locoregional recurrence of breast cancer: univariate and multivariate analysis Int J Radiat Oncol Biol Phhys 1992; 23(2): 285.

95. Early Breast Cancer Trialists' Collaborative Group (EBCTCG), Darby S, McGale P, et al. Effect of radiotherapy after breast-conserving surgery on 10--year recurrence and 15-year breast cancer death: meta-analysis of individual patient data for 10,801 women in 17 randomised trials. Lancet 2011; 378:1707-1716.

96. http://www.cancer.org/cancer/%20breastcancer/detailedguide/breast-cancer-survival-by-stage

97. American Cancer Society. Breast Cancer Facts and Figures 2013-2014. Atlanta, GA: American Cancer Society, 2013. - See more at: http://ww5.komen.org/BreastCancer/BreastFactsReferences.html#sthash. RLb22ACH.dpuf

98. Aebi S, Gelber S, Anderson SJ, et al. Chemotherapy for isolated locoregional recurrence of breast cancer (CALOR): a randomised trial. Lancet Oncol 2014;15:156-163.

Brain metastases

99. Barnholtz-Sloan JS, Sloan AE, Davis FG, et al. Incidence proportions of brain metastases in patients diagnosed (1973 to 2001) in the Metropolitan Detroit Cancer Surveillance System. J Clin Oncol 2004;22(14):2865.

100. Arvold ND, Oh KS, Niemierko A, et al. Brain metastases after breast-conserving therapy and systemic therapy: incidence and characteristics by biologic subtype. Breast Cancer Res Treat 2012;136(1):153.

101. Kennecke H, Yerushalmi R, Woods, R et al. Metastatic behavior of breast cancer subtypes. J Clin Oncol 2010 Jul;28(20);3271-7. Epub 2010 May 24.

102. Sperduto PW, Kased N, Roverge D, et al. Summary report on the graded prognostic assessment: An accurate and facile diagnosis-specific tool to estimate survival for patients with brain metastases. J Clin Oncol 2012: 30(419).

103. Arvold ND, Oh KS, Niemierko A, et al. Brain metastases after breast-conserving therapy and sstemic therapy: incidence and characteristics by biologic subtype. Breast Cancer Res Treat 2012;136(1):153.

104. Kennecke H, Yerushalmi R, Woods, R et al. Metastatic behavior of breast cancer subtypes. J Clin Oncol 2010 Jul;28(20);3271-7. Epub 2010 May 24.

105. Sperduto PW, Kased N, Roverge D, et al. Summary report on the graded prognostic assessment: An accurate and facile diagnosis-specific tool to estimate survival for patients with brain metastases. J Clin Oncol 2012: 30(419).

Leptomeningeal spread

106. Lee S, et al. Leptomeningeal metastases from breast cancer: intrinsic subtypes may affect unique clinical manifestations. Breast Cancer Res Treat 2011 Oct;129(3):809-817. Epub 2011 Jul 23.

Locoregional recurrence

107. EBCTCG Lancet Oncol 378:1707-16, 2011

Local recurrence and chemotherapy

108. Wapnir IL, Price KN, Anderson SJ, Robidoux A, et al. Efficacy of Chemotherapy for ER-Negative and ER-Positive Isolated Locoregional Recurrence of Breast Cancer: Final Analysis of the CALOR Trial. J Clin Oncol. 2018 Apr 10;36(11):1073-1079. doi: 10.1200/JCO.2017.76.5719. Epub 2018 Feb 14.

Node positive: Genomic testing

109. Mook S, Schmidt MK, Viale G, et al. The 7--gene prognosis-signature predicts disease outcome in breast cancer patients with 1-3 positive lymph nodes in an independent validation study. Breast Cancer Res Treat 2009;116:295-302.

110. NCCN clinical practice guidelines in oncology: breast cancer. Available at https://www.nccn.org/professionals/physician_gls/pdf/breast.pdf. Accessed March 19, 2017.

111. Cancer. S1526-8209(14)00112-8, 2014.

112. http://www.cancer.org/cancer/breastcancer/moreinformation/inflammatorybreastcancer/inflammatory-breast-cancer-inflammatory-br-ca-aggressive

TILs

113. Loi S, Drubay D, Adams S et al. Tumor-Infiltrating Lymphocytes and Prognosis: A Pooled Individual Patient Analysis of Early-Stage Triple-Negative Breast Cancers. J Clin Onc 2019 37:7, 559-569.

Management

114. Narod SA, Iqbal J, Giannakeas V, et al. Breast cancer mortality after a diagnosis of ductal carcinoma in situ. JAMA Oncol 2015;1(7):888.

115. Rosner D, Bedwani RN, Vana J et al. Noninvasive breast carcinoma: results of a national survey by the American College of Surgeons. Ann Surg 1980;192(2):139.

116. Kinne DW, Petrek JA, Osborne MP et al. Breast carcinoma in situ. Arch Surg 1989;124(1):33.

117. Goodwin A, Parker S, Ghersi D, et al. Breast 2009;18(3):143.

118. Wapnir IL, Dignam JJ, Fisher B, et al: Long- term outcomes of invasive ipsilateral breast tumor recurrences after lumpectomy in NSABP B-17 and B-24 randomized clinical trials for DCIS.

J Natl Cancer Inst 103:478-488, 2011
119. RT boost: JAMA Oncol. Published online March 30, 2017. doi:10.1001/jamaoncol.2016.6948

7. INVASIVE - MANAGEMENT

Biopsy
1. Brennan ME, Turner RM, Clatto S et al. Ductal carcinoma in situ at core-needle biopsy: meta-analysis of underestimation and predictors of invasive breast cancer. Radiology 2011;260:119-128.
2. https://en.wikipedia.org/wiki/Paget%27s_disease_of_the_breast#/media/File:Extramammary_Paget_disease_-_high_mag.jpg

Management
3. Narod SA, Iqbal J, Giannakeas V, et al. Breast cancer mortality after a dignosis of ductal carcinoma in situ. JAMA Oncol 2015;1(7):888.
4. Rosner D, Bedwani RN, Vana J et al. Noninvasive breast carcinoma: results of a national survey by the American College of Surgeons. Ann Surg 1980;192(2):139.
5. Kinne DW, Petrek JA, Osborne MP et al. Breast carcinoma in situ. Arch Surg 1989;124(1):33.
6. Goodwin A, Parker S, Ghersi D, et al. Breast 2009;18(3):143.
7. Wapnir IL, Dignam JJ, Fisher B, et al: Long- term outcomes of invasive ipsilateral breast tumor recurrences after lumpectomy in NSABP B-17 and B-24 randomized clinical trials for DCIS. J Natl Cancer Inst 103:478-488, 2011
8. Livi L, Meattini I, Marrazzo L, et al. Accelerated partial breast irradiation using intensity-modulated radiotherapy versus whole breast irradiation: 5-year survival analysis of a phase 3 randomised controlled trial. Eur J Cancer. 2015;51:451-463.
9. Meattini I, Marrazzo L, Saieva C, et al. Accelerated partial-breast irradiation compared with whole-breast irradiation for early breast cancer: Long-term results of the randomized phase III APBI-IMRT-Florence Trial. JClin Oncol 2020;38:4175-4183

Nodes
10. Halsted W. The results of radical operations for the cure of carcinoma of the breast. Ann Surg 1907;46(1):1-19.
11. Fisher B, Montague E, Redmond C, et al. Comparison of radical mastectomy with alternative treatments for primary breast cancer. A first report of results from a prospective randomized
12. Cuzick J, Sestak I, Pinder SE, et al: Effect of tamoxifen and radiotherapy in women with locally excised ductal carcinoma in situ: Long-term results from the UK/ANZ DCIS trial. Lancet Oncol 12:21-29, 2011
13. Donker M, Litière S, Werutsky G et al. Breast-conserving treatment with or without radiotherapy in ductal carcinoma in situ: 15-year recurrence rates and outcome after a recurrence, from the EORTC 10853 randomized phase III trial. J Clin Oncol 10: 4054-4059, 2013
14. Neuschatz AC, DiPetrillo T, Safaii H, et al. Margin width as a determinant of local control with and without radiation therapy for ductal carcinoma in situ (DCIS) of the breast. Int J Cancer. 2001;96 suppl:97–104.
15. Silverstein MJ, Buchanan C. Ductal carcinoma in situ: USC/Van Nuys prognostic index and the impact of margin status. Breast. 2003;12(6):457–471.
16. Holland PA, Gandhi A, Knox WF, et al. The importance of complete excision in the prevention of local recurrence of ductal carcinoma in situ. Br J Cancer. 1998;77(1):110–114.
17. Wang SY, Shamliyan T, Virnig BA, Kane R. Tumor characteristics as predictors of local recurrence after treatment of ductal carcinoma in situ: a meta-analysis. Breast Cancer Res Treat.

2011;127(1):1–14.

OncoType DX DCIS
18. http://breast-cancer.oncotypedx.com/en-US/Professional-DCIS
19. Rakovitch E, Nofech-Mozes S, Hanna W, et al. A large prospectively-designed study of the DCIS score: Predicting recurrence risk after local excision for ductal carcinoma in situ patients with and without irradiation. 2014 San Antonio Breast Cancer Symposium. Abstr S5-04.

Hormone receptors
20. http://www.nature.com/nchembio/journal/v2/n4/fig_tab/nchembio0406-175_F1.html

Tamoxifen for DCIS
21. Wapnir IL, Dignam JJ, Fisher B, et al. Long-term outcomes of invasive ipsilateral breast tumor recurrences after lumpectomy in NSABP B-17 and B-24 randomized clinical trials for DCIS. J Natl Cancer Inst. 103(6):478-88, 2011.
22. Allred DC, Anderson SJ, Paik S, et al. Adjuvant tamoxifen reduces subsequent breast cancer in women with estrogen receptor-positive ductal carcinoma in situ: a study based on NSABP protocol B-24. J Clin Oncol. 30(12):1268-73, 2012.
23. Cuzick J, Sestak I, Pinder SE, et al. Effect of tamoxifen and radiotherapy in women with locally excised ductal carcinoma in situ: long-term results from the UK/ANZ DCIS trial. Lancet Oncol. 12(1):21-9, 2011.
24. Staley H, McCallum I, Bruce J. Postoperative tamoxifen for ductal carcinoma in situ. Cochrane Database Syst Rev. 10:CD007847, 2012.
25. Staley H, McCallum I, Bruce J. Postoperative tamoxifen for ductal carcinoma in situ. Cochrane Database Syst Rev 2012; 10:CD007847.
26. Allred DC, Anderson SJ, Paik S, et al. Adjuvant tamoxifen reduces subsequent breast cancer in women with estrogen receptor-positive ductal carcinoma in situ: a study based on NSABP protocol B-24. J Clin Oncol 2012; 30:1268.

Risk does not plateau
27. Solin LJ, Gray R. Hughes LL, et al. Surgical Excision Without Radiation for Ductal Carcinoma in Situ of the Breast: 12-Year Results From the ECOG-ACRIN E5194 Study. JCO.2015.60.8588; published online on September 14, 2015.
28. https://www.nccn.org/professionals/physician_gls/pdf/breast.pdf

Local recurrence
29. Solin LJ, Fourquet A, Vicini FA et al. Long-term outcome after breast-conservation treatment with radiation for mammographically detected ductal carcinoma in situ of the breast Cancer 2005;103(6):1137.
30. Kerlikowske K, Molinari A, Cha I et al. Characteristics associated with recurrence among women with ductal carcinoma in situ treated with lumpectomy. J Natl Cancer Inst 2003;95(22):1692.
31. Allred DC. Ductal carcinoma in situ: terminology, classification, and natural history. J Natl Cancer Inst Monogr 2010;2010(41):134-8.
32. Halverson KJ, Perez CA, Kuske RR, et al. Survival following locoregional recurrence of breast cancer: univariate and multivariate analysis Int J Radiat Oncol Biol Phhys 1992; 23(2): 285.
Subhedar P, Olcese C, Patil S et al. Decreasing Recurrence Rates for Ductal Carcinoma In Situ: Analysis of 2996 Women Treated with Breast-Conserving Surgery Over 30 Years. Breast Oncology; 22(10), 2015.
33. Early Breast Cancer Trialists' Collaborative Group. Effects of Radiotherapy and Surgery in

Early Breast Cancer. An Overview of the Randomized Trials. N Engl J Med. 333:1444-55, 1995.
34. http://dx.doi.org/10.1016/j.ijrobp.2003.12.036
35. Early Breast Cancer Trialists' Collaborative Group (EBCTCG), Darby S, McGale P, Correa C, et al. Effect of radiotherapy after breast-conserving surgery on 10-year recurrence and 15-year breast cancer death: meta-analysis of individual patient data for 10,801 women in 17 randomised trials. Lancet. 2011 Nov 12;378(9804):1707-16. doi: 10.1016/S0140-6736(11)61629-2. Epub 2011 Oct 19.

Surgery: BRCA

36. Howlader N, Noone AM, Krapcho M, et al. (eds). SEER Cancer Statistics Review, 1975-2011, National Cancer Institute. Bethesda, MD, http://seer.cancer.gov/csr/1975_2011/ , based on November 2013 SEER data submission, posted to the SEER web site, April 2014.
37. Antoniou A, Pharoah PD, Narod S, et al. Average risks of breast and ovarian cancer associated with BRCA1 or BRCA2 mutations detected in case series unselected for family history: A combined analysis of 22 studies. American Journal of Human Genetics 2003; 72(5):1117–1130.
38. Chen S, Parmigiani G. Meta-analysis of BRCA1 and BRCA2 penetrance. Journal of Clinical Oncology 2007; 25(11):1329–1333.

Surgery: Nodes

39. Silverstein MJ, Skinner KA, Lomis TJ. Predicting axillary nodal positivity in 2282 patients with breast carcinoma. World J Surg 2001; 25:767.
40. Ravdin PM, De LauertisM, Vendely T et al. Prediction of axillary node status in breast cancer patients by use of prognostic indicators. J Natl Cancer Inst 1994; 86;1771
41. Morrow M, Foster RS Jr. Staging of breast cancer: a new rationale for internal mammary node biopsy. Arch Surg 1981; 116:748.
42. Ravdin PM, De LauertisM, Vendely T et al. Prediction of axillary node status in breast cancer patients by use of prognostic indicators. J Natl Cancer Inst 1994; 86;1771
43. de Freitas R Jr, Costa MV, Schneider SV et al. Accuracy of ultrasound and clinical exmination in the diagnosis of axillary lymph node metastases in breast cancer. Eur J Surg Oncol 1991; 17:240.
44. Lanng C, Hoffman J, Galatius H et al. Assessment of clinical palpation of the axilla as a criterion for performing the sentinel node procedure in breast cancer. Eur J Surg Oncol 2007; 33:281.
45. Fowble B, Solin LJ, Schultz DJ et al. Frequency, sites of relapse, and outcome of regional node failures following conservative surgery and radiation for early breast cancer. Int J Radiat Biol Phys 1989; 17:703.
46. Graversen HP, et al. Breast cancer: risk of axillary recurrence in node-negative patients following partial dissection of the axilla. Eur J Surg Oncol 1988; 14:407.
47. Fisher B, et al. The accuracy of clinical nodal staging and of limited axillary dissection as a determinant of histologic nodal status in carcinoma of the breast. Surg Gynecol Obstet 1981; 152:765.
48. Sanghani M, et al. Impact of axillary lymph node dissection on breast cancer outcome in clinically node negative patients: a systematic review and meta-analysis. Cancer 2009; 115:1613.
49. Louis-Sylvestre C, et al. Axillary treatment in conservative management of operable breast cancer: dissection or radiotherapy? Results of a randomized study with 15 years of follow-up. J Clin Oncol 2004; 22:97.
50. Fisher B, et al. Ten-year results of a randomized clinical trial comparing radical mastectomy and total mastectomy with or without radiation. N Engl J Med 2002; 347:567.
51. Greco C, et al. Randomized clinical trial on the role of axillary radiotherapy in breast conservative management without axillary dissection lesion <1 cm (abstract). Int J Radiat Oncol Biol 1998; 42:250.
52. Krag DN, et al. Sentinel-lymph-node resection compared with conventional axillary-lymph-

node dissection in clinically node-negative patients with breast cancer: overall survival findings from the NSABP B-32 randomised phase 3 trial. Lancet Oncology 2010; 11(10):927–933.

53. Kell M, Burke JM, Barry K, et al. Axillary dissection versus no axillary dissection in women with invasive breast cancer and sentinel node metastasis. JAMA 2011;305(6);569-75.

54. Giuliano AE, Hunt KK, Ballman KV, et al. Axillary dissection vs no axillary dissection in women with invasive breast cancer and sentinel node metastasis: a randomized clinical trial. JAMA: The Journal of the American Medical Association 2011; 305(6):569–575.

55. van Wely BJ, et al. Meta-analysis of ultrasound-guided biopsy of suspicious axillary lymph nodes for the selection of patients with extensive axillary tumour burden in breast cancer. Br J Surg 2015; 102:159.

56. Knauer M, Konstantiniuk P, Haid A, et al. Multicentric breast cancer: a new indication for sentinel node biopsy--a multi-institutional validation study. J Clin Oncol 2006; 24:3374.

57. Boughey J, Suman V, Mittendorf ET, et al. The role of sentinel lymph node surgery in patients presenting with node positive breast cancer (T0-T4), (NN1-N2) who receive neoadjuvant chemotherapy - results from the ACOSOG Z1071. Cancer Res 2012;72(24):94s.

58. https://ascopost.com/issues/january-25-2022/rxponder-update-explores-benefit-of-chemotherapy-in-subgroups/

59. Donker M, van Tienhoven G, Straver M, et al. Radiotherapy or surgery of the axilla after a positive sentinel node in breast cancer (EORTC 10981-22023 AMAROS): a randomised, multi-centre, open-label, phase 3 non-inferiority trial. Lancet Oncol 2014; 15(12):1303-10.

Surgery: Margins

60. http:www.nccn.org/professionals/physicain_gls/pdf/breast.pdf.

61. Singletary SE. Surgical margins in patients with early-stage breast cancer treated with breast conservation therapy. *Am J Surg.* 2002;184:383-393.

62. Houssami N, Macaskill P, Marinovich ML, et al. Meta-analysis of the impact of surgical margins on local recurrence in women with early-stage invasive breast cancer treated with breast coserving surgery. *Eur J Cancer.* 2010;46:3219-3232.

63. Morrow M, Harris JR, Schnitt S. Surgical margins in lumpectomy for breast cancer - bigger is not better [Sounding Board]. *N Engl J Med.* 2012;367:79-82.

Lumpectomy versus Mastectomy

64. Impact of locoregional treatment on the early-stage breast cancer patients: a retrospective analysis. Eur J Cancer. 39(15):2192-9, 2003.

65. Fisher B, Anderson S, Bryant J, Margolese RG, Deutsch M, Fisher ER, Jeong JH, Wolmark N. Twenty-year follow-up of a randomized trial comparing total mastectomy, lumpectomy, and lumpectomy plus irradiation for the treatment of invasive breast cancer. N Engl J Med. 347(16):1233-41, 2002.

66. Litière S, Werutsky G, Fentiman IS, et al. Breast conserving therapy versus mastectomy for stage I-II breast cancer: 20 year follow-up of the EORTC 10801 phase 3 randomised trial. Lancet Oncol. 13(4):412-9, 2012.

67. Blichert-Toft M, Nielsen M, Düring M, et al. Long-term results of breast conserving surgery vs. mastectomy for early stage invasive breast cancer: 20-year follow-up of the Danish randomized DBCG-82TM protocol. Acta Oncol. 47(4):672-81, 2008.

68. Veronesi U, Cascinelli N, Mariani L, et al. Twenty-year follow-up of a randomized study comparing breast-conserving surgery with radical mastectomy for early breast cancer. N Engl J Med. 347(16):1227-32, 2002.

69. Simone NL, Dan T, Shih J, et al. Twenty-five year results of the national cancer institute randomized breast conservation trial. Breast Cancer Res Treat. 132(1):197-203, 2012.

70. Arriagada R, Le MG, Guinebretiere JM, Dunant A, Rochard F, Tursz T. Late local recurrences in a randomised trial comparing conservative treatment with total mastectomy in early breast

cancer patients. Ann Oncol. 14(11):1617-22, 2003.

71. Early Breast Cancer Trialists' Collaborative Group. Effects of Radiotherapy and Surgery in Early Breast Cancer. An Overview of the Randomized Trials. N Engl J Med. 333:1444-55, 1995.

72.Jatoi I, Proschan MA. Randomized trials of breast-conserving therapy versus mastectomy for primary breast cancer: A pooled analysis of updated results. Am J Clin Oncol. 28(3):289-94, 2005.

10. van der Hage JA, Putter H, Bonnema J, et al. on behalf of the EORTC Breast Cancer Group.

Radiation therapy: After mastectomy; after lumpectomy

73. EBCTCG (Early Breast Cancer Trialists' Collaborative Group), McGale P, Taylor C et al. Effect of radiotherapy after mastectomy and axillary surgery on 10-year recurrence and 20-year breast cancer mortality: meta-analysis of individual patient data for 8135 women in 22 randomised trials. Lancet 2014; 383:2127.

73. Darby S, McGale P et al. Effect of radiotherapy after breast-conserving surgery on 10-year recurrence and 15-year breast cancer death: meta-analysis of individual patient data for 10,801 women in 17 randomised trials. Lancet 2011; 378: 1707–1716.

74. Werkhoven EV, Hart G, Tinteren HV et al. Nomogram to predict ipsilateral breast relapse based on pathology review from the EORTC 22881–10882 boost versus no boost trial. Radiother Oncol 2011; 100: 101–107.

75. Bartelink H, Maingon P, Poortmans P et al. Whole-breast irradiation with or without a boost for patients treated with breast-conserving surgery for early breast cancer: 20-year follow-up of a randomised phase 3 trial. Lancet Oncol 2015; 16: 47–56.

76. Clarke M, Collins R, Darby S, et al. Effects of radiotherapy and of differences in the extent of surgery for early breast cancer on local recurrence and 15-year survival: an overview of the randomised trials. Lancet. 2005 Dec 17;366(9503):2087-106.

77. Fisher B1, Anderson S, Bryant J, et al. Twenty-year follow-up of a randomized trial comparing total mastectomy, lumpectomy, and lumpectomy plus irradiation for the treatment of invasive breast cancer. N Engl J Med. 2002 Oct 17;347(16):1233-41.

conserving surgery: updated results of a 2 x 2 randomised clinical trial in patients with low risk of recurrence. Eur J Cancer. 2010 Jan;46(1):95-101.

78. Holli K1, Hietanen P, Saaristo R, et al. Radiotherapy after segmental resection of breast cancer with favorable prognostic features: 12-year follow-up results of a randomized trial. J Clin Oncol. 2009 Feb 20;27(6):927-32.

79. Liljegren G1, Holmberg L, Bergh J, et al. 10-Year results after sector resection with or without postoperative radiotherapy for stage I breast cancer: a randomized trial. J Clin Oncol. 1999 Aug;17(8):2326-33.

80. Winzer KJ, Sauerbrei W, Braun M, et al. Radiation therapy and tamoxifen after breast-conserving surgery: updated results of a 2 x 2 randomized clinical trial in patients with low risk of recurrence. Eur J Cancer 2010;46:95-101.

81. Veronesi U, Marubini E, Mariani L, Radiotherapy after breast-conserving surgery in small breast carcinoma: long-term results of a randomized trial Ann Oncol. 2001 Jul;12(7):997-1003.

Radiation Therapy: Fields and dose

82. Whelan TJ, Olivotto IA, Parulekar WR, et al. Regional nodal irradiation in early-stage breast cancer. N Engl J Med 2015;373:307-316.

83. Poortmans PS, Collette S, Kirkove C, et al. Internal mammary and medial supraclavicular irradiation in breast cancer. N Engl J Med 2015;373:317-327.

84. Burstein HJ, Morrow M. Nodal irradiation after breast-cancer surgery in the rea of effective adjuvant treatment. N Engl J Med 2015;373:379-381.

85. Whelan TJ, Pignol JP, Levine MN et al. Long-term results of hypofractionated radiation therapy for breast cancer. N Engl J Med 2010; 362: 513–520.

86. Bentzen SM, Agrawal RK et al. The UK Standardisation of Breast Radiotherapy (START) trial B of radiotherapy hypofractionation for treatment of early breast cancer: a randomised trial. Lancet 2008; 371: 1098–1107.

87. Bentzen SM, Agrawal RK et al. The UK Standardisation of Breast Radiotherapy (START) trial A of radiotherapy hypofractionation for treatment of early breast cancer: a randomised trial. Lancet Oncol 2008; 9: 331–341.

88. Adams S, Chakravarthy AB, Donach M et al. Preoperative concurrent paclitaxel- radiation in locally advanced breast cancer: pathologic response correlates with five-year overall survival. Breast Cancer Res Treat 2010; 124: 723–732.

89. Bartelink H, Horiot JC, Poortmans P, et al. Impact of a higher radiation dose on local control and survival in breast-conserving therapy of early breast cancer: 10-year results of the randomized boost versus no boost EORTC 22881-10822 trial. J Clin Oncol 2007;25:3259-3265

90. Romestaing P, Lehingue Y, Carrie C, et al. Role of a 10-Gy boost in the conservative treatment of early breast cancer: results of a randomized trial in Lyon, France. J Clin Oncol 1997;15:963-968.

91. Long term survival and local control outcomes from single dose targeted intraoperative radiotherapy during lumpectomy (TARGIT-IORT) for early breast cancer: TARGIT-A randomized clinical trial. *BMJ* 2020; 370:m2836.

92. Bartelink H, Horiot JC, Poortmans P, et al. Impact of a higher radiation dose on local control and survival in breast-conserving therapy of early breast cancer: 10-year results of the randomized boost versus no boost EORTC 22881-10822 trial. J Clin Oncol 2007;25:3259-3265

93. Romestaing P, Lehingue Y, Carrie C, et al. Role of a 10-Gy boost in the conservative treatment of early breast cancer: results of a randomized trial in Lyon, France. J Clin Oncol 1997;15:963-968

94. Jeruss JS, Kuerer HM, Peter D. Beitsch PD et al. Update on DCIS Outcomes from the American Society of Breast Surgeons Accelerated Partial Breast Irradiation Registry Trial. Annals of Surgical Oncology 2011; 18 (1); 65-71.

Accelerated breast radiation therapy

95. Goldberg M, Bridhikitti J, Khan A et al. A Meta-analysis of trials of partial breast irradition. *IJROBP* 2022; 115 (1), 60-72.

96.Breast Cancer Index: NCCN references 8-11

97. Ana Lluch, PhD; Carlos H. Barrios, MD4; Laura Torrecillas, MD, et al. phase III Trial of Adjuvant Capecitabine After Standard Neo-/Adjuvant Chemotherapy in Patients With Early Triple-Negative Breast Cancer (GEICAM/2003-11). *Journal of Clinical Oncology* 38 (3), 2020, 203-213.

98. Brunt A, Haviland J, Sydenham M, et al. Ten-Year Results of FAST: A Randomized Controlled Trial of 5-Fraction Whole-Breast Radiotherapy for Early Breast Cancer. *Journal of Clinical Oncology* 2020 38:28, 3261-3272.

After mastectomy: Radiation therapy

99. Early Breast Cancer Trialists' Collaborative Group (EBCTCG). Effect of radiotherapy after mastectomy and axillary surgery on 10-year recurrence and 20-year breast cancer mortality: meta-analysis of individual patient data for 8135 women in 22 randomised trials. Lancet 2014; 383: 2127–2135.

100. Kyndi M, Overgaard M, Nielsen HM et al. High local recurrence risk is not associated with large survival reduction after postmastectomy radiotherapy in high-risk breast cancer: a subgroup analysis of DBCG 82 b&c. Radiother Oncol 2009; 90: 74–79.

Radiation therapy: Respiratory gating

101. Darby SC, Ewertz M, McGale P et al. Risk of ischemic heart disease in women after radiotherapy or breast cancer N Engl J Med 2013; 368:987-998.

Radiation therapy: Risk of causing cancer
102. Rombouts, AJM; Huising J, Hugen, N et. al. Assessment of Radiotherapy-Associated Angiosarcoma After Breast Cancer Treatment in a Dutch Population-Based Study. JAMA Oncol. Published online January 24, 2019. doi:10.1001/jamaoncol.2018.6643.

Endocrine therapy
103. Paul E. Goss, James N. Ingle, Kathleen I. Pritchard. A randomized trial (MA.17R) of extending adjuvant letrozole for 5 years after completing an initial 5 years of aromatase inhibitor therapy alone or preceded by tamoxifen in postmenopausal women with early-stage breast cancer. J Clin Oncol 34, 2016 (suppl; abstr LBA1).
104. Francis PA Regan MM, Fleming GF et al. Adjuvant ovarian suppression in premenopausal breast cancer. N Engl J Med 2015; 372:436.
105. LHRH-agonists in Early Breast Cancer Overview group. Cuzick J, Ambroisine L, et al. Use of luteinising-hormone-releasing hormone agonists as adjuvant treatment in premenopausal patients with hormone-receptor-positive breast cancer: a meta-analysis of individual patient data from randomised adjuvant trials. Lancet 2007; 369:1711.
106. Tevaarwerk AJ, Wang M, Zhao F, et al. Phase III comparison of tamoxifen versus tamoxifen plus ovarian function suppression in premenopausal women with node-negative, hormone receptor-positive breast cancer (E-3193, INT-0142): a trial of the Eastern Cooperative Oncology Group. J Clin Oncol 2014; 32:3948.
107. Steams V, Ullmer L, Lopez JF, et al. Hot flushes. Lancet 2002;360(9348; 1851.
108. Day R. Quality of life and tamoxifen in a breast cancer prevention trial: a summary of findings from the NSABP P-1 study. National Surgical Adjuvant Breast and Bowel Project. Ann NY Acad Sci 2001;949:143.
109. Jin Y, Hayes DF, Robarge JD et al. Estrogen receptor genotypes influence hot flash prevalence and composite score before and after tamoxifen therapy. J Clin Oncol 2008;26(36):5849.
110. Slamon DJ, Neven P, Chia S, et al. Phase III randomized study of ribociclib and fulvestrant in hormone receptor-positive, human epidermal growth factor receptor 2-negative advanced breast cancer: MONALEESA-3. J Clin Oncol. 36(24):2465-2472, 2018.
111. Slamon DJ, Neven P, Chia S, et al. Overall survival with ribociclib plus fulvestrant in advanced breast cancer. N Engl J Med. 382(6):514-524, 2020.
112. Davies C, Godwin J, Gray R et al. Relevance of breast cancer hormone receptors and other factors to the efficacy of adjuvant tamoxifen: patient-level meta-analysis of randomised trials. Lancet 2011;378(9793):771.
113. Fisher B, Constatino JP, Wikerham DL. Tamoxifen for prevention of breast cancer: report of the National Surgical Adjuvant Breast and Bowel Project P-1 Study. J Natl Cancer Inst 1998; 90:1371-88.
114. Curtis RE, Freedman DM, Sherman ME, Fraumeni JF Jr. Risk of malignant mixed mullerian tumors after tamoxifen therapy for breast cancer. J Natl Cancer Inst 2004;96(1):70.
115. Braithwaite RS, Chlebowski RT, Lau J, et al. Meta-analysis of vascular and neoplastic events associated with tamoxifen. J Gen Intern Med 2003;18(11):937.
116. Reis SE, Constantino JP, Wickerham DL et al. Cardiovascular effects of tamoxifen in women with and without heart disease: breast cancer prevention trial. National Surgical Adjuvant Breast and Bowel Project Breast Cancer Prevention Trial Investigators. J Natl Cancer Inst 2001;93(1):16.
117. Fisher B, Constantino JP, Wickerham DL et al. Tamoxifen for the prevention of breast cancer: current status of the National Surgical Adjuvant Breast and Bowel Project P-1 study. J Natl Cancer Inst 2005;97(22):1652.
118. Rastelli AL, Taylor ME, Gao F, Armamento-Villareal R, Jamalabadi-Majidi S, Napoli N, El-

lis MJ. Vitamin D and aromatase inhibitor-induced musculoskeletal symptoms (AIMSS): a phase II, double-blind, placebo-controlled, randomized trial. Breast Cancer Research and Treatment. Online June 2011.

119. Gianni L, Panzini I, Li S et al. Ocular toxicity during adjuvant chemoendocrine therapy for early breast cancer: results from the International Breast Cancer Study Group trials. Cancer 2006; 106(3):505.

120. Bradbury BD, Lash TL, Kaye JA et al. Tamoxifen and cataracts: a null association. Breast Cancer Res Treat 2004;87(2):189.

121. Pierce LJ, Hutchins LF, Green SR et al. Sequencing of tamoxifen and radiotherapy after breast-conserving surgery in early breast cancer. J Clin Oncol 2005;23:24.

122. Early Breast Cancer Trialists' Collaborative Group (EBCTCG), DowsettM, Forbes JF et al. Aromatase inhibitors versus tamoxifen in early breast cancer: patient-level meta-analysis of the randomised trials. Lancet 2015;386:1341.

123. Kidwell KM, Harte SE, Hayes DF et al. Patient-reported symptoms and discontinuation of adjuvant aromatase inhibitor therapy. Cancer 2014; 120:2403.

124. Amir E, Seruga B, Niraula S et al. Toxicity of adjuvant endocrine therapy in postmenopausal breast cancer patients; a systematic review and meta-analysis. J Natl Cancer Inst 2011;103:1299.

125. Ahn PH, Vu HT, Lannin D et al. Sequence of radiotherapy with tamoxifen in conservatively managed breast cancer does not affect local relapse rates. J Clin Oncol 2005;23:17.

126. Harris EE, Christensen VJ, Hwang WT et al. Impact of concurrent versus sequential tamoxifen with radiation therapy in early-stage breast cancer patients undergoing breast conservation treatment. J Clin Oncol 2005;23:11.

127. Ruhstaller T, Giobbie-Hurder A, Colleoni M, et al. Adjuvant letrozole and tamoxifen alone or sequentially for postmenopausal women with hormone receptor-positive breast cancer: Long-term follow-up of the BIG 1-98 trial. J Clin Oncol 2019;37(2):105-114. Extending tamoxifen to ten years improves disease-free survival.

Herceptin

128. Piccart-Gebhart MJ, Procter M, Leyland-Jones B et al. Trastazumab after adjuvant chemotherapy in HER2-positive breast cancer. N Engl J Med 2005;353:1659.

129. Lamon D Eiermann W, Robert N et al. Adjuvant trastazumab in HER2-positive breast cancer. N Eng J Med 2011;365:1273.

130. NCCN Clinical Practice Guidelines in Oncology (NCCN Guidelines). Breast Cancer (version 2.2016. https://www.nccn.org/professionals/physician_gls/pdf/breast.pdf (Accessed on June 12, 2016).

131. Moja L, Tagliabue L, Balduzzu S et al. Trastazumab containing regiment for early breast cancer. Cochrane Database Syst Rev 2012:4:CD006243.

132. Perez E, Romond E, Suman V et al. Trastazumab plus adjuvant chemotherapy for human epidermal growth factor receptor 2-positive breast cancer: planned joint analysis of overall survival from NSABP B-31 and NCCTG N9831: J Clin Oncol 2014; 32:3744.

133. Gianni L, Dafni U, Gelber RD et al. Treatment with trastazumab for 1 year after adjuvant chemotherapy in patients with HER2-positive early breast cancer: a 4-year follow-up of a randomised controlled trial. Lancet Oncol 2011; 12:236.

134. Goldhirsch A, Gelber RD, Oiccart-Gebhart MJ et al. 2 years versus 1 year of adjuvant trastazumab for HER2-positive breast cancer (HERA): an open-label, randomised controlled trial. Lancet 2013; 14:741.

135. Pivot X, Romieu G, Debled M et al. 6 months versus 12 months of adjuvant trastazumab for HER2-positive early breast cancer (PHARE): a randomised phase 3 trial. Lancet Oncol 2013; 14:741.

136. Pivot X, Suter T, Nabholtz JM et al. Cardiac toxicity events in the PHARE trial, an adjuvant trastazumab randomised phase III study. Eur J Cancer 2015;51:1660.

137. Perez EA, Romond EH, Suman VJ et al. Four-year follow-up of trastuzumab plus adjuvant chemotherapy for operable human epidermal growth factor receptor 2-positive breast cancer: joint analysis of data from NCCTG N9831 and NSABP B-31. J Clin Oncol 2011;29:336.

CAR-T cell therapy for brain metastases

138. https://www.healio.com/hematology-oncology/breast-cancer/news/online/%7B68f57e59-2188-475c-af92-e2daa99b5fb3%7D/trial-to-assess-car-t-cell-therapy-for-her2-positive-metastatic-breast-cancer?utm_source=selligent&utm_medium=email&utm_campaign=hematology%20oncology%20news&m_bt=1690795913719 Accessed 22 Dec 2022.

Genomic testing

139. https://www.prosigna.com/ Accessed 22 Dec 2022.

140. https://myriad.com/ Accessed 22 Dec 2022.

141. https://www.lynparzahcp.com/ Accessed 22 Dec 2022.

142. Fan C, Oh DS, Wessels L, et al. Concordance among gene-expression-based predictors for breast cancer. N Engl J Med. 355(6):560-9, 2006.

143. Koboldt DC, Fulton RS, McLellan MD, et al. For the Cancer Genome Atlas Network. Comprehensive molecular portraits of human breast tumours. Nature. 490(7418):61-70, 2012.

144. Kohler BA, Sherman RL, Howlader N, et al. Annual report to the nation on the status of cancer, 1975-2011, featuring incidence of breast cancer subtypes by race/ethnicity, poverty, and state. J Natl Cancer Inst. 107(6), 2015.

145. Albain KS, Barlow WE, Shak S, MD Prognostic and Predictive Value of the 21-Gene Recurrence Score Assay in a Randomized Trial of Chemotherapy for Postmenopausal, Node-Positive, Estrogen Receptor-Positive Breast Cancer. Lancet Oncol. 2010 January; 11(1): 55–65.

146. Long-term outcomes for neoadjuvant versus adjuvant chemotherapy in early breast cancer: meta-analysis of individual patient data from ten randomised trials
Early Breast Cancer Trialists' Collaborative Group (EBCTCG). 11 Dec 2017.

147. Sparano JA, Gray RJ, Makower DF, et al. Adjuvant Chemotherapy Guided by a 21-Gene Expression Assay in Breast Cancer. N Engl J Med 2018; 379:111-121.

95. RxPONDER

148. Cardoso R, van't Veer LJ, Bogaerts J et al. 70-Gene Signature as an Aid to Treatment Decisions in Early-Stage Breast Cancer. N Engl J Med 2016; 375:717-29.

149. Following the 2016 publication of MINDACT, the 2017 ASCO guidelines were updated to indicate favorable results in patients with 1-3 positive lymph nodes. FDA 510(k) clearance (K201902).

150. Cardoso, F et al. N Engl J Med 2016; 375: 717-29.

151. Knauer M et al. Breast Cancer Res Treat. 2010 Apr; 120(3): 655-61.

152. Sgroi DC, Carney E, Steffel L, et al. Prediction of late disease recurrence and extended adjuvant letrozole benefit by the HOXB13/IL 17BR biomarker. J Natl Cancer Inst 2013; 105(14):1036.

153. Gnant M, Filipits M, Greil R, et al. Predicting distant recurrence in receptor-positive breast cancer patients with limited clinicopathological risk: using the PAM50 Risk of Recurrence score in 1478 postmenopausal patients of the ABCSG-8 trial treated with adjuvant endocrine therapy alone. Ann Oncol 2014;25(2);339-45.

154. Krop I, Ismaila N, Andrew F, et al. Use of biomarkers to guide decisions on adjuvant systemic therapy for women with early-stage invasive breast cancer: American Society of Clinical Oncology Clinical Practice Guideline Focused Update. J Clin Oncol 2017;35(24):2838.

Older patients and chemo

155. Low-Intensity Adjuvant Chemotherapy for Early Breast Cancer in Older Women. Oncology. Dec 2022.

Residual cancer after neoadjuvant chemotherapy
156. Masuda N, Lee S, Ohtani, S et al. Adjuvant capecitabine for breast cancer after preoperative chemotherapy. N Engl J Med 2017; 376:2147-2159.
PARP inhibitor (Olaparib)
157. Tutt ANJ et al. Adjuvant olaparib for patients with BRCA1- or BRCA2-mutated breast cancer. N Engl J Med 2021; 384:2394-2405.

CDK4/6 inhibitors
158. Loibl S, Marmé F, Martin M, et al. Palbociclib for Residual High-Risk Invasive HR-Positive and HER2-Negative Early Breast Cancer-The Penelope-B Trial. J Clin Oncol. 2021;39(14):1518-1530.
159. Johnston S, Harbeck, R, Hegg, M et al on behalf of the monarchE Committee Members and Investigators. Journal of Clinical Oncology 2020 38:34, 3987-3998

Side effects
160. Lagos R et al. Towards diagnostic imaging of ChemoBrain phenomenon" RSNA 2012; Abstract LL-MIS-TU2A.

Scalp cooling for chemotherapy-induced hair loss
161. Rugo H et al.: 2016 MASCC/ISOO International Symposium. Presented June 23, 2016.

Triple negative breast cancer
162. University of Colorado Anschutz Medical Campus. "Finally, targeted therapies for triple-negative breast cancer: Promising clinical trials of IMMU-132, vantictumab and atezolizumab against TNBC." ScienceDaily. ScienceDaily, 4 June 2016.
163. Dent R, Trudeau M, Pritchard KI et al. Triple-negative breast cancer; Clinical features and
164. National Comprehensive Cancer Network (NCCN). NCCN Clinical practice guidelines in oncology: Breast cancer V.1.2016. http://www.nccn.org/, 2016.

Fertility
165. National Comprehensive Cancer Network (NCCN). NCCN Clinical practice guidelines in oncology: Breast cancer V.1.2016. http://www.nccn.org/, 2016.
166. Jeruss JS, Woodruff TK. Preservation of fertility in patients with cancer. N Engl J Med. 360(9):902-11, 2009.
167. American College of Obstetricians and Gynecologists' Committee on Gynecologic Practice: Committee Opinion No. 584: oocyte cryopreservation. Obstet Gynecol. 123(1):221-2, 2014.
168. Lambertini M, Boni L, Michelotti A, et al. for the GIM Study Group. Ovarian suppression with triptorelin during adjuvant breast cancer chemotherapy and long-term ovarian function, pregnancies, and disease-free survival: a randomized clinical trial. JAMA. 314(24):2632-40, 2015.
169. Munhoz RR, Pereira AA, Sasse AD, et al. Gonadotropin-releasing hormone agonists for ovarian function preservation in premenopausal women undergoing chemotherapy for early-stage breast cancer: a systematic review and meta-analysis. JAMA Oncol. 2(1):65-73, 2016.

Aromatase inhibitors and pre-menopausal women
170. Pagani O, Regan MM, Walley BA, et al. for the TEXT and SOFT Investigators and the International Breast Cancer Study Group. Adjuvant exemestane with ovarian suppression in premenopausal breast cancer. N Engl J Med. 371(2):107-18, 2014.

Vaginal dryness
171. Runowicz CD et al. American Cancer Society/American Society of Clinical Oncology Breast

540

Radiation therapy: Modern techniques reduce complications
172. Meric F, Bucholz TA, Mirza NQ et al. Long-term complications associated with breast-conservation surgery and radiotherapy. Ann Surg Oncol 2002;9(6):543.
173. Management of symptomatic vulvovaginal atrophy: 2013 position statement of The North American Menopause Society. Menopause 2013; Sep:20(9):888-902; quiz 903-904.
174. Meric F, Bucholz TA, Mirza NQ et al. Long-term complications associated with breast-conservation surgery and radiotherapy. Ann Surg Oncol 2002;9(6):543.
175. Schaapveld M, Visser O, Louwman M et al. Risk of new primary non breast cancers after breast cancer treatment: A Dutch population-based study. J Clin Oncol 2008;26(8):1239-1246.
176. Whelan TJ, Olivotto I, Ackerman I, et al. NCIC-CTG MA.20: an intergroup trial of regional nodal irradiation in early breast cancer. Program and abstracts of the 2011 American Society of Clinical Oncology Annual Meeting; June 3-7, 2011; Chicago, Illinois. Abstract LBA1003.
177. Darby S, McGale P, Correa C, Taylor C, et al. Effect of radiotherapy after breast-conserving surgery on 10-year recurrence and 15-year breast cancer death: meta-analysis of individual patient data for 10,801 women in 17 randomised trials. Lancet. 2011 Nov 12;378(9804):1707-16. doi:

14. RELAPSE

Locoregional recurrence
178. https://www.nccn.org/professionals/physician_gls/pdf/breast.pdf
32. Port ER, Garcia-Etienne CA, Park J, et al. Reoperative sentinel lymph node biopsy: a new frontier in the management of ipsilateral breast tumor recurrence. Ann Surg Oncol 2007; 14(8):2209-14.
179. Intra M, Viale G, MD, Vila J, et al. Second axillary sentinel lymph node biopsy for breast tumor recurrence: Experience of the European Institute of Oncology. Ann Surg Oncol (2015) 22:2372–2377.
180. Newman L ed. Surgical Oncology Clinics of North America. Breast Cancer. July 2014.
181. EBCTCG Lancet Oncol 378:1707-16, 2011
182. Masuda N, Lee S, Ohtani, S et al. Adjuvant capecitabine for breast cancer after preoperative chemotherapy. N Engl J Med 2017; 376:2147-2159. 10.1016/S0140-6736(11)61629-2. Epub 2011 Oct 19.
183. https://www.nccn.org/professionals/physician_gls/pdf/breast.pdf
184. Early Breast Cancer Trialists' Collaborative Group (EBCTCG). Lancet. 2011; 378(9804): 1707–1716.

15. METASTASES

Cancer cells travel in gangs
185. https://www.fredhutch.org/en/news/releases/2016/02/shedding-new-light-on-breast-cancer-metastasis.html
186. PNAS 2016; published ahead of print February 1, 2016, doi:10.1073/pnas.1508541113.

Coping & prognosis

187. https://www.bcna.org.au/secondary-breast-cancer/finding-out-your-cancer-has-spread/

188. Brain K, Willams B, Iredale R et al. Psychological distress in men with breast cancer. J Clin Oncol 2006;24:95.

189. Lobbezoo DJ, van Kampen RJ, Voogd AC, et al. Prognosis of metastatic breast cancer: are there differences between patients with de novo and recurrent metastatic breast cancer? Br J Cancer. 112(9):1445-51, 2015.

190. Lippman ME. Chapter 74: Management summary for the care of patients with metastatic breast cancer, in Harris JR, Lippman ME, Morrow M, Osborne CK. Diseases of the Breast, 5th edition. Lippincott Williams and Wilkins, 2014.

191.Gennari A, Conte P, Rosso R, et al. Survival of metastatic breast carcinoma patients over a 20-year period: a retrospective analysis based on individual patient data from six consecutive studies. Cancer 2005;104(8):1742.

192. Greenberg PA, Hortobagyi GN, Smith TL, et al. Long-term follow-up of patients with complete remission following combination chemotherapy for metastatic breast cancer. J Clin Oncol 1996;14(8):2197.

193. Kelly BE, Soon YY, Tattersall MH, Stockler MR. How long have I got? Estimating typical, best-case, and worst-case scenarios for patients starting first-line chemotherapy for metastatic breast cancer: a systematic review of recent randomized trials. J Clin Oncol 2011;29(4):456.

194. Stockler M, Wilcken NR, Ghersi D, and Simes RJ. Systematic review of chemotherapy and endocrine therapy in metastatic breast cancer. Cancer Treat Rev 2000;26(3):151.

195. Swenerton KD, Legha SS, Smith T, et al. Prognostic factors in metastatic breast cancer treated with combination chemotherapy. Cancer Res 1979;39(5):1552.

196. Yamamoto N, Watanabe T, Katsumata N, et al. Construction and validation of a practical prognostic index for patients with metastatic breast cancer. J Clin Oncol 1998;16(7):2401.

197. Clark GM, Sledge GW Jr, Osborne CK, et al. Survival from first recurrence: relative importance of prognostic factors in 1,015 breast cancer patients. J Clin Oncol 1987;5(1):55.

198. Leivonen MK, Kalima TC. Prognostic factors associated with survival after breast cancer recurrence. Acta Oncol 1991;30(5):583.

199. Wilcken N, Hornbuckle J, Ghersi D. Chemotherapy alone versus endocrine therapy alone for metastatic breast cancer. Cochrane Database Syst Rev 2003;(2).

200. Wilcken N, Hornbuckle J, Ghersi D. Chemotherapy alone versus endocrine therapy alone for metastatic breast cancer. Cochrane Database Syst Rev. 2003;2:CD002747.

201. Johnston SRD, Schiavon G. Treatment algorithms for hormone receptor-positive advanced breast cancer: going forward in endocrine therapy – overcoming resistance and introducing new agents. Am Soc Clin Oncol Educ Book. 2013;2013:e28.

202. Mauriac L, Romieu G, Bines J. Activity of fulvestrant versus exemestane in advanced breast cancer patients with or without visceral metastases: data from the EFECT trial. Breast Cancer Res Treat. 2009;117(1):69–75.

Metastases and CDK 4/6 inhibitors

203. Slamon DJ, Neven P, Chia S, et al. Phase III randomized study of ribociclib and fulvestrant in hormone receptor-positive, human epidermal growth factor receptor 2-negative advanced breast cancer: MONALEESA-3. J Clin Oncol. 36(24):2465-2472, 2018.

204. Slamon DJ, Neven P, Chia S, et al. Ribociclib plus fulvestrant for postmenopausal women with hormone receptor-positive, human epidermal growth factor receptor 2-negative advanced breast cancer in the phase III randomized MONALEESA-3 trial: updated overall survival. Ann Oncol. 32(8):1015-1024, 2021.

205. Sledge GW Jr, Toi M, Neven P, et al. MONARCH 2: abemaciclib in combination with fulvestrant in women with HR+/HER2- advanced breast cancer who had progressed while receiving endocrine therapy. J Clin Oncol. 35(25):2875-2884, 2017.

206. Hortobagyi GN, Stemmer SM, Burris HA, et al. Ribociclib as first-line therapy for HR-positive, advanced breast cancer. N Engl J Med. 375(18):1738-1748, 2016.

207. Hortobagyi GN, Stemmer SM, Burris HA, et al. Overall survival with ribociclib plus letrozole in advanced breast cancer. N Engl J Med. 386(10):942-950, 2022.

208. Goetz MP, Toi M, Campone M, et al. MONARCH 3: abemaciclib as initial therapy for advanced breast cancer. J Clin Oncol. 35(32):3638-3646, 2017.

209. https://www.komen.org/breast-cancer/metastatic/metastatic/cdk4-6-inhibitors-for-metastatic-breast-cancer/ . Accessed Dec 15, 2022.

Immunotherapy for metastases

210. Cortes J, Rugo HS, Cescon DW, et al. for the KEYNOTE-355 investigators. Pembrolizumab plus chemotherapy in advanced triple-negative breast cancer. N Engl J Med 387(3):217-226, 2022.

211. https://www.komen.org/breast-cancer/metastatic/metastatic/immunotherapy-for-metastatic-

PARP inhibitor for metastases

212. https://www.medicalnewstoday.com/articles/parp-inhibitor

HER2 positive metastases

213. Cortés J, Kim S, Chung W, et al. M.D.,Trastuzumab Deruxtecan versus Trastuzumab Emtansine for Breast Cancer. N Engl J Med 2022; 386:1143-1154.**Occult**

214. Halsted W. The Results of Radical Operations for the Cure of Carcinoma of the Breast* Ann Surg. 1907 Jul; 46(1): 1–19.

215. Foroudi F, Tiver KW. Occult breast carcinoma presenting as axillary metastases. Int J Radiat Oncol Biol Phys. 2000;47(1):143.

216. Walsh R, Kornguth P, Soo M, et al. Axillary lymph nodes: mammographic, pathologic, and clinical correlation. AJR Am J Roentgenol. 1997;168(1):33.

217. Copeland E and McBride C. Axillary metastases from unknown primary sites. Ann Surg 1973 Jul;178(1):25-7.

Predicting response

218. Swenerton KD, Legha SS, Smith T et al. Prognostic factors in metastatic breast cancer treated with combination chemotherapy. Cancer Res 1979;39:1552.

219. Ahmann DL, Schaid DJ, Ingle JN, et al. A randomized trial of cyclophosphamide, doxorubicin, and prednisone versus cyclophosphamide, 5-fluorouracil, and prednisone in patients with metastatic breast cancer. Am J Clin Oncol 1991; 14:179.

220. White J, Kearins O, Dodwell D, et al. Male breast carcinoma: increased awareness needed. Breast Cancer Res 2011; 13(5):219.

221. Siegel R, Ward E, Brawley O, Jemal A. Cancer statistics, 2011: the impact of eliminating socioeconomic and racial disparities on premature cancer deaths. CA Cancer J Clin 2011;61(4);212.

222. Hortobagyi GN, Smith TL, Legha SS et al. Multivariate analysis of prognostic factors in metastatic breast cancer. J Clin Oncol 1983;776.

Work-up

223. https://www.nccn.org/professionals/physician_gls/pdf/breast.pdf

Bone-protecting drugs

224. Lipton, A, Fizazi, K, Stopeck, AT. Superiority of denosumab to zoledronic acid for prevention of skeletal-related events: a combined analysis of 3 pivotal, randomised, phase 3 trials.

European Journal of Cancer 1990;48 (16): 3082–92.

225. Rosen LS, Gordon D, Kaminski M, et al. Zoledronic acid versus pamidronate in the treatment of skeletal metastases in patients with breast cancer or osteolytic lesions of multiple myeloma: a phase III, double-blind, comparative trial. Cancer J 2001;7:377-387.

226. Rosen LS, Gordon DH, Dugan W, et al. Zoledronic acid is superior to pamidronate for the treatment of bone metastases in breast carcinoma patients with at least one osteolytic lesion. Cancer 2004;100:36-43.

227. Gralow J, Barlow WE, Paterson AHG, et al. Phase III trial of bisphosphonates as adjuvant therapy in primary breast cancer: SWOG/Alliance/ECOG-ACRIN/NCIC Clinical Trials Group/NRG Oncology study S0307. J Clin Oncol 33, 2015 (suppl; abstr 503).

228. Aapro M, Abrahamsson PA, Body JJ, et al. Guidance on the use of bisphosphonates in solid tumours: recommendations of an international expert panel. Ann Oncol. 19(3):420-32, 2008.

229. Rathbone EJ, Brown JE, Marshall HC, et al. Osteonecrosis of the jaw and oral health-related quality of life after adjuvant zoledronic acid: an adjuvant zoledronic acid to reduce recurrence trial subprotocol (BIG01/04). J Clin Oncol. 31(21):2685-91, 2013.

Spinal cord compression

230. https://en.wikipedia.org/wiki/Spinal_cord_compression#/media/File:Diagram_showing_a_tumour_causing_spinal_cord_compression_CRUK_081.svg

Reducing harm from whole brain radiotherapy

231. Day J, Zienius K, Gehring K et al. Interventions for preventing and ameliorating cognitive deficits in adults treated with cranial irradiation. Cochrane Database Syst Rev 2014; CD011335

232. Brown OR, Pugh S, Laack NN et al. Memantine for the prevention of cognitive dysfunction in patients receiving whole-brain radiotherapy: a randomized, placebo-controlled trial. Neuro Oncol 2013; 15:1429.

233. Eichenbaum H, Cohen NJ (1993). Memory, Amnesia, and the Hippocampal System. MIT Press.

234. Squire, LR; Schacter DL (2002). The Neuropsychology of Memory. Guilford Press.

Breast cancer cells masquerade as neurons to sneak into the brain

235. PNAS, DOI: 10.1073/pnas.1322098111

Brain metastases treatment

236. Patchell RA, Tibbs PA, Regine WF, et al. Postoperative radiotherapy in the treatment of single metastases to the brain: a randomized trial. JAMA 1998;280:1485-1489.

237. Paek SH, Audu PB, Sperling MR, et al. Reevaluation of surgery for the treatment of brain metastases: review of 208 patients with single or multiple brain metastases treated at one institution with modern neurosurgical techniques. Neurosurgery 2005;56:1021-1034.

238. Stark AM, Tscheslog H, Buhl R, et al. Surgical treatment for brain metastases: prognostic factors and survival in 177 patients. Neurosurg Rev 2005;28:115-119.

239. Karlsson B, Hanssens P, Wolff R, et al. Thirty years' experience with Gamma Knife surgery for metastases to the brain. J Neurosurg 2009;111:449-457.

240. Kased N, Binder DK, McDermott MW, et al. Gamma Knife radiosurgery for brain metastases from primary breast cancer. Int J Radiat Oncol Biol Phys 2009;75:1132-1140.

241. Bindal RK, Sawaya R, Leavens ME et al. Reoperation for recurrent metastatic brain tumors. J Neurosurg 1995; 83:600.

Distant spread; Diagram

242. https://en.m.wikipedia.org/wiki/Breast_cancer#/media/File%3ADiagram_showing_stage_4_

breast_cancer_CRUK_228.svg

Choosing Wisely campaign

243. http://www.choosingwisely.org/societies/american-society-for-radiation-oncology/

244. Aoyama H, Shirato H, Tago M, et al. Stereotactic radiosurgery plus whole-brain radiation therapy vs stereotactic radiosurgery alone for treatment of brain metastases: a randomized controlled trial. JAMA 2006;295:2483-2491.

245. Tsao M, Xu W, Sahgal A. A meta-analysis evaluating stereotactic radiosurgery, whole-brain radiotherapy, or both for patients presenting with a limited number of brain metastases. Cancer 212;118:2486- 2493.

246. Cooper JS, Steinfeld AD, Lerch IA. Cerebral metastases: value of reirradiation in selected patients. Radiology 1990;174:883-885.

247. Sadikov E, Bezjak A, Yi QL, et al. Value of whole brain re- irradiation for brain metastases--single centre experience. Clin Oncol (R Coll Radiol) 2007;19:532-538.

Re-recurrence in brain: Treatment

248. Wong WW, Schild SE, Sawyer TE, Shaw EG. Analysis of outcome in patients reirradiated for brain metastases. Int J Radiat Oncol Biol Phys 1996;34:585-590.

249. Chao ST, Barnett GH, Vogelbaum MA et al. Salvage stereotactic radiosurgery effectively treats recurrences from whole-brain radiation therapy. Cancer 2008; 113:2195.

Leptomeningeal spread

250. Morikawa A, Jordan L, Rozner R, et al. Characteristics and Outcomes of Patients With Breast Cancer With Leptomeningeal Metastasis. Clin Breast Cancer 17(1): 23-28.

Any role for breast surgery for those with metastases

251. Badwe RA, Parmar V, Hawaldar RW. Surgical removal of primary tumor in metastatic breast cancer: Impact on health-related quality of life (HR-QOL) in a randomized controlled trial (RCT). J Clin Oncol 32:5s, 2014 (suppl; abstr 1124).

252. Soran A, Ozmen V, Ozbas S. A randomized controlled trial evaluating resection of the primary breast tumor in women presenting with de novo stage IV breast cancer: Turkish Study (Protocol MF07-01). J Clin Oncol 34, 2016 (suppl; abstr 1005).

253. King TA, Lyman J, Gonen M, et al: A prospective analysis of surgery and survival in stage IV breast cancer (TBCRC 013). 2016 ASCO Annual Meeting. Abstract 1006. Presented June 4, 2016.

Bone-hardening drugs

254. Dhesy-Thind S et al. Use of adjuvant bisphosphonates in postmenopausal women with early-stage breast cancer: A cancer care Ontario and American Society of Clinical Oncology clinical practice guideline. J Clin Oncol 2017 Mar 6

Breast surgery for those with metastases

255. Badwe RA, Parmar V, Hawaldar RW. Surgical removal of primary tumor in metastatic breast cancer: Impact on health-related quality of life (HR-QOL) in a randomized controlled trial (RCT). J Clin Oncol 32:5s, 2014 (suppl; abstr 1124).

256. Soran A, Ozmen V, Ozbas S. A randomized controlled trial evaluating resection of the primary breast tumor in women presenting with de novo stage IV breast cancer: Turkish Study (Protocol MF07-01). J Clin Oncol 34, 2016 (suppl; abstr 1005).

257. King TA, Lyman J, Gonen M, et al: A prospective analysis of surgery and survival in stage IV breast cancer (TBCRC 013). 2016 ASCO Annual Meeting. Abstract 1006. Presented June 4, 2016.

Oligometastases

258. Weichselbaum, R.The 46th David A. Karnofsky Memorial Award Lecture: Oligometastasis—From Conception to Treatment. *Journal of Clinical Oncology* 36, no. 32 (November 10 2018) 3240-3250.

259. Milano MT, Katza AW, Zhong H. Oligometastatic breast cancer treated with hypofractionated stereotactic radiotherapy: Some patients survive longer than a decade. Radiotherapy and Oncology 131, 45-51.

260. Early Breast Cancer Trialists' Collaborative Group (EBCTCG). Effect of radiotherapy after breast-conserving surgery on 10-year recurrence and 15-year cancer death: meta-analysis of individual patient data for 10 801 women in 17 randomised trials. The Lancet 2011; 378 (9804): 1707-16.

261. Schmid P, Adams S, Rugo H. et al. Atezolizumab and Nab-Paclitaxel in Advanced Triple-Negative Breast Cancer. N Engl J Med 2018; 379: 2108-2121.

262. Schmid P, Cortes J, Dent R, et al: KEYNOTE-522: Phase 3 study of neoadjuvant pembrolizumab plus chemotherapy versus placebo plus chemotherapy, followed by adjuvant pembrolizumab versus placebo for early-stage triple-negative breast cancer. ESMO Virtual Plenary. Abstract VP7-2021. Presented July 15, 2021.

263. Saura C, Oliveira M, Feng YH, et al. Neratinib Plus Capecitabine Versus Lapatinib Plus Capecitabine in HER2-Positive Metastatic Breast Cancer Previously Treated With ≥ 2 HER2-Directed Regimens: Phase III NALA Trial. J Clin Oncol. 2020;38(27):3138-3149.

16. PHYLLODES

1. Geisler DP, Boyle MJ, Malnar KF et al. Phylloides tumors of the breast: a review of 32 cases. Am Surg 2000; 66(4):360.

2. Birch JM, Alston RD, McNally RJ, et al. Relative frequency and morphology of cancers in carriers of germline TP53 mutations Oncogene 2001;20(34):4621.

3. Calhoun K, Lawton TJ, Kim JM et al. Phylloides tumors. In Diseases of the breast, Harris J, Lippman ME, Osborn CK, Morrow M (eds). Lippincott Williams and Wilkins. 2010, 781.

4. Geisler DP, Boyle MJ, Malnar KF et al. Phylloides tumors of the breast: a review of 32 cases. Am Surg 2000; 66(4):360.

5. Birch JM, Alston RD, McNally RJ, et al. Relative frequency and morphology of cancers in carriers of germline TP53 mutations Oncogene 2001;20(34):4621.

6. Telli ML, Horst KC, Guardino AE et al. Phylloides tumors of the breast: natural history, diagnosis, and treatment. J Natl Compr Cancer Netw 2007; 5(3):324.

7. Norris HJ, Taylor HB. Relationship of histologic features to behavior of cystosarcoma phylloides. Analysis of ninety-four cases. Cancer 1967;20(12):2090.

8. Jacklin RK, Ridgway PF, Ziprin P et al. Optimising preoperative diagnosis in phylloides tumour of the breast. J Clin Pathol 2006; 59(5):454.

9. Wurdinger S, Herzog AB, Fischer DR et al. Differentiation of phylloides tumors from fibroadenomas on MRI. AJR Am J Roentgenol 2005; 185(5):1317.

10. Belkacemi Y, Bousquet G, Marsiglia H et al. Phylloides tumor of the breast. Int J Radiat Oncol Biol Phys 2008; 70(2):492.

11. Dillon MF, Quinn CM, McDermott EW et al. Needle core biopsy in the diagnosis of phyllodes neoplasm. Surgery 2006; 140(5):779

12. Lee AH. Recent developments in the histological diagnosis of spindle cell carcinoma, fibromatosis and phyllodes tumour of the breast. Histopathology 2008; 52(1):45.

Surgery; local control

13. Spitaleri G, Toesca A, Botteri E et al. Breast phylloides tumor: a review of literature and a single center retrospective series analysis. Crit Rev Oncol Hematol 2013; 88:427.

14. Chen WH, Cheng SP, Tzen CY et al. Surgical treatment of phyllodes tumors of the breast: retrospective review of 172 cases. J Surg Oncol 2005; 91:185.

15. Macdonald OK, Lee CM, Tward JD, et al. Malignant phyllodes tumor of the female breast: association of primary therapy with cause-specific survival from the Surveillance, Epidemiology, and End Results (SEER) program. Cancer 2006; 107(9): 2127.

16. Barth RJ Jr. Histologic features predict local recurrence after breast conserving therapy of phyllodes tumors. Breast Cancer Res Treat 1999; 57:291.

17. Barth RT Jr, Wells WA, Mitchell SE, Cole BF. A prospective, multi-institutional study of adjuvant radiotherapy after resection of malignant phyllodes tumors. Ann Surg Oncol 2009; 16:2288.

18. Belkacemi Y, Bousquet G, Marsiglia H et al. Phylloides tumor of the breast. Int J Radiat Oncol Biol Phys 2008; 70(2):492.

19. Jang JH Choi MY, Lee SK et al. Clinicopathologic risk factors for the local recurrence of phyllodes tumors of the breast. Ann Srug Oncol 2012; 19(8): 2612.

Endocrine therapy

20. Telli ML, Horst KC, Guardino AE et al. Phyllodes tuors of the breast: natural history, diagnosis, and treatment. J Natl Compr Canc Netw 2007; 5:324.

21. Tse GM, Lee CS, Kung FY et al. Hormonal receptors expression in epithelial cells of mammary phyllodes tumors correlates with pathologic grade of the tumor: a multicenter study of 143 cases. Am J Clin Pathol 2002; 118:552.

Survival

22. Confavreux C, Lurkin A, Mitton N t al. Sarcomas and malignant phyllodes tumours of the breast - a retrospective study. Eur J Cancer 2006; 42:2715.

23. Lee AH, Hodi Z, Ellis IO, Elston CW. Histologic features useful in the distinction of phyllodes tumour and fibroadenoma on needle core biopsy of the breast. Histopathology 2007; 51(3):336.

24. https://commons.wikimedia.org/wiki/File:Phylloidestumor_der_Mamma_-_Mammographie.jpg

Recurrence

24. Reinfuss M, Mitus J, Duda K et al. The treatment and prognosis of patients with phyllodes tumor of the breast: an analysis of 170 cases. Cancer 1996; 77:910.

25. Telli ML, Horst KC, Guardino AE et al. Phyllodes tuors of the breast: natural history, diagnosis, and treatment. J Natl Compr Canc Netw 2007; 5:324.

26. National Comprehensive Cancer Network (NCCN). NCCN clinical practice guidelines in oncology (NCCN Guidelines). Breast Cancer. Version 2.2016. www.nccn.org [Accessed on July 15, 2016)

17. MALE BREAST CANCER

Surgery type

1. Cutuli B, Lacroze M, Dilhuydy JM et al. Male breast cancer: results of the treatments and prognostic factors in 397 cases. Eur J Cancer 1995;31A(12): 1960.

2. Digenis AG, Ross CB, Morrison JG, et al. Carcinoma of the male breast: a review of 41 cases. South Med J 1990;83(10):1162.

3. Gough DB, Donohue JH, Evans MM, et al. A 50-year experience of male breast cancer. Surg Oncol 1993;2(6):325101. Golshan M, Rusby J, Dominguez R, et al. Breast conservation for male breast carcinoma. Breast 2007;16(6):653.

Sentinel node
4. Lyman GH, Giuliano AE, Somerfield MR et al. American Society of Clinical Oncology guideline recommendations for sentinel lymph node biopsy in early-stage breast cancer. J Clin Oncol 2005;23(30):7703.
5. Gentilini O, Chagas E, Zurrida S et al. Sentinel lymph node biopsy in male patients with early breast cancer. Oncologist 2007;12(5):512.

Endocrine ("anti-estrogen") therapy
6. Giordano SH, Perkins GH, Broglio K, et al. Adjuvant systemic therapy for male breast carcinoma. Cancer 2005;104(11):2359.

19. SPECIAL

Pregnancy-related breast cancer
1. Clark RM, Chua T: Breast cancer and pregnancy: the ultimate challenge. Clin Oncol (R Coll Radiol) 1 (1): 11-8, 1989.
2. Yang WT, Dryden MJ, Gwyn K, et al.: Imaging of breast cancer diagnosed and treated with chemotherapy during pregnancy. Radiology 239 (1): 52-60, 2006.
3. Middleton LP, Amin M, Gwyn K, et al.: Breast carcinoma in pregnant women: assessment of clinicopathologic and immunohistochemical features. Cancer 98 (5): 1055-60, 2003.
4. Middleton LP, Amin M, Gwyn K, et al.: Breast carcinoma in pregnant women: assessment of clinicopathologic and immunohistochemical features. Cancer 98 (5): 1055-60, 2003.
5. Elledge RM, Ciocca DR, Langone G, et al.: Estrogen receptor, progesterone receptor, and HER-2/neu protein in breast cancers from pregnant patients. Cancer 71 (8): 2499-506, 1993.
6. Petrek JA, Dukoff R, Rogatko A: Prognosis of pregnancy-associated breast cancer. Cancer 67 (4): 869-72, 1991.
7. Barnavon Y, Wallack MK: Management of the pregnant patient with carcinoma of the breast. Surg Gynecol Obstet 171 (4): 347-52, 1990.
8. Litton JK and Theriault RL. Chapter 65: Breast cancer during pregnancy and subsequent pregnancy in breast cancer survivors, in Harris JR, Lippman ME, Morrow M, Osborne CK. Diseases of the Breast, 5th edition. Lippincott Williams and Wilkins, 2014.
9. Germann N, Goffinet F, Goldwasser F. Anthracyclines during pregnancy: embryo-fetal outcome in 160 patients. Ann Oncol 2004;15:146-150.
10. Johnson PH, Gwyn K, Gordon N, et al. The treatment of pregnant women with breast cancer and the outcomes of the children exposed to chemotherapy in utero [abstract]. J Clin Oncol 2005;23(Suppl 16):Abstract 540.
11. Doll DC, Ringenberg QS, Yarbro JW. Antineoplastic agents and pregnancy. Semin Oncol 1989;16:337-346.
12. Ebert U, Loffler H, Kirch W. Cytotoxic therapy and pregnancy. Pharmacol Ther 1997;74:207-220.
13. Hoover HC Jr: Breast cancer during pregnancy and lactation. Surg Clin North Am 70 (5): 1151-63, 1990.
14. Rugo HS: Management of breast cancer diagnosed during pregnancy. Curr Treat Options Oncol 4 (2): 165-73, 2003.
15. Gwyn K, Theriault R: Breast cancer during pregnancy. Oncology (Huntingt) 15 (1): 39-46; discussion 46, 49-51, 2001.
16. Clark RM, Chua T: Breast cancer and pregnancy: the ultimate challenge. Clin Oncol (R Coll

Radiol) 1 (1): 11-8, 1989.

17. Barnavon Y, Wallack MK: Management of the pregnant patient with carcinoma of the breast. Surg Gynecol Obstet 171 (4): 347-52, 1990.

Occult

18. Bhatia SK, Saclarides TJ, Witt TR, et al. Hormone receptor studies in axillary metastases from occult breast cancers. Cancer 1987;59:1170-1172.

19. Bleicher RJ, Morrow M. MRI and breast cancer: role in detection, diagnosis, and staging. Oncology (Williston Park) 2007;21:1521-1528, 1530; discussion 1530, 1532-1523.

20. Stomper PC, Waddell BE, Edge SB, Klippenstein DL. Breast MRI in the Evaluation of Patients with Occult Primary Breast Carcinoma. Breast J 1999;5:230-234.

24. Varadarajan R, Edge SB, Yu J, et al. Prognosis of occult breast carcinoma presenting as isolated axillary nodal metastasis. Oncology 2006;71:456-459.

25. Schelfout K, Kersschot E, Van Goethem M, et al. Breast MR imaging in a patient with unilateral axillary lymphadenopathy and unknown primary malignancy. Eur Radiol 2003;13:2128-2132.

Breast lymphoma

26. Joks M, Myśliwiec K, and Lewandowski, K. Primary breast lymphoma – a review of the literature and report of three cases. Arch Med Sci. 2011 Feb; 7(1): 27–33.

27. 1. Jeanneret-Sozzi W, Taghian A, Epelbaum R, et al. Primary breast lymphoma: patient profile, outcome and prognostic factors. A multicentre Rare Cancer Network study. BMC Cancer. 2008;8:86.

28. Jeanneret-Sozzi W, Taghian A, Epelbaum R, et al. Primary breast lymphoma: patient profile, outcome and prognostic factors. A multicentre Rare Cancer Network study. BMC Cancer. 2008;8:86.

29. Arber DA, Simpson JF, Weiss LM, Rappaport H. Non-Hodgkin's lymphoma involving the breast. Am J Surg Pathol. 1994;18:288–95.

30. Aviles A, Delgado S, Nambo MJ, Neri N, Murillo E, Cleto S. Primary breast lymphoma: results of a controlled clinical trial. Oncology. 2005;69:256–60.

31. Bobrow LG, Richards MA, Happerfield LC, et al. Breast lymphomas: a clinicopathologic review. Hum Pathol. 1993;24:274–8.

32. Brogi E, Harris NL. Lymphomas of the breast: pathology and clinical behavior. Semin Oncol. 1999;26:357–64.

33. Cohen Y, Goldenberg N, Kasis S, Shpilberg D, Oren M. Primary breast lymphoma. Harefuah. 1993;125:24–6. 63.

34. Joks, M, Myśliwiec K, Lewandowski K. Primary breast lymphoma – a review of the literature and report of three cases. Arch Med Sci. 2011 Feb; 7(1): 27–33.

35. Domchek SM, Hecht JL, Fleming MD, Pinkus GS, Canellos GP. Lymphomas of the breast: primary and secondary involvement. Cancer. 2002;94:6–13.

36. Ha CS, Dubey P, Goyal LK, Hess M, Cabanillas F, Cox JD. Localized primary non-Hodgkin lymphoma of the breast. Am J Clin Oncol. 1998;21:376–80.

37. Kuper-Hommel MJ, Snijder S, Janssen-Heijnen ML, et al. Treatment and survival of 38 female breast lymphomas: a population-based study with clinical and pathological reviews. Ann Hematol. 2003;82:397–404.

38. Mattia AR, Ferry JA, Harris NL. Breast lymphoma. A B-cell spectrum including the low grade B-cell lymphoma of mucosa associated lymphoid tissue. Am J Surg Pathol. 1993;17:574–87.

39. Ryan G, Martinelli G, Kuper-Hommel M, et al. Primary diffuse large B-cell lymphoma of the breast: prognostic factors and outcomes of a study by the International Extranodal Lymphoma Study Group. Ann Oncol. 2008;19:233–41.

40. Topalovski M, Crisan D, Mattson JC. Lymphoma of the breast. A clinicopathologic study of primary and secondary cases. Arch Pathol Lab Med. 1999;123:1208–18.
41. Barista I, Baltali E, Tekuzman G et al. Primary breast lymphomas - a retrospective review of twelve cases. Acta Oncol 2000;39(2): 135.
42. Jennings WC, Baker RS, Murray SS, et al. Primary breast lymphoma: the role of mastectomy and the importance of lymph node status. Ann Surg. 2007;245:784–9.
43. Buchanan CL, Morris EA, Dorn PL, et al. Utility of breast magnetic resonance imaging in patients with occult primary breast cancer. Ann Surg Oncol 2005;12:1045-1053.
44. Olson JA, Morris EA, Van Zee KJ, et al. Magnetic resonance imaging facilitates breast conservation for occult breast cancer. Ann Surg Oncol 2000;7:411-415.
45. Joks M, Myśliwiec K,2 and Lewandowski, K. Primary breast lymphoma – a review of the literature and report of three cases. Arch Med Sci. 2011 Feb; 7(1): 27–33.
46. 1. Jeanneret-Sozzi W, Taghian A, Epelbaum R, et al. Primary breast lymphoma: patient profile, outcome and prognostic factors. A multicentre Rare Cancer Network study. BMC Cancer. 2008;8:86.

Paget disease
47. Harris JR, Lippman ME, Morrow M, Osborne CK, editors. Diseases of the Breast. 4th ed. Philadelphia: Lippincott Williams & Wilkins; 2009.
48. Caliskan M, Gatti G, Sosnovskikh I, et al. Paget's disease of the breast: the experience of the European Institute of Oncology and review of the literature. Breast Cancer Research and Treatment 2008;112(3):513–521.
49. Kanitakis J. Mammary and extramammary Paget's disease. Journal of the European Academy of Dermatology and Venereology 2007;21(5):581–590.
50. Kawase K, Dimaio DJ, Tucker SL, et al. Paget's disease of the breast: there is a role for breast-conserving therapy. Annals of Surgical Oncology 2005;12(5):391–397.
51. Marshall JK, Griffith KA, Haffty BG, et al. Conservative management of Paget disease of the breast with radiotherapy: 10- and 15-year results. Cancer 2003;97(9):2142–2149.
52. Sukumvanich P, Bentrem DJ, Cody HS, et al. The role of sentinel lymph node biopsy in Paget's disease of the breast. Annals of Surgical Oncology 2007;14(3):1020–1023.
53. Laronga C, Hasson D, Hoover S, et al. Paget's disease in the era of sentinel lymph node biopsy. American Journal of Surgery 2006;192(4):481–483.
54. Chen CY, Sun LM, Anderson BO. Paget disease of the breast: changing patterns of incidence, clinical presentation, and treatment in the U.S. Cancer 2006;107(7):1448–1458.
55. Ashikari R, Oark K, Huvos AG et al. Paget's disease of the breast. Cancer 1970; 26:680.
56. Nance, FC, DeLoacj DH, Welsh RA et al. Paget's disease of the breast. Ann Surg 1970; 171:864.

Pregnancy
57. Clark RM, Chua T: Breast cancer and pregnancy: the ultimate challenge. Clin Oncol (R Coll Radiol) 1 (1): 11-8, 1989.
58. Harvey JC, Rosen PP, Ashikari R, et al.: The effect of pregnancy on the prognosis of carcinoma of the breast following radical mastectomy. Surg Gynecol Obstet 153 (5): 723-5, 1981.
59. Petrek JA: Pregnancy safety after breast cancer. Cancer 74 (1 Suppl): 528-31, 1994.
60. von Schoultz E, Johansson H, Wilking N, et al.: Influence of prior and subsequent pregnancy on breast cancer prognosis. J Clin Oncol 13 (2): 430-4, 1995.
61. Kroman N, Mouridsen HT: Prognostic influence of pregnancy before, around, and after diagnosis of breast cancer. Breast 12 (6): 516-21, 2003.
62. Malamos NA, Stathopoulos GP, Keramopoulos A, et al.: Pregnancy and offspring after the appearance of breast cancer. Oncology 53 (6): 471-5, 1996 Nov-Dec.
63. Gelber S, Coates AS, Goldhirsch A, et al.: Effect of pregnancy on overall survival after the

diagnosis of early-stage breast cancer. J Clin Oncol 19 (6): 1671-5, 2001.

64. Gwyn K, Theriault R: Breast cancer during pregnancy. Oncology (Huntingt) 15 (1): 39-46; discussion 46, 49-51, 2001.

65. Rugo HS: Management of breast cancer diagnosed during pregnancy. Curr Treat Options Oncol 4 (2): 165-73, 2003.

Pregnancy after treatment: Safe?

66. Valachis A, Tsali L, Pesce LL et al. Safety of pregnancy after primary breast carcinoma in young women: a meta-analysis to overcome bias of healthy mother effect studies. Obstet Gynecol Surg 2010; 65:786.

67. Azim HA Jr, Sabtoro L, Pavlidis N et al. Safety of pregnancy following breast cancer diagnosis: a meta-analysis of 14 studies. Eur J Cancer 2011;47:74.

Inflammatory breast cancer

68. Tai P, Yu E, Shiels R et al. Short- and long-term causes-specific survival of patients with inflammatory breast cancer. BMC Cancer 2005: 5:137.

69. Hance KW, Anderson WF, Devesa SS et al. Trends in inflammatory breast carcinoma incidence and survival: the surveillance, epidemiology, and end results program at the National Cancer Institute. J Natl Cancer Inst 2005; 97:966.

70. Anderson WF, Schairer C, Chen BE te al. Epidemiology of inflammatory breast cancer (IBF). Breast Dis 2005-2006; 22:9.

71. Bristol IK, Woodward WA, Strom EA et al. Locoregional treatment outcomes after multimodality management of inflammatory breast cancer. Int J Radiat Oncol Biop Phys 2008; 72:474.

Young

72. https://www.cdc.gov/cancer/breast/young_women/index.htm

73. Tai P, Yu E, Shiels R, et al. Short- and long-term cause-specific survival of patients with inflammatory breast cancer. BMC Cancer 2005; 5:137.

74. Hance KW, Anderson WF, Devesa SS et al. Trends in inflammatory breast carcinoma incidence and survival: the surveillance, epidemiology, and end results program at the National Cancer Institute. J Natl Cancer Inst 2005; 97:966.

75. Anderson WF, Schairer C, Chen BE te al. Epidemiology of inflammatory breast cancer (IBF). Breast Dis 2005-2006; 22:9.

76. https://www.cdc.gov/cancer/breast/young_women/index.htm

77. Valachis A, Tsali L, Pesce LL, Polyzos NP. Safety of pregnancy after primary breast carcinoma in young women: a meta-analysis to overcome bias of healthy mother effect studies. Obstet Gynecol Surv 2010 Dec;65(12):786-93. ance KW, Anderson WF, Devesa SS et al. Trends in inflammatory breast carcinoma incidence and survival: the surveillance, epidemiology, and end results program at the National Cancer Institute. J Natl Cancer Inst 2005; 97:966.

78. Anderson WF, Schairer C, Chen BE te al. Epidemiology of inflammatory breast cancer (IBF). Breast Dis 2005-2006; 22:9.

79. Bristol IK, Woodward WA, Strom EA et al. Locoregional treatment outcomes after multimodality management of inflammatory breast cancer. Int J Radiat Oncol Biop Phys 2008; 72:474.

20. SPECIAL

Lymphedema
1. Ozaslan C, Kuru B. Lymphedema after treatment of breast cancer. *Am J Surg* 2004; 187(1): 69-72.
2. Erickson VS, Pearson ML, Ganz PA et al. Arm edema in breast cancer patients. J Natl Cancer Inst 2001;93(2):96.

Follow-up
3. GLOBOCON 2008 Update http:www.iarc.fr/en/media-centre/iarcnews/2011/globocon2008-prev.php
4. https://academic.oup.com/jnci/advance-article/doi/10.1093/jnci/djab202/6423212
5. DeSantis CE, Lin CC, Mariotto AB et al. Cancer treatment and survivorship statistics, 2014. CA Cancer J Clin 2014; 64(4): 252.
6. Rojas MP, Telaro E, Russo A et al. Follow-up strategies for women treated for early breast cancer. Cochrane Database Syst Rev 2005.
7.Kwan ML, Kushi LH, Weltzien E et al. Alcohol consumption and breast cancer recurrence and survival among women with early stage breast cancer: the life after cancer epidemiology study. J Clin Oncol 2010; 28(29): 4410.
8. Lyman GH, Greenleee H, Bohike K et al. Integrative therapies during and after breast cancer treatment: ASCO endorsement of the SIO clinical practice guideline. J Clin Oncol 2018; 36(25):2647.

Hot flashes
9. Paddock, Catharine. Acupuncture reduces hot flashes, night sweats in menopause. Medical News Today. MediLexicon, Intl., 25 May 2016. Web.

Fertility; pregnancy after breast cancer
10. Iqbal J, Amir E, Rochon PA et al. Association of the timing of pregnancy with survival in women with breast cancer. JAMA Oncol 2017;3(5):659.
11. Valachis A, Tsali L, Pesce LL et al. Safety of pregnancy after primary breast carcinoma in young
12. Cariati M, Bains SK, Grootendorst MR et al. Adjuvant taxanes and the development of breast cancer-related arm lymphoedema. *Br J Surg* 2015; 102(9): 1071-1078.
13. McDuff SGR, Mina AI, Brunelle CL et al. Timing of lymphedema after treatment of breast cancer: when are patients most at risk? Int J Radiat Oncol Biol Phys 2019103(1):62.
14. Bloomquist K, Oturai P, Steele ML et al. Heavy-load lifting: Acute response in breast cancer survivors at risk for lymphedema. Med Sci Sports Exer 2018;50(2):187.
15. Moseley Al, Loller NB. Exercise for limb edema: Evidence that it is beneficial. J Lymphoedema 2008;3:51.
16. Schmitz KH, Ahmed Rl, Troxel A, et al. Weight lifting in women with breast-cancer-related lymphedema. N Engl J Med 2009;361(7):664.
17. Ahmed RL, Thomas W, Yee D, Schmitz KH. Randomized controlled trial of weight training and lymphedema in breast cancer survivors. J Clin Oncol 2006;24(18):2765.
18. Ezzo J, Manheimer E, McNeely ML, et al. Manual lymphatic drainage for lymphedema following breast cancer treatment. Cochrane Database Syst Rev 2015.
19. Didem K, Ufuk YS, and Sumre A. The comparison of two different physiotherapy methods in treatment of lymphedema after breast surgery. Breast Cancer Res Treat 2005;93(1):49.
20. Dayes IS, Whelan TJ, Julian JA et al. Randomized tiral of decongestive lymphatic drainage for the treatment of lymphedema in women with breast cancer. J Clin Oncol 2013;31(30):3758-63.

19. Ezzo J, Manheimer E, McNeely ML, et al. Manual lymphatic drainage for lymphedema following breast cancer treatment. Cochrane Database Syst Rev 2015.
20. DiSipio T, Rye S, Newman B, Hayes S. Incidence of unilateral arm lymphoedema after breast cancer: a systematic review and meta-analysis. Lancet Oncol 2013;14(6):500.
21. Cancer. 2012 Mar 15;118(6):1710-7. doi: 10.1002/cncr.26459. Epub 2011 Sep 1. Pretreatment fertility counseling and fertility preservation improve quality of life in reproductive age women with cancer.
22. Letourneau J, Ebbel E, Katz P. Pretreatment fertility counseling and fertility preservation improve quality of life in reproductive age women with cancer. Cancer. 2012;118(6):1710-7.

Printed in Great Britain
by Amazon